AN ATLAS OF PRIMATE GROSS ANATOMY

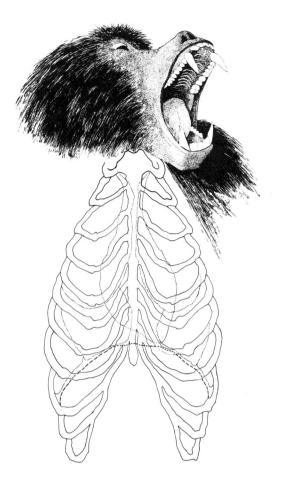

AN ATLAS OF

Baboon,

Daris R. Swindler and Charles D. Wood

PRIMATE GROSS ANATOMY

Chimpanzee, and Man

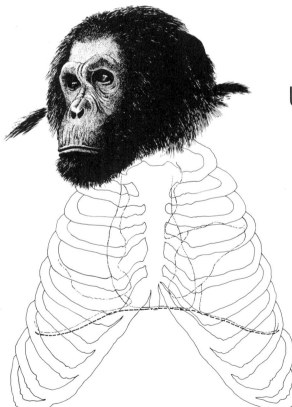

UNIVERSITY OF WASHINGTON PRESS

SEATTLE AND LONDON

Designed by Audrey Meyer

Library of Congress Cataloging in Publication Data

Swindler, Daris Ray.
  An atlas of primate gross anatomy.

  Bibliography: p.
  1. Antomy, Human—Atlases. 2. Baboons—
Anatomy—Atlases. 3. Chimpanzees—Anatomy—Atlases.
I. Wood, Charles D., 1941-   joint author.
II. Title, DNLM: 1. Anatomy, Comparative—Atlases.
2. Baboons—Anatomy and histology—Atlases.
3. Chimpanzees—Anatomy and histology—Atlases.
4. Primates—Anatomy and histology—Atlases.
QS17 S978a 1973
QM25.S915   599'.884'044   73-6909
ISBN 0-295-95261-X

To Wilton M. Krogman and Melvin K. Knisely, who have fostered teaching and research in so many students through the years.

DARIS R. SWINDLER

To my wife, Nancy, and our first six years.

CHARLES D. WOOD

FOREWORD

It is always difficult to speak for a work which, a few pages farther on, is prepared to speak for itself. This is all the more true when the work speaks eloquently through gracious pictures and succinct text. I was tempted therefore to postpone comment until an invitation to review this work might provide an opportunity to laud its usefulness and, after a careful search, to disclose some minor real or imagined blemish. But it is also tempting to be associated (as signatory of the foreword) with a work one had hoped for before it was conceived, valued as it unfolded, and followed with much enthusiasm to its final embodiment in a volume such as this.

Anatomy is a useful science. It is the handmaiden of surgery and its study is the initiation ceremony of medical education. The typical medical student, usually in company with three companions, more or less completely dissects an adult human cadaver. This activity provides the concrete instance on which he projects the general descriptions of his textbook of anatomy. But a pediatrician dealing with young children or a dentist with a practice among both sexes intuitively translates the discrepancies between some particular old male cadaver that he has dissected and a young or female subject by reference to the general accounts of typical human anatomy of the textbooks.

More overt concern with anatomic variability as such takes several directions: (1) the study of differences between individuals as seen in series of cadavers or skeletal parts from various places; (2) the study of temporal variation through examination of different age groups and especially of fetuses at different stages of development; and (3) the comparative study of different species. Individual variability provides the most immediate low-level extension of anatomical knowledge from the form in which it is learned to the case in which it must be applied. Comparative anatomy, on the other hand, is the method for the development of wide anatomical principles. Insofar as these principles are to be applied to the explanation of human anatomy, however, the comparative study of anatomy of the primates is of greatest immediate interest. Edward Tyson, M.D., F.R.S. (1650-1708), was the father of primatology. His *Orang-Outang, Sive Homo Sylvestris* (London, 1699) is the first comparative anatomy of an anthropoid ape. The relationship of apes to man continued to stimulate an interest in primate dissection, and proponents of the theory of natural selection (among them Charles Darwin and Thomas H. Huxley) relied heavily on the results of such studies.

In the years since then the need for suitable animals for the experimental study of physiological and pathological processes has demanded attention to man's nearest relatives, the monkeys and apes. Any surgical work on these forms has to be based on a knowledge of their anatomy. Largely because of its availability, the rhesus macaque was the first species studied repeatedly and in various ways. In 1933 C. G. Hartman and W. L. Straus, Jr., edited the *Anatomy of the Rhesus Monkey* (Williams and Wilkins, Baltimore); it remains the key work on the anatomy of that species.

Over the years the comparative frame of reference has widened. More different species, especially various Old World monkeys, have been the subject of study, and the need has grown among both students of human evolution and those engaged in experimental biology for a reliable and easy-to-use reference on primate anatomy. Such a work would have to illustrate fully the gross anatomy of several species of primates. Since all the Old World monkeys follow one basic pattern and the great apes are similar to each other, however, it could be limited to a few species and the text could be brief. When Daris Swindler first told me that he had under way a series of dissections of baboons, I enthusiastically encouraged him to publish an atlas of their anatomy in which this anatomy could be directly compared with that of the great apes and man. The African great apes, the gorilla and chimpanzee, are of almost equal theoretical interest; but the chimpanzee was selected because it is more available to biologists for study and indeed was more available to the authors. They were sensitive to the needs for conservation of the subjects of their study, and the anatomy of the chimpanzee, in the pages which follow, is based on a smaller number of specimens than that of the baboon. The human anatomy is, of course, informed by the much wider experience of generations of anatomical scholarship involving thousands of dissections.

Now the orangutan and gorilla are threatened species, the chimpanzee is also plagued by the clearing of forests, and the baboon and all other primates are also limited to shrinking domains as natural areas are despoiled by burgeoning human exploitation. One reason the higher primates are so valuable in respect to research on public health is that they are so similar to us as to be susceptible to human infectious diseases. Incursions of human occupation may entail the threat of human disease as well as those of slaughter, capture, and deprivation of natural habitat. The study of nonhuman primate behavior and, for that matter, an understanding of primate physiology and anatomy are now urgent. An appreciation of the value of primatology can lead to a demand for adequate care and protection. We must guarantee the continuation of their evolutionary lines. My good wishes of a long and useful life for Swindler and Wood's volume do not extend to the hope that it will outlive its subjects. Quite the contrary, I hope they will flourish together and not the last of them mankind, whose self-understanding will be enriched by the encouragement this volume will provide to understanding man's place in nature.

GABRIEL W. LASKER
Wayne State University
Detroit, Michigan

PREFACE

In 1933, Carl G. Hartman and William L. Straus, Jr., edited *The Anatomy of the Rhesus Monkey (Macaca mulatta)*, originally published by Williams and Wilkins. Within a few years the book was out of print. In 1961, Hafner Publishing Company reprinted the book, making it available once again to the scientific community. The work is still one of the most widely quoted sources in the field of nonhuman primate anatomy. Another invaluable source of nonhuman primate anatomy is W. C. Osman Hill's series entitled, *Primates: Comparative Anatomy and Taxonomy,* published by Interscience Publishers. There is, of course, voluminous literature on the anatomy of particular systems in individual species, and one only has to consult the anatomical and primatological journals to affirm the importance of nonhuman primates to basic and clinical research.

In spite of this vast literature, there are few works which cover in one book the gross anatomy of more than one species. Also, there is a notable lack of good regional illustrations of the different anatomical systems of any species of nonhuman primates. Therefore, several years ago we set out to rectify this situation by producing an atlas of the gross anatomy of three species of primates. It was our intent to produce an anatomical work which would be useful to anthropologists, human and comparative anatomists, physicians, dentists, and other workers in the biological and health sciences. It was also our desire to produce a volume which could be used by students as well as by seasoned researchers.

The first task was to select the species to be used in the comparisons. Several different genera were considered before the final decision was made to select the baboon *(Papio cynocephalus),* the chimpanzee *(Pan troglodytes),* and man *(Homo sapiens).* The precise zoological classification of the baboon and chimpanzee is still debated by experts. Most agree that the generic names *Papio* and *Pan* are correct, and that the latter is represented by two species, *troglodytes* and *paniscus* (Hill 1967a, 1967b; Napier and Napier 1967; Thorington and Groves 1970). The taxonomy of the baboon is more complicated, and we have followed the recent studies of Buettner-Janusch, Thorington and Groves, and Maples (1966, 1970, 1972) in designating the olive baboon from Kenya, *Papio cynocephalus.* On the other hand, equally competent students would suppress the specific name, *cynocephalus,* and replace it with *anubis* (Hill 1959, 1967b; Napier and Napier 1967). Indeed, Thorington and Groves believe that all savanna and hamadryas baboons represent a single polytypic species, that is, a single gene pool, whose correct specific name should be *hamadryas.* However, for the present, they recommend the use of *cynocephalus* since they feel that *hamadryas* would only increase an already confused situation (1970). The systematics of the baboon is obviously difficult and carking at the present time. We do know that all specimens used in the atlas came from Kenya, and we have retained the name *Papio cynocephalus.*

The baboon and chimpanzee were chosen because both are so widely used today in basic and clinical research that a detailed and comprehensive investigation of the gross anatomy of these primates would be beneficial to a broad audience of scientific investigators. In addition, these two animals represent very different grades of locomotor adaptations. The baboon is a terrestrial primate, a quadruped living most of its life on the ground. The chimpanzee, on the other hand, is a brachiator, which progresses through the trees by swinging arm over arm; when on the ground, however, the chimpanzee becomes a knuckle-walker (Tuttle 1965). The anatomy of these two primates, especially the muscle-bone relations, reflects these opposed modes of locomotor behavior. The third primate, man, was selected for two reasons. First, man is the only truly bipedal primate and consequently he manifests the anatomical arrangements associated with this type of locomotion. Second, because comparative anatomists, especially primate anatomists, usually compare the anatomy of nonhuman primates with that of man, he has been included to facilitate such studies.

We believe the uniqueness of the present work is the regional presentation in one volume of the gross anatomy of three primates. The regional plan was adopted because the majority of laboratory courses in primate anatomy are based on regional dissections. Systematic anatomy, however, is not neglected, and illustrations depicting the general organization of the arterial distribution, superficial vein and cutaneous nerve patterns appear at the beginning of several sections. Also, muscle-bone maps and tables of muscle origin, insertion, and innervation were prepared by Robert M. George, Jr., and are included in Parts 9 and 10. The format of the book is such that an illustration of *Papio* appears on the left-hand page and illustrations of *Homo* and *Pan* on the right-hand page. Thus, the student can quickly and accurately compare the anatomical structures of a region in all three primates without turning a page.

The text was written by Daris R. Swindler and the illustrations were prepared by Charles D. Wood, unless otherwise noted. The correlation of text and illustrations required the assistance of many people in order to give the reader a visual and verbal description of the major anatomical structures in a particular region. The illustrations of *Papio* and *Pan* have been drawn from original dissections of twenty-two baboons and six chimpanzees, and represent composite illustrations based upon the specimens. The illustrations of *Homo* represent composites redrawn from numerous human atlases to correspond with the drawings of *Papio* and *Pan*. All illustrations are of the animals' right sides.

By using a number of specimens of each species we believe the illustrations represent an accurate picture of the "normal" pattern of anatomy of these primates. The anatomical variation is greater in some regions and systems than in others, so we have included inserts on many of the plates to demonstrate these quantitative data. Undoubtedly students using this book will encounter specimens varying in one anatomical region or another from the "normal" pattern presented here. Such discrepancies are to be expected since they simply reflect intraspecific variability. However, to restrict the book to reasonable length we have considered only the more frequent variations.

This work is not designed to replace or supplant a textbook of anatomy, but rather to highlight the salient morphological features of a region and the major differences and similarities of the three species illustrated. Additionally, anatomic information of other primates is included in the text to enhance the comparative value of the material. Relevant books and articles which should meet the requirements of the more advanced students appear in the bibliography.

The terminology used in the plates is *Nomina anatomica*, 1966. The terminology of human anatomy was selected because it seemed appropriate for the majority of anatomical structures illustrated. In some instances, the labels on the plates of *Papio* and *Pan* designate structures which are not present in *Homo*. These terms have been Latinized to maintain the style of *Nomina anatomica*. It was decided to write the text using the English translation of *Nomina anatomica*.

DARIS R. SWINDLER

Professor, Department of Anthropology,
University of Washington
Research Affiliate, Regional Primate Research Center,
University of Washington

CHARLES D. WOOD

Director of Medical Illustration,
The Mason Clinic, Seattle
Research Affiliate, Regional Primate Research Center,
University of Washington

Seattle, Washington
1972

ACKNOWLEDGMENTS

We wish to thank the following persons for their assistance in the preparation of dissections: Doctors Ann McCoy Beck, Arno Weiss, John Albers, Robert Simmons, and Carol Davis. We are further indebted to Robert M. George, Jr., graduate student, Department of Anthropology, University of Washington, for preparing the majority of the dissections as well as the bone maps and tables of muscle origin and insertion. In addition, Mr. George participated with the authors in numerous conferences regarding the organization of the atlas.

In the summer of 1967, the authors visited Dr. William L. Straus, Jr., Department of Anatomy, Johns Hopkins University Medical School, and Dr. George Erikson, Department of Anatomy, Brown University Medical School. The format of the atlas was discussed, and many helpful criticisms and suggestions were offered by these two scholars.

The authors wish to express their most sincere gratitude to two distinguished gentlemen, Dr. Theodore C. Ruch, former director of the Regional Primate Research Center at the University of Washington, and Dr. Orville A. Smith, the present director of the center. Their unfailing assistance and encouragement during the period from 1968 to 1971 permitted the successful completion of the project. Without the understanding and tireless effort of these two men the atlas would certainly have been delayed several more months, if not indefinitely.

We wish to acknowledge the value of Theodore Ruch's *Bibliographia primatologica* (1941). The book was of unprecedented assistance in locating sources published prior to 1941. We are also indebted to the personnel of the Primate Information Center of the Regional Primate Research Center, University of Washington, for their inexhaustible patience in helping us locate references, particularly the more abstruse ones.

We also wish to thank Dr. Lloyd Dillingham and Timothy Bauer, supervisory veterinarian and research technician, respectively, at the Regional Primate Research Center, for supplying us with different baboon specimens. Their assistance enables us to check on numerous anatomical details in a much greater number of animals.

We are grateful to John Edwards and Lewis Tarrant, graduate students, Department of Anthropology, University of Washington, for reading sections of the manuscript and making many constructive suggestions. Mr. Tarrant also helped with lead-lining and labeling, two onerous chores in the preparation of a work of this nature. We also received assistance from Carol Fahrenbruch and Dana Swindler, Bruce Swindler, and Geoffrey Swindler during the final stages of preparing the atlas.

We were particularly fortunate in soliciting the aid of three excellent artists, Jean Pajot Smith, Pauline Green, and Adriano U. Graziotti. Special thanks are due Johsel Namkung, senior photographer, Department of Pathology, University of Washington Medical School, for photographic assistance.

We wish to extend special thanks to Janet Nobel for proofreading the sections on the lower limb, abdomen, and thorax, and to Kathleen Schmidt, who read proof on the entire manuscript. Both ladies made many helpful corrections.

We wish to thank Dr. Gabriel W. Lasker, Department of Anatomy, Wayne State University School of Medicine, for his early interest in our project and his continued concern and thoughtful and provocative criticisms. Dr. Lasker also read the manuscript, and his suggestions were most valuable.

The assistance of Roberta Swindler with the typescript, lead-lining, and labeling is hereby gratefully noted.

The illustrations of *Papio* and *Pan* were based upon dissections of the animals and are original drawings. Those of *Homo* are original but represent composites drawn from numerous human anatomy texts and atlases to coincide with the anatomical region illustrated in *Papio* and *Pan*. Thus, many sources have contributed to the final project.

The authors wish to acknowledge the support of the National Institutes of Health from 1964 to 1969. Without this grant, LM 00686 (formerly GM 12635), the atlas would not have been possible. In addition, National Institutes of Health grant RR 00166 has supported portions of the work during the last two years as well as subsidizing the final publication.

CONTENTS

Part 1 Osteology

Part 2 Head and Neck

Part 1

OSTEOLOGY

PLATE 1

Frontal View of Skull

Viewed anteriorly, the cerebral cranium, or forehead, of *Homo* stands out in marked contrast to this region in *Papio* and *Pan*. This difference reflects the great development of the frontal lobes of the brain in *Homo*. The supraorbital ridges, whether large or small, are marked either by supraorbital foramina or sulci. In the examples shown, all three species possess the grooves rather than the foramina.

The orbits are separated by broad interorbital partitions, and the lacrimal bone lies within the orbital margin in the three animals. The nasal bones are extremely long and attenuated in *Papio* and they normally achieve contact with the frontal bones. In both *Papio* and *Pan* the nasal bones fuse soon after birth, whereas the internasal suture remains patent much longer in *Homo*. The premaxillary element is present in all three primates, but the suture between it and the maxilla is obliterated early in prenatal life in *Homo*. It remains open for several years in the other forms, serving as an important growth site in the cercopithecoids (Moore 1949). The large maxilla is flattened dorsally in *Papio* and is usually perforated by several infraorbital foramina. The number varies from three to ten foramina per side. In *Papio,* the lateral wall of the maxilla presents a deeply excavated region termed the maxillary fossa. The size and depth of the fossa varies a great deal among adult *Papio*.

The mandible is heavy and massive in *Papio*. Anteriorly the symphysis is narrow and rough, presenting two vertically coursing ridges overlying the roots of the central incisors. A large middle symphyseal foramen may be present in *Papio*.

Observe the tremendous tusklike canines of *Papio* with the deep mesial grooves coursing along the crown of the teeth. These, it may be noted, pass onto the roots in these animals.

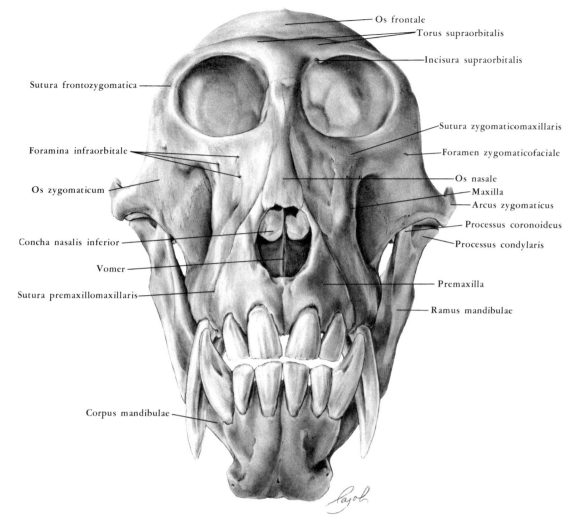

Papio

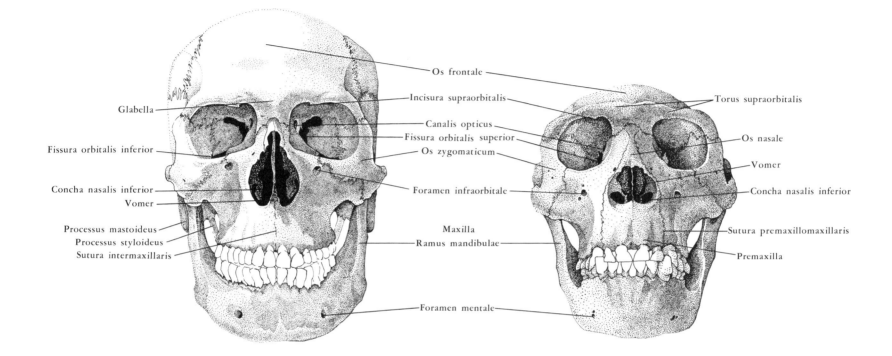

Glabella

Fissura orbitalis inferior

Concha nasalis inferior

Vomer

Processus mastoideus

Processus styloideus

Sutura intermaxillaris

Os frontale

Incisura supraorbitalis

Canalis opticus

Fissura orbitalis superior

Os zygomaticum

Foramen infraorbitale

Maxilla

Ramus mandibulae

Foramen mentale

Torus supraorbitalis

Os nasale

Vomer

Concha nasalis inferior

Sutura premaxillomaxillaris

Premaxilla

Homo

Pan

PLATE 2

Lateral View of Skull

In *Papio* differential growth causes the facial skeleton of
the adult to be long relative to the cranial portion of the
skull (Zuckerman 1926; Krogman 1930; Freedman 1957).
As Hill (1970) points out, *Papio* has the greatest amount
of prognathism of any of the living cercopithecoids.
The basicranial axis is flexed so that this large facial part
lies below the anterior part of the brain case. The foramen
magnum lies more on the basal portion of the skull. Both
of these evolutionary processes reach their maximum
expression in the skulls of modern man.

The neurocranial or brain case is much larger in *Homo*.
The forehead is vertical and the occipital region is
rounded. The teeth and jaws are reduced. These
evolutionary changes are well documented, and the
interested reader need only consult any of a dozen or
more readily available textbooks in physical anthropology
for the complete story.

The supraorbital ridges are pronounced in *Papio* and
Pan, slight in *Homo*. The number of infraorbital and
mental foramina is usually multiple in *Papio*, reduced in
Pan and *Homo*. The articulation at pterion is between the
frontal and temporal bones in *Papio* and *Pan*, parietal and
sphenoid in *Homo*. The mastoid process is appreciably
larger in *Homo*. The shallow glenoid fossa of *Papio* and
Pan is obvious in this view. In addition, note the long,
well-developed postglenoid process in *Pan*, and
particularly in *Papio*. Finally, compare the flattened malar
bone of *Papio* with its vertically oriented counterpart
in *Pan* and *Homo*.

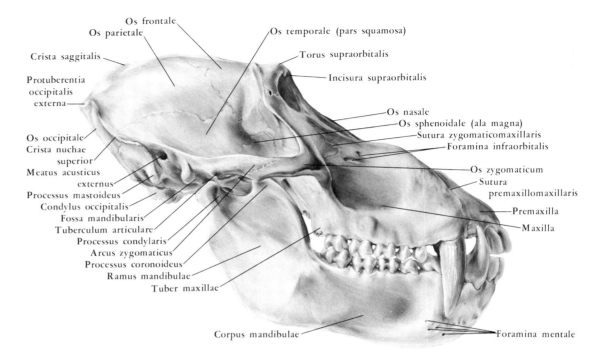

Papio

4

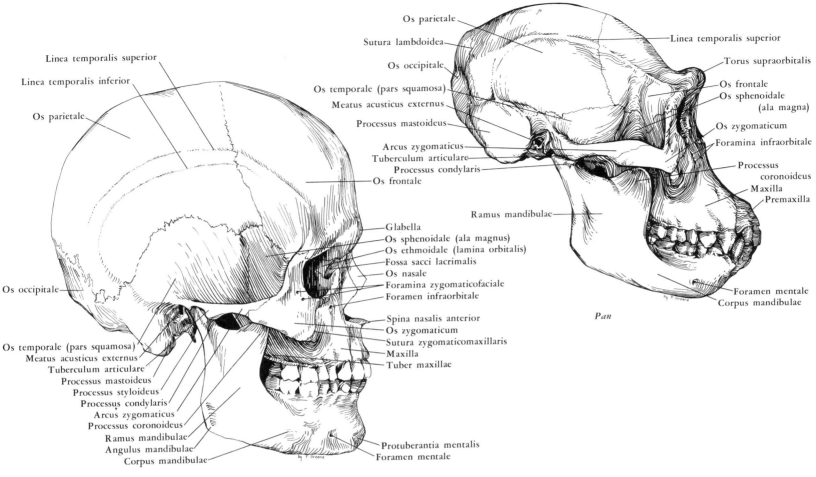

Linea temporalis superior
Linea temporalis inferior

Os parietale

Os occipitale

Os temporale (pars squamosa)
Meatus acusticus externus
Tuberculum articulare
Processus mastoideus
Processus styloideus
Processus condylaris
Arcus zygomaticus
Processus coronoideus
Ramus mandibulae
Angulus mandibulae
Corpus mandibulae

Os frontale

Glabella
Os sphenoidale (ala magnus)
Os ethmoidale (lamina orbitalis)
Fossa sacci lacrimalis
Os nasale
Foramina zygomaticofaciale
Foramen infraorbitale

Spina nasalis anterior
Os zygomaticum
Sutura zygomaticomaxillaris
Maxilla
Tuber maxillae

Protuberantia mentalis
Foramen mentale

Homo

Os parietale
Sutura lambdoidea
Os occipitale
Os temporale (pars squamosa)
Meatus acusticus externus
Processus mastoideus
Arcus zygomaticus
Tuberculum articulare
Processus condylaris

Ramus mandibulae

Linea temporalis superior
Torus supraorbitalis
Os frontale
Os sphenoidale
(ala magna)
Os zygomaticum
Foramina infraorbitale
Processus
coronoideus
Maxilla
Premaxilla

Foramen mentale
Corpus mandibulae

Pan

PLATE 3

Basilar View of Skull

A variety of bones, openings, processes, and projections are seen from this view of the skull.

From the anterior end, the most obvious difference is the tremendously elongated palate with its parallel sides in *Papio*. In the midline of the palate opposite the canines is the very large incisive fossa of *Papio*. The opening is much reduced in *Pan* and *Homo*. The nasal spine extends distally well beyond the tooth row in *Papio*, while its free end lies about tangential to the distal border of the third molar in *Homo*. In this feature, *Pan* is intermediate.

In *Papio* the medial pterygoid plates are minute compared with the large, quadrangular lateral plates, which are sharply inclined distolaterally. At the anterior end of the medial plate a small hamular process projects inferiorly. The pterygoid fossa is between the two plates and, according to Hill (1970), the fossa is wider in females than in males.

The foramen lacerum is completely obliterated in *Papio*, but is present in *Pan* and *Homo*. The foramen ovale lies between the sphenoid and rostral part of the petrosal in *Papio*; in *Homo* it perforates the great wing of the sphenoid, while in *Pan* it is located entirely within the temporal bone. Just lateral and slightly distal to the oval opening is the passage for the middle meningeal vessels in *Homo*. This passage is the foramen spinosum, which is absent in *Papio*, the meningeal vessels being transmitted through the foramen ovale. Note that the foramen spinosum is present in *Pan* as an opening in the squamous part of the temporal bone.

The petrous temporal presents a well-formed bony process near its apex in *Papio*. There is really not a comparable development in *Pan* or *Homo*. The circular carotid canal is present in *Papio*, penetrating the inferior surface of the petrous temporal. Just distolateral to this opening is the styloid process, which is longest in *Homo*, and near its base is the stylomastoid foramen.

There are mastoid processes in all three primates, but they are much better developed in *Homo*.

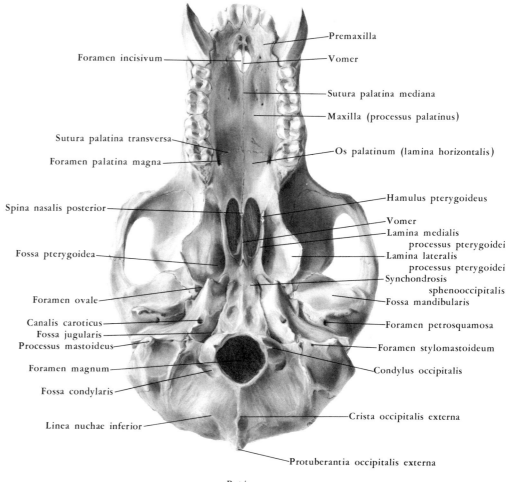

Papio

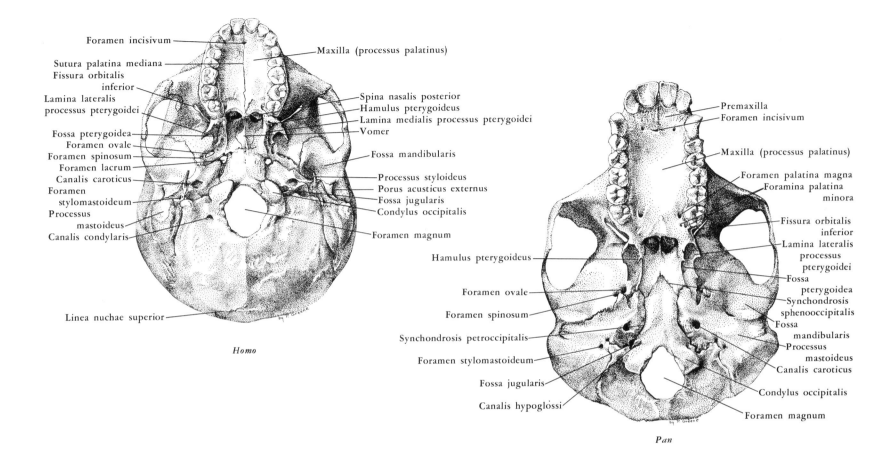

Foramen incisivum

Sutura palatina mediana
Fissura orbitalis
inferior
Lamina lateralis
processus pterygoidei

Fossa pterygoidea
Foramen ovale
Foramen spinosum
Foramen lacrum
Canalis caroticus
Foramen
stylomastoideum
Processus
mastoideus
Canalis condylaris

Linea nuchae superior

Maxilla (processus palatinus)

Spina nasalis posterior
Hamulus pterygoideus
Lamina medialis processus pterygoidei
Vomer

Fossa mandibularis

Processus styloideus
Porus acusticus externus
Fossa jugularis
Condylus occipitalis

Foramen magnum

Homo

Premaxilla
Foramen incisivum

Maxilla (processus palatinus)

Foramen palatina magna
Foramina palatina
minora

Fissura orbitalis
inferior
Lamina lateralis
processus
pterygoidei
Fossa
pterygoidea
Synchondrosis
sphenooccipitalis
Fossa
mandibularis
Processus
mastoideus
Canalis caroticus

Condylus occipitalis

Foramen magnum

Hamulus pterygoideus

Foramen ovale

Foramen spinosum

Synchondrosis petroccipitalis

Foramen stylomastoideum

Fossa jugularis

Canalis hypoglossi

Pan

PLATE 4

Dorsal View of Skull

The posterior region of the skull appears quite differently among the three primates. In *Papio* the junction between the parietal and occipital bones is much more acute than the rounded, globular configuration presented by *Pan* and even more so by *Homo*. The planum occipitale is flattened in *Papio* and convex in *Pan* and *Homo*. Its surface usually presents several crests. In the midline is the external occipital protuberance from which a raised, often well-defined median ridge extends to the posterior rim of the foramen magnum. These structures give attachment to the ligamentum nuchae in *Papio* and *Homo,* the latter being absent in *Pan.*

The superior nuchal lines arch laterally from the external occipital protuberance. In *Papio* the line is elevated into a well-formed ledge, which passes laterally toward the squamous portion of the temporal bone and the mastoid process. In the region lying cranial to the external auditory meatus, the superior nuchal ledge becomes confluent with the root of the zygomatic arch. At this juncture, the zygomatic arch broadens to pass anteriorly as a strong bar of bone.

There are usually inferior nuchal lines, but these are better developed in *Homo,* being either slightly indicated or absent in *Papio.*

Note the vertebral artery passing through the transverse foramina of the cranial five or six cervical vertebrae on its way to join its companion vessel just inside the foramen magnum, where they form the basilar artery (see Plate 46).

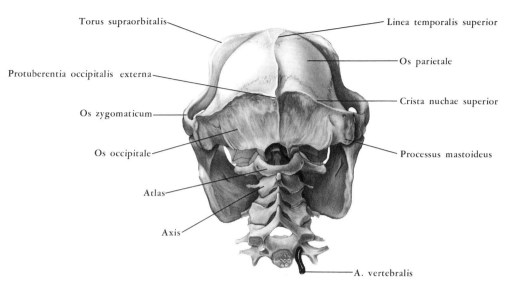

Papio

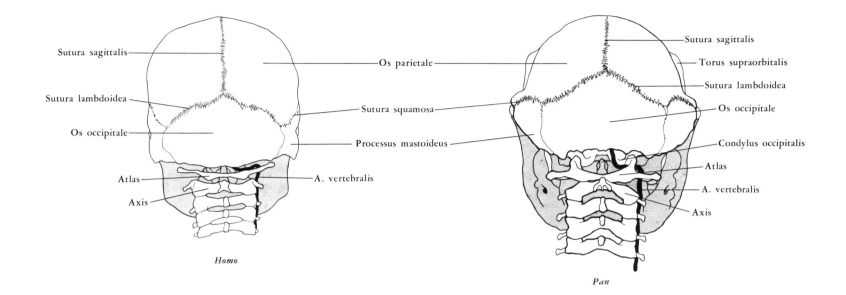

Sutura sagittalis

Sutura lambdoidea

Os occipitale

Atlas

Axis

Os parietale

Sutura squamosa

Processus mastoideus

A. vertebralis

Homo

Sutura sagittalis

Torus supraorbitalis

Sutura lambdoidea

Os occipitale

Condylus occipitalis

Atlas

A. vertebralis

Axis

Pan

PLATE 5

Hyoid Bone

The hyoid bone of *Papio* is typical of cercopithecoids, albeit larger than in most members of the taxon. The anterior surface of the body is very convex, and often there is a median ridge running craniocaudally. The cranio-caudal length of the corpus is much greater in *Papio* than in the other two primates, particularly when compared with the narrow horseshoe-shaped configuration presented by *Homo.* In *Papio* and *Pan* the corpus presents a deeply excavated pharyngeal surface, which is referred to as a hyoid bulla (Kelemen 1969). This recess receives the expanded laryngeal air sacs of these primates.

The greater cornu (thyrohyal) is large in all three species and projects from the cranioposterior surface of the body. It terminates posteriorly as a small tubercle.

The lesser cornu (hypohyal) is a small projection from the cranial border of the hyoid between the corpus and greater cornu. It may be ossified or remain partly or completely cartilaginous in the three primates. In *Pan* it is hardly perceptible, being merely a slight elevation (Schultz 1969). The gorilla likewise has a small hypohyal (Raven 1950). For a recent description of the primate hyoid bone, see Hilloowala 1970.

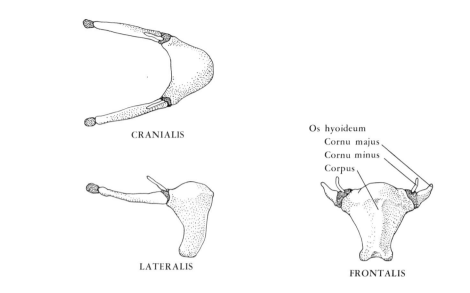

CRANIALIS

LATERALIS

Os hyoideum
Cornu majus
Cornu minus
Corpus

FRONTALIS

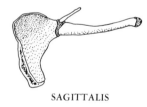

SAGITTALIS

Papio

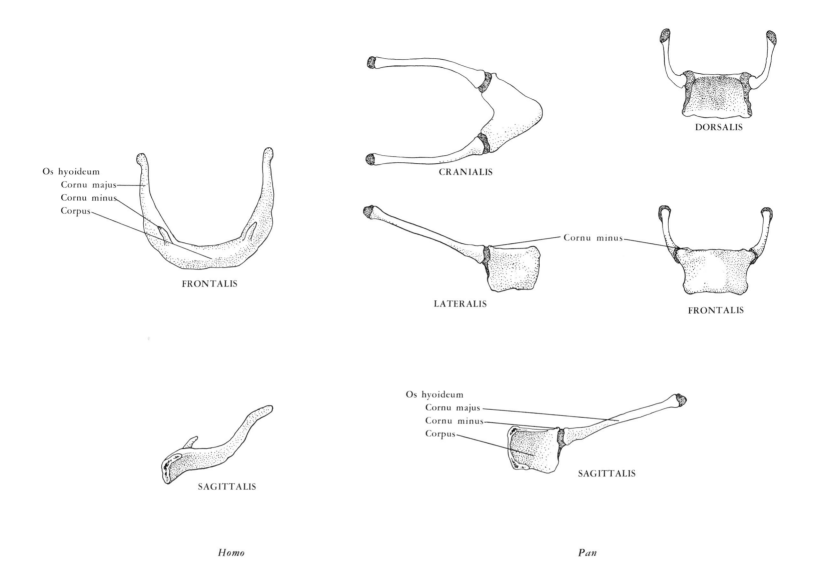

CRANIALIS

DORSALIS

Os hyoideum
Cornu majus
Cornu minus
Corpus

FRONTALIS

Cornu minus

LATERALIS

FRONTALIS

Os hyoideum
Cornu majus
Cornu minus
Corpus

SAGITTALIS

SAGITTALIS

Homo

Pan

PLATE 6

Vertebral Column

The vertebral column affords attachment to muscles, assists in the support of the trunk, and helps to protect the spinal cord. It is divided into various regions which differ in many respects.

The vertebral formula varies in these three species as shown here. All 3 have 7 cervical vertebrae; indeed, 7 is the typical number in mammals. The thoracic region is more variable, consisting of anywhere from 11 to 14 vertebrae in these animals (Schultz 1961). According to the same authority, the averages are 12.5 in *Papio,* 13.2 in *Pan,* and 12.0 in *Homo.* The differences result from shifting at the thoracolumbar border where the most cranial lumbar vertebra becomes incorporated into the thoracic series. Note that there are 13 thoracic vertebrae shown here for *Papio*; the thirteenth is the transitional member of the series.

The number of lumbar vertebrae varies among these primates between 3 and 7 according to Schultz's data (1961). The averages are 6.4 in *Papio,* 3.6 in *Pan,* and 5.0 in *Homo.* There is a tendency to reduce the number of lumbar segments in the Pongidae; indeed, it is not rare for *Pan* to have only 3 lumbar vertebrae. *Homo* is conservative in the lumbar region, maintaining 5 lumbars in 90 percent of the cases (Schultz 1961), and as a result his trunk is more flexible.

The sacral region has also been subject to its own phylogenetic transgressions. In these groups, the numbers fluctuate between 3 and 8. The averages are 3.2 in *Papio,* 5.7 in *Pan,* and 5.2 in *Homo.* It is well known that the majority of short-tailed primates tend to have higher numbers of sacral vertebrae.

The greatest variation in the number of vertebrae occurs in the caudal or coccygeal region, ranging from 2 to 26 with averages of 19.4 in *Papio,* 3.3 in *Pan,* and 4.0 in *Homo.*

The total number of vertebrae in primates runs from 29 to 63, the highest numbers occurring among platyrrhines and the lowest number among gibbons. Thus, there is a great deal of variability within the vertebral regions of a genus, as well as intergenerically.

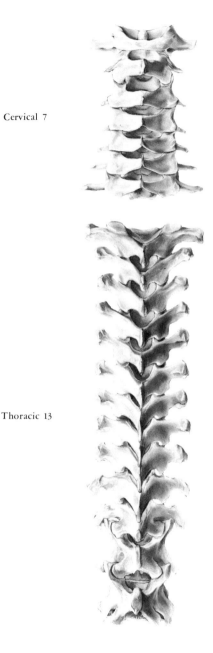

Cervical 7

Thoracic 13

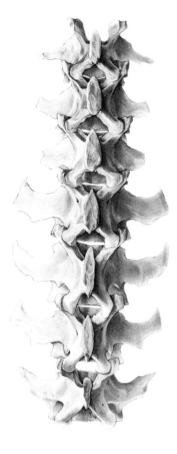

Lumbar 7

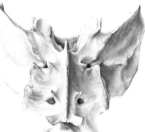

Sacral 3

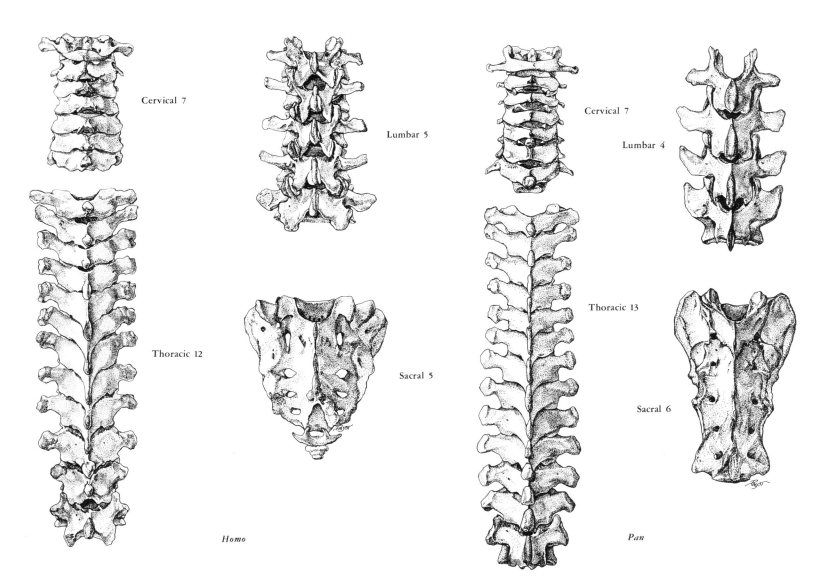

Cervical 7

Lumbar 5

Cervical 7

Lumbar 4

Thoracic 12

Sacral 5

Thoracic 13

Sacral 6

Homo

Pan

PLATE 7

Atlas Vertebra

The atlas is noticeable in one respect: it lacks a body. The two lateral masses are connected by the anterior and posterior arches. The transverse processes extend laterally from each lateral mass. Note that the transverse processes of the atlas extend much farther laterally than those of the vertebrae immediately caudal. In fact, one can palpate these structures in *Homo* by placing one's index finger on the lateral side of the neck just caudal to the ear lobe and posterior to the mandibular ramus.

The ventral arch is thicker and shorter than the dorsal one, especially in *Papio*. Both arches present roughened elevations in their medial sections, the ventral and dorsal tubercles. The ventral tubercle is the most pronounced, and in *Papio* it is in the form of an elongated, hooklike process projecting caudal to the centrum. Dorsal to the tubercle is the concave facet which articulates with the dens of the axis. The posterior tubercle represents the rudimentary spinous process.

Each transverse process is perforated by the transverse foramen, which is large in *Pan* and *Homo*. The opening is more restricted in *Papio* and is actually somewhat hidden by the superior articular process. A groove for the vertebral artery is continuous with the sulcus and passes medially along the cranial surface of the posterior arch. It also houses the first (suboccipital) cervical nerve. The groove may be a foramen or a canal as shown in *Pan*.

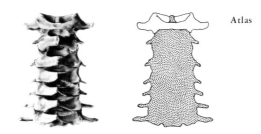

Atlas

Vertebrae Cervicales

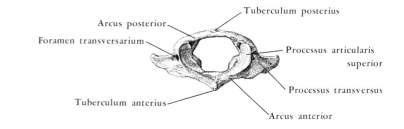

Tuberculum posterius

Arcus posterior

Foramen transversarium

Processus articularis superior

Processus transversus

Tuberculum anterius

Arcus anterior

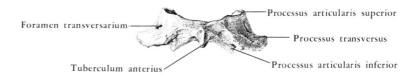

Foramen transversarium

Processus articularis superior

Processus transversus

Tuberculum anterius

Processus articularis inferior

Papio

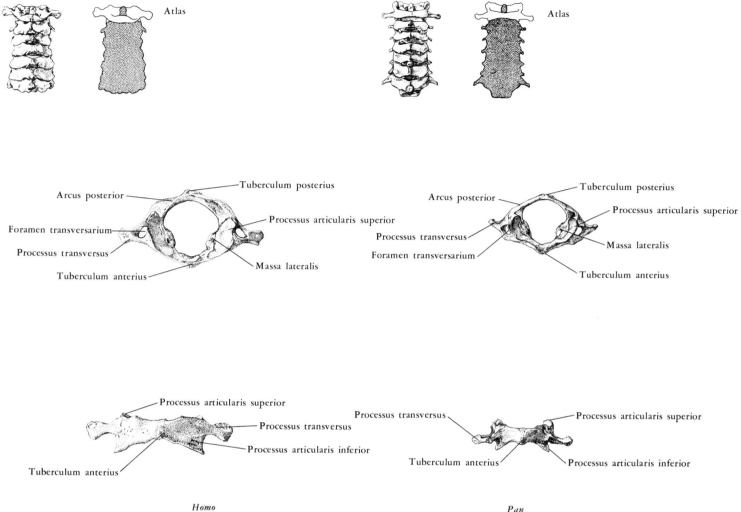

Atlas

Atlas

Arcus posterior — Tuberculum posterius

Processus articularis superior

Foramen transversarium

Processus transversus

Tuberculum anterius — Massa lateralis

Arcus posterior — Tuberculum posterius

Processus articularis superior

Processus transversus

Foramen transversarium

Massa lateralis

Tuberculum anterius

Processus articularis superior

Processus transversus

Processus articularis inferior

Tuberculum anterius

Processus transversus

Processus articularis superior

Tuberculum anterius

Processus articularis inferior

Homo

Pan

PLATE 8

Axis Vertebra

The second cervical vertebra is the axis, the pivot upon which the atlas rotates the head. It is immediately recognizable by the dens, which is the body of the atlas. The dens is a rather large, bluntlike process presenting a smooth, oval facet on its ventral surface for articulation with the atlas. The superior articular facets lie opposite the dens and face somewhat ventrolaterally.

The transverse processes are small projections from the body and lamina. They are not grooved and end abruptly as short, blunt tips. They are much more expanded dorsoventrally in *Papio* than in the other forms. The transverse foramen is present near the base of the process.

The spinous process is a large extension from the posterior arch. In *Homo* the tip is bifid, but there is no suggestion of a bipartite structure in *Papio*. According to Sonntag (1924), the spinous process of the axis is the only cervical spine of pongids displaying a bifurcated tip.

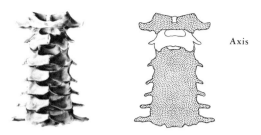

Axis

Vertebrae cervicales

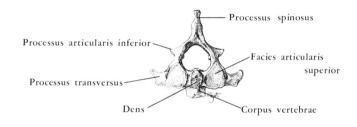

Processus spinosus

Processus articularis inferior

Facies articularis superior

Processus transversus

Dens

Corpus vertebrae

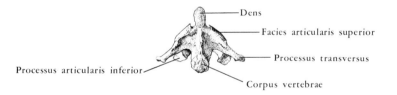

Dens

Facies articularis superior

Processus transversus

Processus articularis inferior

Corpus vertebrae

Papio

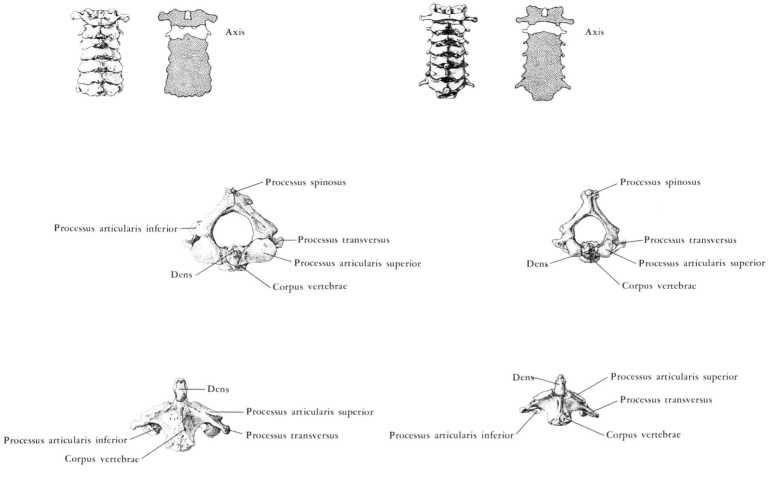

Axis

Axis

Processus spinosus

Processus articularis inferior

Processus transversus

Processus articularis superior

Dens

Corpus vertebrae

Processus spinosus

Dens

Processus transversus

Processus articularis superior

Corpus vertebrae

Dens

Processus articularis superior

Processus transversus

Processus articularis inferior

Corpus vertebrae

Homo

Dens

Processus articularis superior

Processus transversus

Processus articularis inferior

Corpus vertebrae

Pan

PLATE 9

Typical Cervical Vertebra

A typical cervical vertebra includes the third to sixth
segments. The centra are rather small, and in *Papio* their
greatest dimension is transverse, whereas in *Pan* and
Homo their configuration tends to be round or oval.

 The spinous processes are short and bifid in *Homo,* but
terminate as a single point in *Papio* and *Pan.* Their
general length is increased only in *Pan.* These processes
are directed more caudally in *Homo* than in most other
groups of primates.

 The transverse processes are well formed and present
the transverse foramina. These openings are rarely present
in the seventh cervical vertebra except in *Homo,* where
they are frequently encountered at least unilaterally
(Schultz 1961). When present in *Homo,* the foramen does
not often transmit the vertebral artery. Each transverse
process ends in two tubercles, the anterior and posterior,
which are particularly well developed in *Papio.* There is a
well-marked sulcus on the cranial surface separating
the tubercles. The cervical nerves leave the spinal cord
through these grooves. When in articulation, these grooves
form the intervertebral foramina.

 The seventh cervical is atypical in that it has
characteristics common to both cervical and thoracic
vertebrae. The spinous process is longer than all other
cervical spines, and in *Homo* it is called the vertebra
prominens. It is not bifid, ending instead in a blunt
tubercle. The transverse processes are large and end
bluntly rather than bifidly. As mentioned above, it may or
may not possess the transverse foramen.

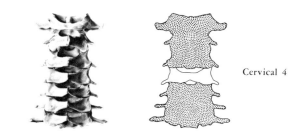

Cervical 4

Vertebrae Cervicales

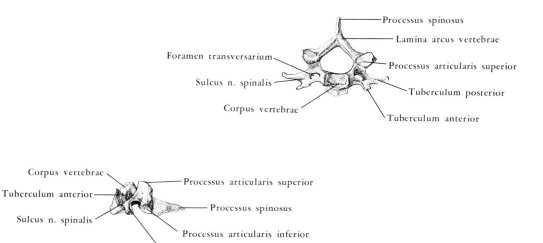

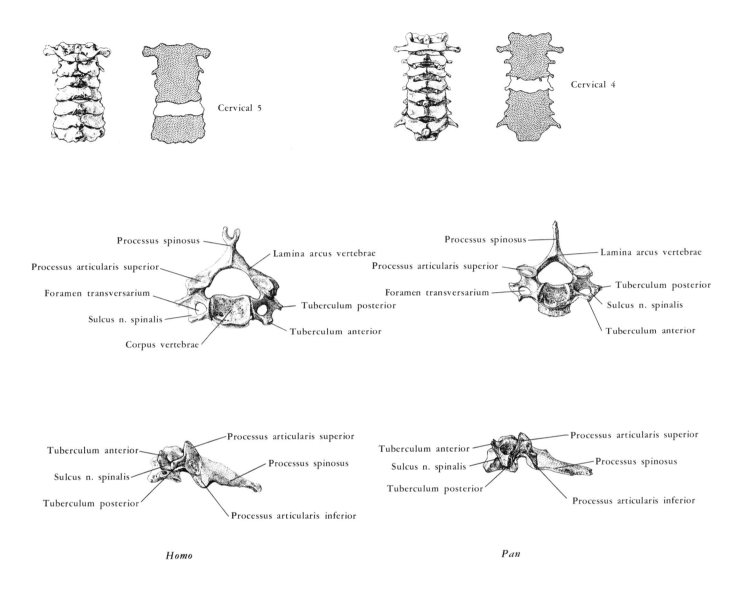

Cervical 5

Cervical 4

Processus spinosus — Lamina arcus vertebrae

Processus articularis superior —

Foramen transversarium —

Sulcus n. spinalis — Tuberculum posterior

Corpus vertebrae — Tuberculum anterior

Processus spinosus — Lamina arcus vertebrae

Processus articularis superior —

Foramen transversarium — Tuberculum posterior

Sulcus n. spinalis

Tuberculum anterior

Tuberculum anterior — Processus articularis superior

Sulcus n. spinalis — Processus spinosus

Tuberculum posterior — Processus articularis inferior

Homo

Tuberculum anterior — Processus articularis superior

Sulcus n. spinalis — Processus spinosus

Tuberculum posterior

Processus articularis inferior

Pan

PLATE 10

Typical Thoracic Vertebra

The centra of thoracic vertebrae are strongly constructed and their greatest diameter is dorsoventral. There are two costal facets on each side of the centrum, which receive the ribs in the living.

The vertebral arch consists of the lamina and pedicles. The latter connect with the body to outline the vertebral foramen. This foramen is smaller than it is in the cervical region; in *Pan* and *Homo* it is circular, whereas in *Papio* it is more triangular. Also, the pedicles are much shorter in *Papio* than in the other forms.

The spinous process is long, terminating in a single tubercle. In *Papio* it is much more compressed than in the other animals. At the same time, the lamina and transverse processes project horizontally in *Papio* and *Pan,* whereas they are inclined much more dorsally in *Homo,* creating a gutter or troughlike condition when the vertebrae are articulated. The transverse process presents a smooth articular facet at its end, which articulates with the tubercle of the rib.

Several atypical thoracic vertebrae can be defined. For example, in *Homo* the first, ninth, tenth, eleventh, and twelfth are usually placed in this category. The distinguishing features generally relate to the number, type, and position of the costal pits. In general, the more caudal vertebrae have but a single costal facet on the body which tends to migrate toward the pedicle. Commensurate with this positional shift is the gradual disappearance of the transverse costal facet. In *Papio* the caudal three transverse processes lack the facets.

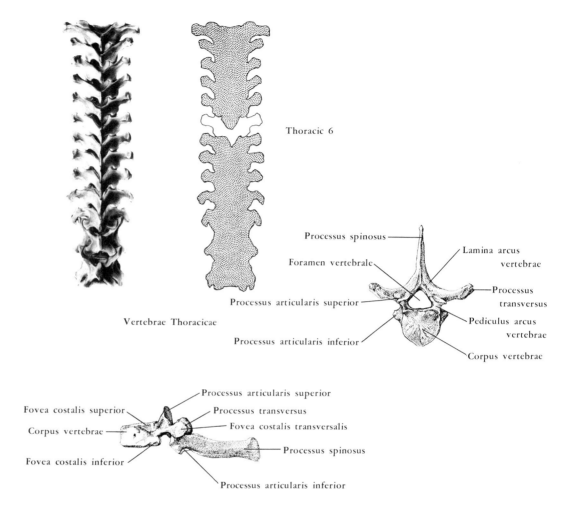

Thoracic 6

Vertebrae Thoracicae

Papio

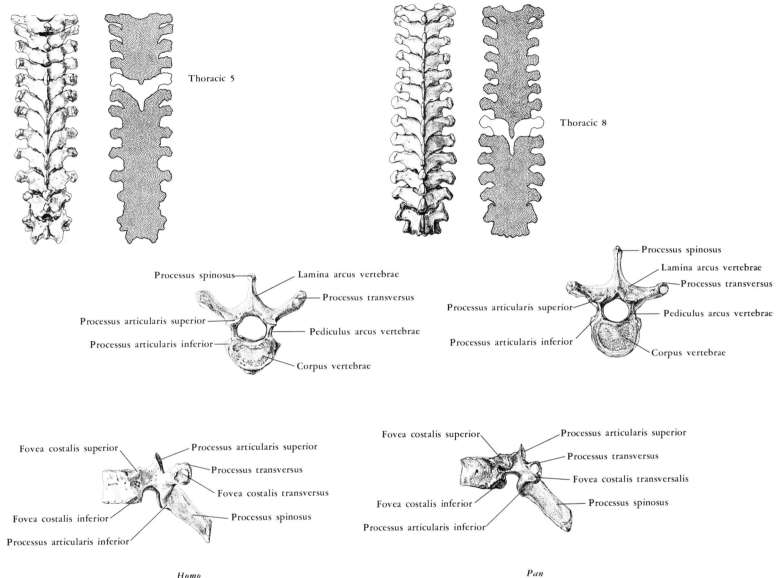

Thoracic 5

Thoracic 8

Processus spinosus — Lamina arcus vertebrae

Processus transversus

Processus articularis superior — Pediculus arcus vertebrae

Processus articularis inferior — Corpus vertebrae

Processus spinosus

Lamina arcus vertebrae

Processus transversus

Processus articularis superior — Pediculus arcus vertebrae

Processus articularis inferior — Corpus vertebrae

Fovea costalis superior — Processus articularis superior

Processus transversus

Fovea costalis transversus

Fovea costalis inferior — Processus spinosus

Processus articularis inferior

Homo

Fovea costalis superior — Processus articularis superior

Processus transversus

Fovea costalis transversalis

Fovea costalis inferior — Processus spinosus

Processus articularis inferior

Pan

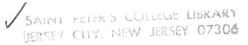

PLATE 11

Typical Lumbar Vertebra

The lumbar segment of the column is massive and the individual vertebrae are large. They can be distinguished from cervical and thoracic vertebrae by the absence of transverse foramina and costal facets.

The body is large, and in *Papio* it is wider dorsoventrally, while in *Pan* and *Homo* its greatest diameter is transverse. The pedicles and lamina are strongly constructed. The former pass almost straight dorsally, and the latter are much heavier than the thoracic lamina. The configuration of the vertebral foramen is triangular. Its dimensions are greater than those in the thoracic region, but do not surpass the cervical foramina. The spinous processes are heavy quadrilateral structures projecting horizontally in *Papio* and in *Homo*, but decidedly caudally in Pan.

A large mammillary process (metapophysis) sits astride the dorsal surface of each superior articular process. The transverse processes are long, slender projections which gradually increase in size from cranial to caudal. This progression is more marked in *Papio* than it is in the other animals. The small elevation at the base of each transverse process visible in the figures, is the accessory process (anapophysis). These processes are quite pronounced in *Papio* and also occur on the twelfth thoracic vertebra.

In *Papio,* note the prominent ventral mid-sagittal keel on the centrum. This is present on all thoracic and lumbar centra in cercopithecoids; only traces are present in pongids, and it is normally absent in *Homo* (Straus 1963). The ventral longitudinal ligament of the vertebral column attaches to it.

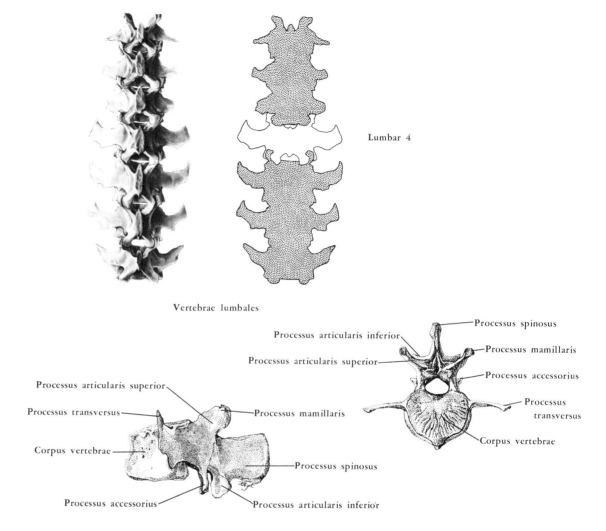

Lumbar 4

Vertebrae lumbales

Papio

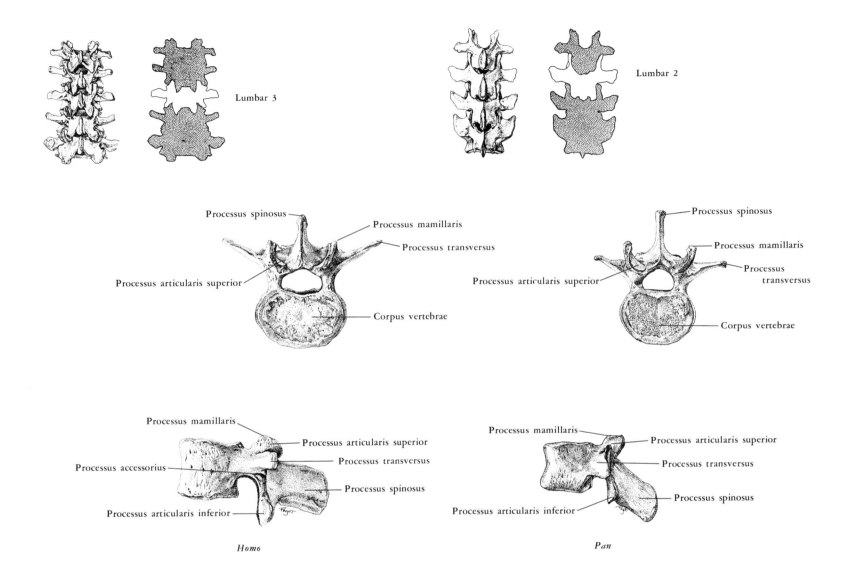

Lumbar 3

Lumbar 2

Processus spinosus

Processus mamillaris

Processus transversus

Processus articularis superior

Corpus vertebrae

Processus spinosus

Processus mamillaris

Processus transversus

Processus articularis superior

Corpus vertebrae

Processus mamillaris

Processus articularis superior

Processus transversus

Processus accessorius

Processus spinosus

Processus articularis inferior

Homo

Processus mamillaris

Processus articularis superior

Processus transversus

Processus spinosus

Processus articularis inferior

Pan

PLATE 12

Bony Thorax

The bony thorax is formed by the thoracic vertebrae, the ribs with their costal cartilages, and the sternum. The thorax is more slender and elongated in *Papio* than in *Pan* and *Homo,* and the chest, therefore, is much narrower in relation to its sagittal diameter in the first than in the last two animals. The change in thoracic shape is correlated with the locomotor habits of the animal, and especially in upright *Homo* these modifications have tended to shift the center of gravity nearer the vertebral column (Schultz 1961; Campbell 1966). The shape of the thorax is broad in all Hominoidea but, as pointed out by Schultz (1961), it is quite differently constructed in *Homo* than it is in *Pan:* in *Homo* the thorax is barrel-shaped, whereas in *Pan* it is almost funnel-shaped.

There are 13 pairs of ribs in *Pan* and 12 pairs in *Papio* and *Homo.* Of these, 7.1 reach the sternum directly in *Pan* and *Homo,* while 7.9 achieve direct sternal contact in *Papio* (Schultz 1961). The remaining ribs in all three primates either connect by cartilage with the rib immediately cranial to it or they are floating.

The sternum in *Papio* is composed of eight segments, which usually remain separated by cartilage even in the adult animal. In *Homo,* and to a lesser extent in *Pan,* the segments forming the body of the sternum fuse into a single bone in the adult. Occasionally in old age the body of the sternum unites with the manubrium and forms a single piece of bone (Schultz 1930). Note the extremely long and narrow sternum of *Papio* compared with the relatively short and broad sternum of *Homo.* Of all the Hominoidea, *Pan* has the narrowest sternum; indeed, it is not much wider than in many of the lower primates.

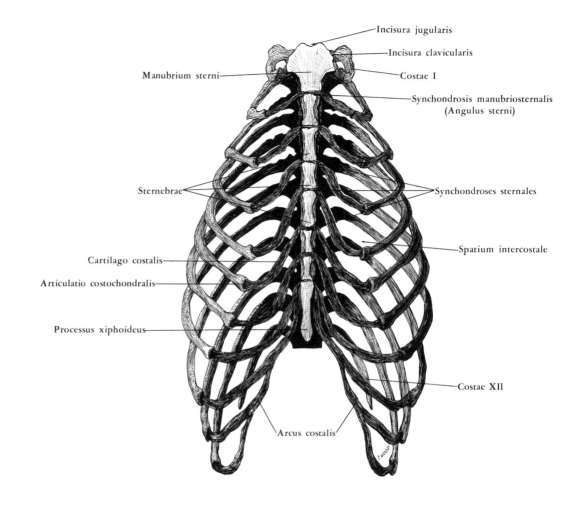

Papio

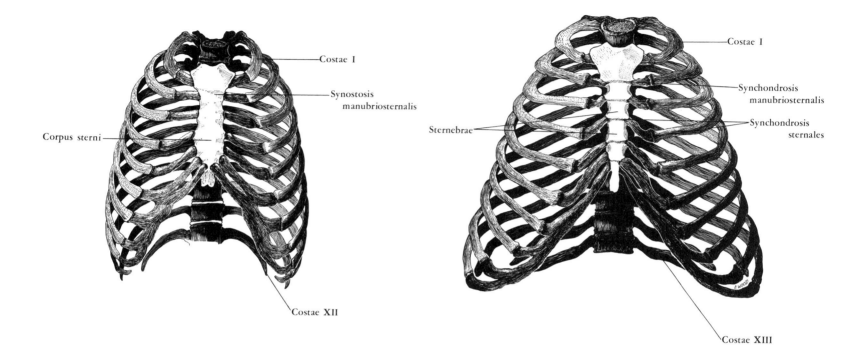

Costae I

Synostosis
manubriosternalis

Corpus sterni

Costae XII

Homo

Costae I

Synchondrosis
manubriosternalis

Sternebrae

Synchondrosis
sternales

Costae XIII

Pan

PLATE 13

Right Clavicle

The skeleton of the upper limb is adapted primarily to the functions of quadrupedal locomotion in *Papio* and of brachiation and prehension in *Pan* and *Homo*. The pectoral girdle consists of two bones, the clavicle and the scapula.

The clavicle extends from the manubrium sterni to the acromion of the scapula. In this position, it connects the skeleton of the upper limb with that of the trunk. Its chief function is that of a prop or strut, holding the upper member away from the side of the trunk and thereby maintaining excellent conditions for free movement of the upper limb. The clavicle is found in all primates.

The clavicle is approximately S-shaped in these primates, being flattened laterally while presenting a blunt or prismatic medial extremity. The lateral end is particularly broad and flat in *Homo*. The medial end articulates with the sternum, forming the important sternoclavicular joint, which takes part in all movements of the pectoral girdle.

The conoid tubercle is present in all three animals; however, it is much more pronounced in *Pan* (a similar condition was reported by Sonntag [1924]). This eminence serves for the attachment of the conoid ligament, a subdivision of the coracoclavicular ligament.

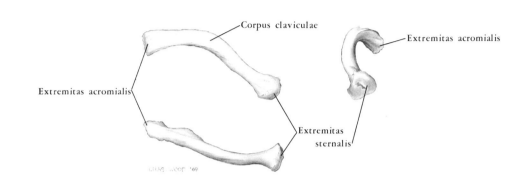

Papio

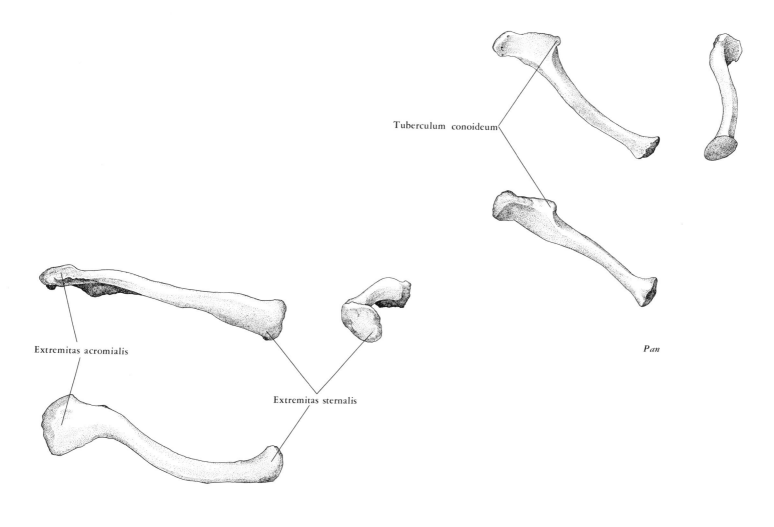

Tuberculum conoideum

Pan

Extremitas acromialis

Extremitas sternalis

Homo

PLATE 14

Right Scapula

The major differences in the scapula are associated with locomotor patterns. The quadrupedal scapula of *Papio* is narrow craniocaudally, resulting in a relatively short vertebral border, whereas the cranial and axillary borders are elongated. This shape can be ascertained from the scapular index—143 in *Papio* and 63 in *Homo*—whereby, according to Schultz (1930), the higher the index becomes, the narrower the scapula. The scapular spine is well formed and divides the dorsal surface into a quadrilateral supraspinous fossa and a triangular infraspinous fossa. Laterally the spine becomes thicker and bends medially as the acromion. The coracoid process is short, narrow, and cylindrical, bends sharply in a ventrocaudal direction, and has a short, thick base. For an excellent study of the coracoid process in primates, see Martin and O'Brien 1938. The glenoid cavity is noticeably concave from cranial to caudal, with the cranial portion jutting forward to overhang the caudal two-thirds of the cavity. The subscapular fossa is only slightly concave and is deepest at its lateral end. There are usually several bony crests near the vertebral border marking the attachments of the subscapularis muscle.

The most noticeable difference between the quadrupedal scapula of *Papio* and the scapulae of *Pan* and *Homo* is the relatively long vertebral border of the latter two animals. The result of an extension of the scapula in a craniocaudal direction, this change provides for more efffective leverage in rotating the scapula and permits elevation of the arm to its fullest extent. The acromion and coracoid processes are proportionately larger in *Pan* and *Homo,* while the glenoid cavity is broader and more shallow.

For detailed discussions of the locomotor functions of the shoulder girdle consult Frey 1923; Napier 1961; Erikson 1963; and Oxnard 1963, 1968.

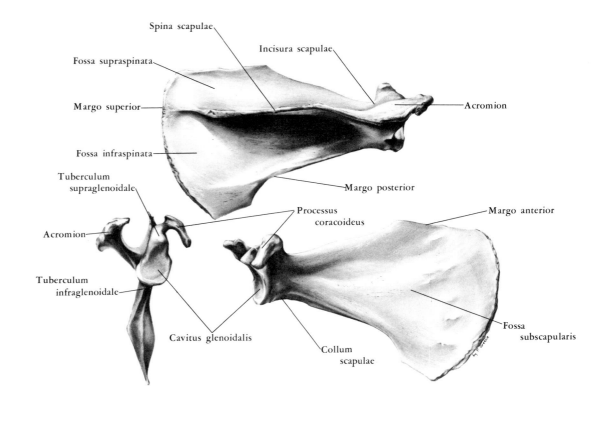

Papio

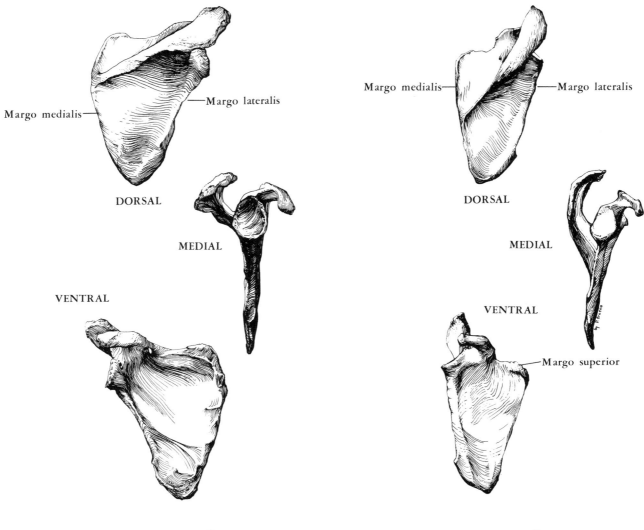

Margo medialis—
—Margo lateralis

DORSAL

MEDIAL

VENTRAL

Margo medialis—
—Margo lateralis

DORSAL

MEDIAL

VENTRAL

—Margo superior

Homo

Pan

PLATE 15

Right Humerus

In *Papio* the humerus displays a marked ventral convexity along the proximal third of the shaft. This bowing is accentuated by the powerful development of the deltoid tuberosity, which is located relatively higher on the humeral shaft than in *Pan* or *Homo*. In those two forms, the deltoid tuberosity is less prominent and situated relatively lower along the straighter humeral shaft. This development is associated with better abduction of the arm in the Hominoidea.

The humeral head is oriented dorsally in *Papio,* while in *Pan* and *Homo* the head is more medial for articulation with the scapula in its new position on the thorax. The greater and lesser tuberosities are well developed and separated by a wide sulcus in *Papio*. The greater tuberosity rises cranial to the summit of the humeral head; and the crest of the greater tuberosity, which is distinctly marked, forms the ventral margin of the shaft in its proximal third. In *Pan* and *Homo* the greater tuberosities do not rise cranial to the humeral head, and the greater and lesser tuberosities are separated by a deep, narrow sulcus. In both animals the crest of the greater tuberosity is much less prominent than in *Papio.*

The supinator crest is strongly developed along the lateral border of the distal portion of the shaft in all three animals. The capitulum is globular, and the trochlear surface is clearly defined in the three groups, although what Gregory (1949) has referred to as the "outer lip" or ridge of the trochlea is more sharply demarcated in *Pan* and *Homo*. He feels that this structure is associated with a greater range of supination at the elbow joint. The large medial rim of the trochlea, so well formed on the ventral surface, disappears as it is followed onto the dorsal surface of the humerus in *Papio*. In *Pan* and *Homo* it remains distinct, forming the medial boundary of the joint. The coronoid and radial fossae are very shallow in *Papio,* but in *Pan* and *Homo* (especially the coronoid fossa) are much deeper and are separated by a bony ridge.

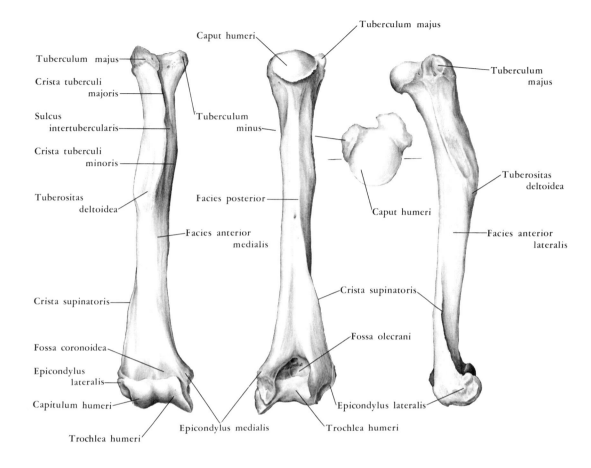

Papio

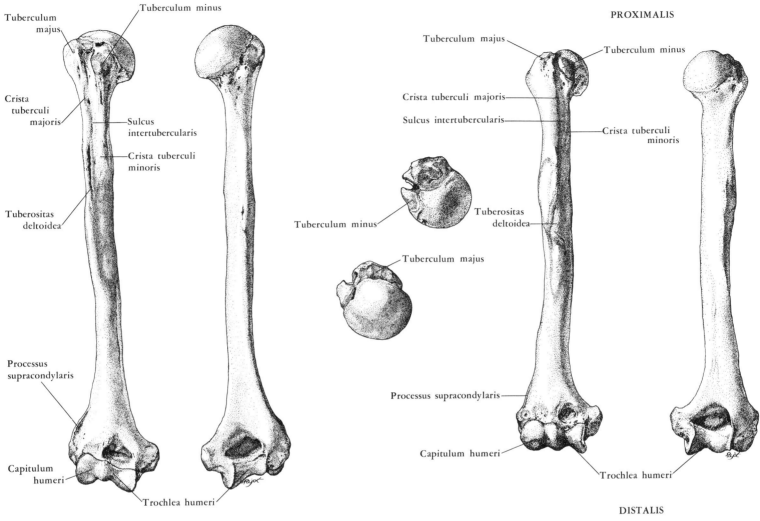

Tuberculum minus

Tuberculum majus

Crista tuberculi majoris

Sulcus intertubercularis

Crista tuberculi minoris

Tuberositas deltoidea

Processus supracondylaris

Capitulum humeri

Trochlea humeri

Homo

Tuberculum majus

Tuberculum minus

Crista tuberculi majoris

Sulcus intertubercularis

Crista tuberculi minoris

Tuberculum minus

Tuberositas deltoidea

Tuberculum majus

Processus supracondylaris

Capitulum humeri

Trochlea humeri

DISTALIS

Pan

PLATE 16

Right Ulna

In *Papio* the ulna is a long, straight bone tapering gradually from a large, roughened olecranon proximally to a small, narrow head distally. In *Pan* and *Homo* it is more curved, especially in the former. The olecranon is relatively long in most genera of Old World monkeys, particularly in *Papio;* but at the same time it is more constricted between its proximal surface and the sigmoid notch in these genera than in the Hominoidea. The less projecting olecranon of the Hominoidea permits a more complete extension at the elbow joint by bringing the triceps muscle closer to the fulcrum of the joint (Le Gros Clark 1960). In *Papio* the proximal aspect of the olecranon presents a laterally compressed contour with two depressions separated by a transverse bony ridge. *Pan* and *Homo* show a much broader olecranon with no transverse crest.

The trochlear notch is bordered medially by a sharply demarcated ridge which is continued ventrally into a prominent coronoid process in *Papio*. The radial notch is at the level of the coronoid process and is composed of a large dorsal and a small ventral portion. In *Pan* and *Homo* the medial ridge of the trochlear notch is present; however, it passes ventrally into a much broader coronoid process. The radial notch is made up of a single articular facet, which lies lateral to the coronoid process. Just dorsal to the dorsal segment of the radial notch in *Papio* is a longitudinal depression coursing approximately one-third of the distance along the ulna shaft. This groove is absent in *Homo* and *Pan*. In general, the proximal portion of the ulna is more compressed mediolaterally (flatter) in *Papio* than in *Pan* or *Homo*. According to Hill (1966), this is apparently associated with terrestrial quadrupedism.

The distal end of the ulna is represented by the head of the styloid process. The head is narrow in *Papio,* being only slightly wider in diameter than the neck, whereas in *Pan* and *Homo* the head is expanded into a rounded, globular contour much broader than the neck. The styloid process is relatively long and prominent in *Papio,* decreases in size in *Pan,* and reaches its smallest dimension in *Homo*.

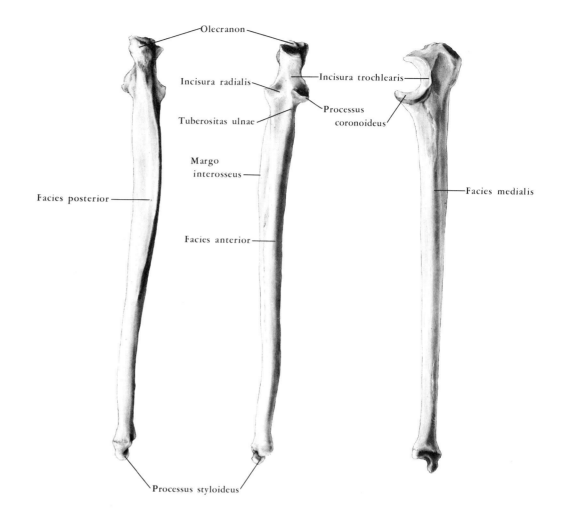

PROXIMALIS

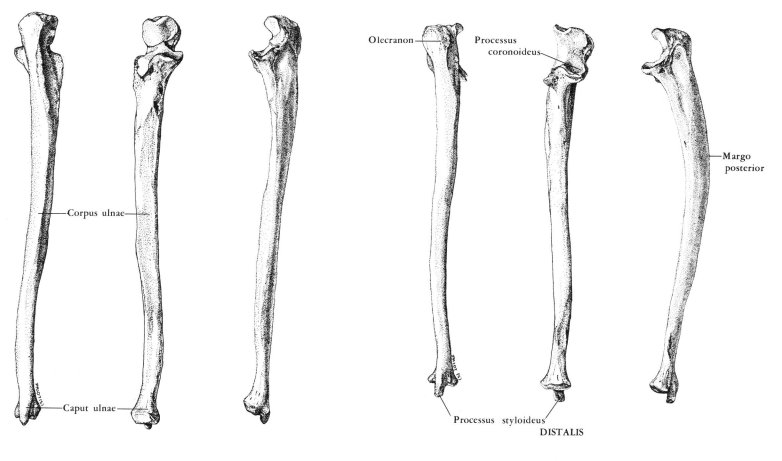

Olecranon

Processus coronoideus

Corpus ulnae

Margo posterior

Caput ulnae

Processus styloideus

DISTALIS

Homo

Pan

PLATE 17

Right Radius

The radius and ulna are separate in all members of the Anthropoidea. The radius is always bowed to some degree in *Papio, Pan,* and *Homo,* with its greatest curvature exemplified by *Pan.* The proximal end of the shaft is more compressed in *Papio* than in *Pan* or *Homo,* and the entire interosseous border is sharper and better delineated. Between this border and the rounded lateral border is a longitudinal groove occupying the middle third of the shaft in *Papio.* This sulcus is absent in *Pan* and *Homo.*

The radial head is rounded and discoidal, sitting at an oblique angle upon a cylindrical neck in *Papio.* Thus, the radial head is higher medially than laterally. In *Pan* the neck is exceedingly long, rounded, and constricted relative to the broad, flattened head; in *Homo* the head and neck are more nearly equal in breadth. A noticeable difference among these three bones is the position of the bicipital tuberosity. In *Papio* it is more proximal than in either *Pan* or *Homo,* a condition which increases the length of the power arm of the forearm lever in the latter forms (Campbell 1966).

The distal end of the shaft is expanded in the three bones, although less so, relative to the shaft in *Papio.* The styloid process is well developed, being somewhat longer and definitely more pointed in *Papio.* Dorsally, the expanded surface displays several broad, shallow depressions between raised bony crests in the three animals. In all three, the lateral tubercle is the most pronounced. The facet for the head of the ulna is flat and only slightly developed in *Papio,* whereas in *Pan* and *Homo* the facet is semilunar in contour, having definite dorsoventral boundaries. This is the most obvious difference in the distal ends of these three bones.

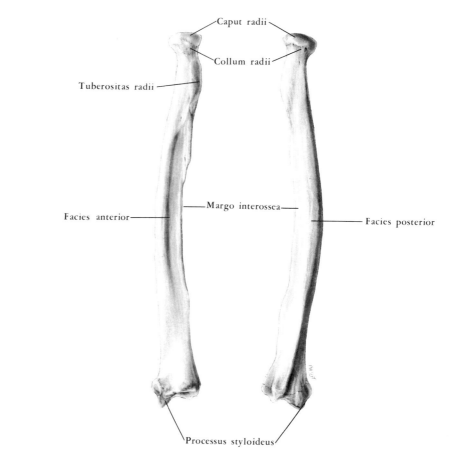

Papio

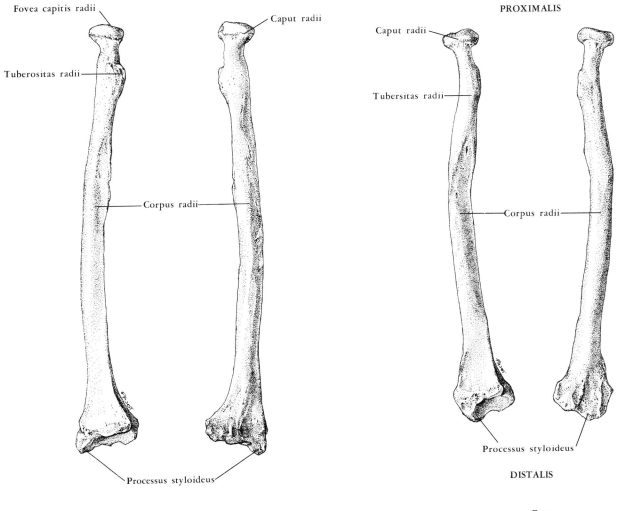

Fovea capitis radii

Caput radii

Tuberositas radii

Caput radii

Tubersitas radii

Corpus radii

Corpus radii

Processus styloideus

Processus styloideus

Homo

Pan

PLATE 18

Right Dorsal Hand

In the carpus, an os centrale is present in *Papio* as well as in all other genera of Old World monkeys (see Plate 19). It articulates with the scaphoid of the proximal row and with the capitate, trapezium, and trapezoid of the distal row. This bone is absent in adult *Pan* and *Homo,* having fused with the scaphoid during fetal life (Le Gros Clark 1960). The remaining eight carpal bones are similar in the three genera, differing more in size than in details of morphology.

The metacarpals are long, narrow bones with enlarged proximal and distal ends. The metacarpals of *Papio* are long compared with the length of the digits, whereas in many genera of Old World monkeys they are short (Napier 1962). The major difference in the phalanges is represented by the terminal phalanx: in *Papio* this is a slender, narrow bone almost coming to a point, while in *Pan* and especially in *Homo* it is a broad, flat bone. On the whole, the hand/foot of *Papio* is rather long and narrow compared with the hand of *Pan* and *Homo.* The digital formula in the three animals is III > IV > II > V > I, characteristic of all primates except certain prosimians in which the fourth finger may be the longest (Schultz 1926).

The thumb is variably developed among all primates. In Old World monkeys it varies in length from a small, atrophied nodule *(Colobus)* to a relatively long, well formed structure *(Macaca* and *Papio).* According to Napier (1962), true opposibility of the thumb "appears for the first time among the living primate in Old World monkeys" (p. 60). He attributes this function to the well-developed carpometacarpal joint, which is concavoconvex in shape. In addition, there is a fair range of movement at the metacarpophalangeal joint. Opposibility is some-what limited in the living Pongidae, particularly in the gibbon and orang, because of an abbreviated thumb. In *Pan* the tip of the terminal phalanx of the thumb although somewhat longer, does not reach the metacarpophalangeal joint of the index finger. In *Homo* it passes distal to this joint, and the greatest range of functional capability (opposibility) is represented.

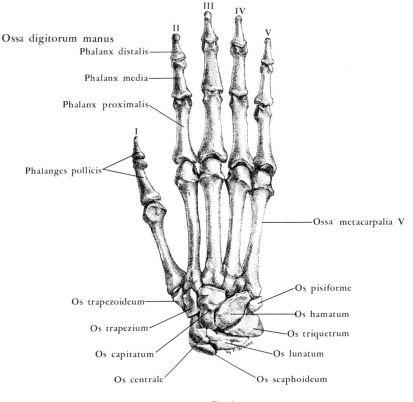

Papio

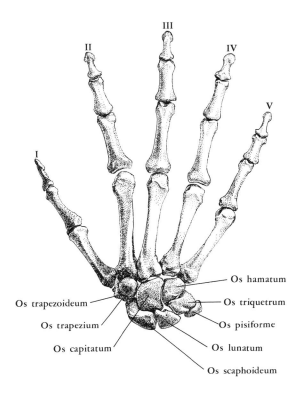

II   III   IV

I   V

Os trapezoideum ——
Os trapezium ——
Os capitatum ——

—— Os hamatum
—— Os triquetrum
—— Os pisiforme
—— Os lunatum
—— Os scaphoideum

Homo

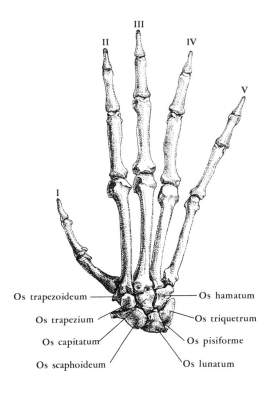

II   III   IV

I   V

Os trapezoideum ——
Os trapezium ——
Os capitatum ——
Os scaphoideum ——

—— Os hamatum
—— Os triquetrum
—— Os pisiforme
—— Os lunatum

Pan

PLATE 19

Right Ventral Hand

There is little to be added concerning the bones of the hand. The various articular facets are easily observed in this volar presentation, and the differences are in size and proportion rather than in morphology.

In *Homo* the capitate is the largest bone of the carpus, whereas in *Papio* it is not as large as the hamate. Also, the middle section of the capitate is much more constricted than in *Pan* or *Homo*. The hamate presents a hooklike process, the hamulus in all three animals. The pisiform is small, but in *Pan* it is elongated and presents a shallow medial curve, which articulates with the hamate.

The metacarpals, particularly the third, are very long in *Papio*. Note the extremely short metacarpal of the pollex in *Pan*, especially when it is compared with the other metacarpal bones.

The terminal phalanges in *Pan* and *Homo* are broad, flat bones with slightly concave palmar surfaces. In *Papio* they are narrow and more constricted in their middle parts.

Note the location of the sesamoid bones in *Papio*. There are frequently five sesamoid bones in *Homo*—two at the metacarpophalangeal joint of the thumb, one at the interphalangeal joint of the pollex, and one each at the metacarpophalangeal articulations of the second and fifth fingers.

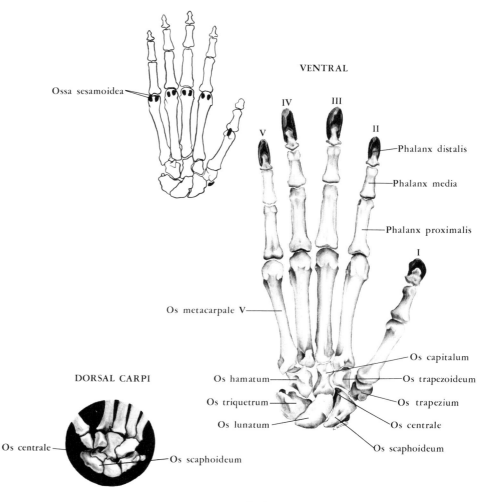

VENTRAL

Ossa sesamoidea

Phalanx distalis

Phalanx media

Phalanx proximalis

Os metacarpale V

DORSAL CARPI

Os hamatum

Os triquetrum

Os lunatum

Os capitalum

Os trapezoideum

Os trapezium

Os centrale

Os scaphoideum

Os centrale

Os scaphoideum

Papio

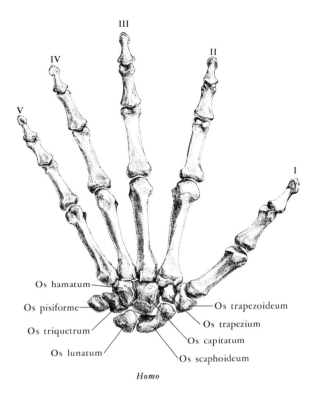

Os hamatum
Os pisiforme
Os triquetrum
Os lunatum
Os trapezoideum
Os trapezium
Os capitatum
Os scaphoideum

Homo

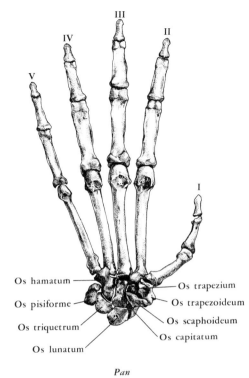

Os hamatum
Os pisiforme
Os triquetrum
Os lunatum
Os trapezium
Os trapezoideum
Os scaphoideum
Os capitatum

Pan

PLATE 20

Right Lateral Hip Bone

The most striking osteological feature exemplified by this view is the broader ilium in *Homo*, which is the widest ilium among the primates. Indeed, Straus (1929) pointed out that the width always exceeds the height by at least one-fourth in adult *Homo*. The dorsal expansion of the human ilium with the commensurate extension of the iliac crest affords a much larger area of attachment for the muscles involved in bipedal walking and maintaining the trunk in the erect attitude (Plates 120 and 121). Washburn (1950) pointed out the evolutionary significance of this morphologic modification for *Homo*. In *Homo* the gluteus maximus has become an extensor of the thigh rather than an abductor of the thigh as in nonhuman primates. The reorientation of the primary function of these muscles has been extremely important in the evolution of the human stride.

The gluteal surface of the ilium in *Papio* presents a craniocaudal concavity extending from the iliac crest to the corpus of the ilium. It is bounded by a bony elevation along the dorsal border of the ilium. The concavity is also present in *Pan*, although wider in a dorsoventral direction. This area provides attachment for the well-developed gluteus medius muscle (Plate 121). For *Papio*, Waterman (1929) correlated this muscle-bone complex with the free lateral rotation of the pelvis evinced by terrestrial quadrupeds.

Another conspicuous anatomical feature from this view is the elongated body of the ischium and the corresponding separation of the ischial tuberosity from the acetabulum in *Papio* and *Pan*. The reverse situation is present in *Homo*, and this approximation of ischium to acetabulum has increased the mechanical advantage of the posterior thigh extensors in balancing the pelvis upon the lower extremity (Le Gros Clark 1960).

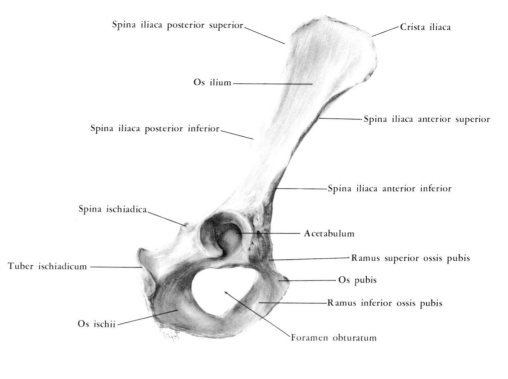

Papio

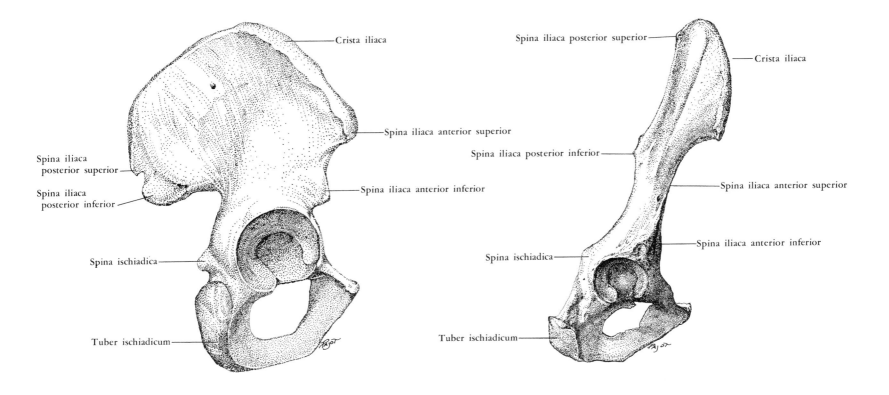

Crista iliaca

Spina iliaca anterior superior

Spina iliaca
posterior superior

Spina iliaca
posterior inferior

Spina iliaca anterior inferior

Spina ischiadica

Tuber ischiadicum

Homo

Spina iliaca posterior superior

Crista iliaca

Spina iliaca posterior inferior

Spina iliaca anterior superior

Spina iliaca anterior inferior

Spina ischiadica

Tuber ischiadicum

Pan

PLATE 21

Right Medial Hip Bone

The medial view offers several interesting points of contrast. The sciatic notch is much deeper and more acute in *Homo,* while it is no more than an elongated depression along the dorsal border of the ilium in *Papio* and *Pan.* The appearance of a true notch in *Homo* occurred *pari passu* with the dorsal expansion of the ilium.

The acetabular border of the ilium is much straighter in nonhuman primates than it is in *Homo.* There are two bony elevations present on the ventral border of the ilium in all three forms. In *Homo* these are designated as the anterior superior and anterior inferior iliac spines. The same terms are used for nonhuman primates, but whether they are homologous is questionable (Benton and Gavan 1960; also Plate 116).

The sacral articular surface is more extensive in *Homo* and lies closer to the acetabulum, a condition which makes for greater stability in bipedal *Homo* (Le Gros Clark 1960).

The pubis is extremely elongated in *Papio* and presents a long symphysial surface, which is proportionately longer than in all other primates (Hill 1970). The surface is also very narrow when compared with the other two animals.

As mentioned earlier, the ischium of *Papio* is massive with a relatively long and expanded corpus. The ischial spine is a narrow projection which is much broader in *Pan* and *Homo.* The more extensive development of the spine in the latter forms, especially in *Homo,* accentuates the lesser sciatic notch.

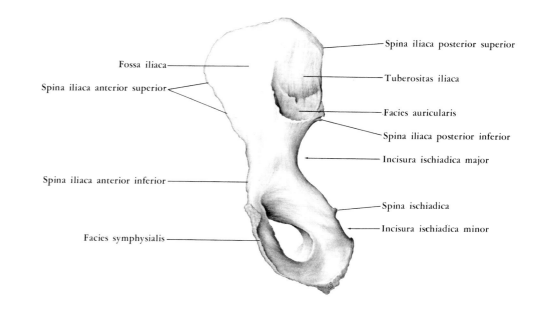

Fossa iliaca

Spina iliaca anterior superior

Spina iliaca anterior inferior

Facies symphysialis

Spina iliaca posterior superior

Tuberositas iliaca

Facies auricularis

Spina iliaca posterior inferior

Incisura ischiadica major

Spina ischiadica

Incisura ischiadica minor

Papio

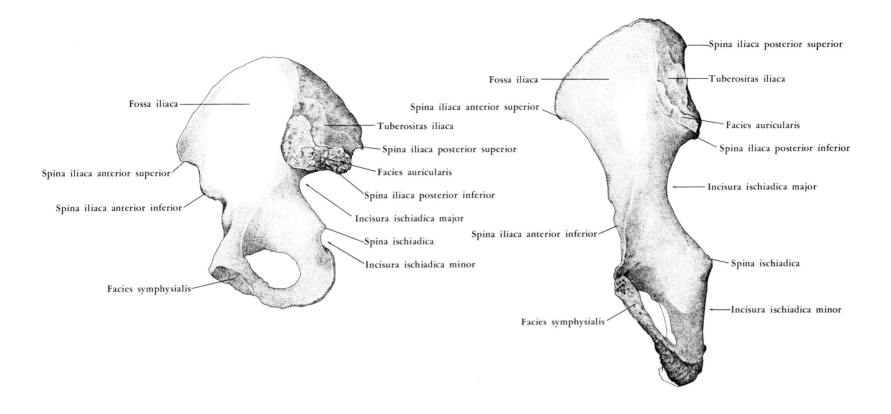

Fossa iliaca

Spina iliaca anterior superior

Spina iliaca anterior inferior

Facies symphysialis

Spina iliaca anterior superior

Tuberositas iliaca

Spina iliaca posterior superior

Facies auricularis

Spina iliaca posterior inferior

Incisura ischiadica major

Spina ischiadica

Incisura ischiadica minor

Homo

Spina iliaca posterior superior

Fossa iliaca

Tuberositas iliaca

Facies auricularis

Spina iliaca posterior inferior

Incisura ischiadica major

Spina iliaca anterior inferior

Spina ischiadica

Incisura ischiadica minor

Facies symphysialis

Pan

PLATE 22

Ventral Pelvis

In *Papio* the innominate bones are elongated craniocaudally and the transverse diameter of the pelvis is narrow. The pubic symphysis normally includes both pubis and ischium, while the sacrum is composed of two or three sacral vertebrae. In *Pan*, and especially in *Homo*, there is a relatively greater expansion of the ilium. The union at the symphysis is between the two pubic bones and the sacrum is usually made up of five sacral vertebrae.

The subpubic angle is wide and presents a more rounded contour in *Homo* than in the other two forms. In *Homo* this angle is a reliable criterion for establishing the sex of an unknown pelvis. The wider the angle, the more likelihood the specimen is female.

The acetabula are directed more dorsolaterally in *Papio* and *Pan*, whereas in *Homo* they are oriented caudoventrally.

The ischial tuberosities are extremely well developed in all cercopithecoids. Note the large triangular development of the processes in *Papio* with their broad, roughened surfaces showing an everted lateral margin. This flattened base forms the bony support for the overlying ischial callosities that are a hallmark of the Old World monkeys. These hard pads are used for sitting, as well as for sleeping in the sitting position. *Pan* and *Homo* completely lack such expanded ischial tuberosities.

The iliac fossa, a feature which Straus (1929) found only in *Homo*, is well depicted, and the much more medially oriented iliac surfaces are clearly observable. The most outstanding impression one gains from this view is the breadth, shallowness, and great capacity of the human pelvis compared to the elongated and narrow pelvis of the nonhuman primates.

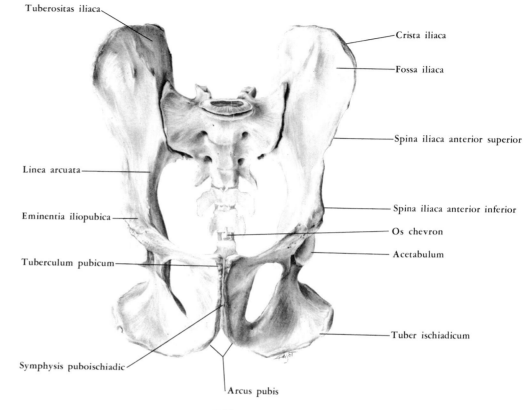

Tuberositas iliaca

Crista iliaca

Fossa iliaca

Spina iliaca anterior superior

Linea arcuata

Spina iliaca anterior inferior

Eminentia iliopubica

Os chevron

Acetabulum

Tuberculum pubicum

Tuber ischiadicum

Symphysis puboischiadic

Arcus pubis

Papio

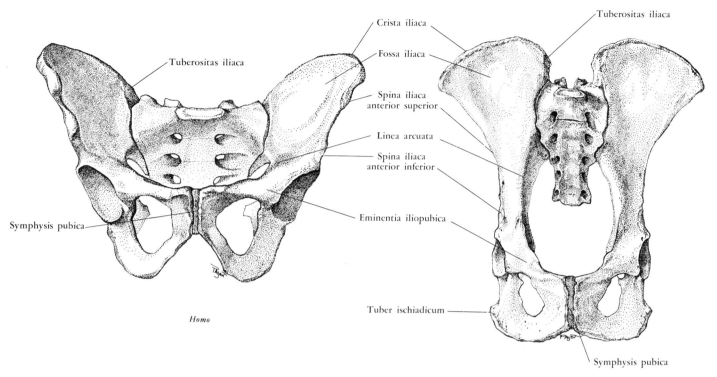

Tuberositas iliaca

Crista iliaca

Fossa iliaca

Spina iliaca
anterior superior

Linea arcuata

Spina iliaca
anterior inferior

Eminentia iliopubica

Symphysis pubica

Homo

Tuberositas iliaca

Tuber ischiadicum

Symphysis pubica

Pan

PLATE 23

Right Femur

The femoral shaft is curved in the sagittal plane with an anterior convexity in all three primates. Such bowing is usually more pronounced in hominoids than in terrestrial monkeys. The shafts present cylindrical contours throughout most of their length.

The proximal femur includes the head, neck, and trochanters. In *Papio* the head is a somewhat flattened hemisphere whereas in *Pan* and *Homo* it is much more globular. The neck in *Papio* is short and presents a flat ventral surface. A noticeable difference is the extension of the greater trochanter proximal to the upper limit of the head in *Papio*. The lesser trochanter is prominent on all three femurs, being more anteroposteriorly compressed in *Papio*. The gluteal tuberosity, or third trochanter, is more prominent in *Papio,* being only occasionally developed in *Pan* and *Homo*.

The trochanteric fossa is deeply excavated in *Papio,* and the intertrochanteric crest connecting the greater and lesser trochanters presents an undulating medial border. The fossa is less deep in *Pan* and *Homo* and far less extensive, being merely a rounded indentation occupying the medial surface of the greater trochanter. The medial border of the intertrochanteric crest is smooth.

The fovea capitis is a rough depression inferoposterior to the center of the head in *Papio* and *Homo,* while its position in *Pan* is more superoposterior. Its form and depth are variable in all three primates.

The intertrochanteric line is not well marked in either *Papio* or *Pan* when compared with the eminence in *Homo*.

The linea aspera is well developed in all three primates but reaches its maximum expression in *Homo*. There it forms an elevated keel in the middle third of the shaft before diverging into the medial and lateral lips, which extend to the condyles. The medial lip terminates as the adductor tubercle, a small sharp projection on the cranial surface of the medial condyle. The lateral lip is usually more prominent and ends on the lateral condyle. Between the two lines is the broad, flat popliteal surface. In *Papio* and *Pan* these ridges are poorly marked, especially the medial one. The adductor tubercle is not present in *Papio;* however, it is present in *Pan* (Plate 118).

The medial and lateral condyles are prominent in the three primates, and in each the medial projects more distally than the lateral. The lateral surface of the lateral condyle is deeply excavated, especially in *Pan,* for the attachment of the popliteus tendon. The intercondylar fossa is relatively wider in *Pan*. In all three, the intercondylar line is sharp.

The patella surface is more prominent on its lateral aspect. *Papio* and *Homo* display a median vertical groove, which is absent in *Pan*.

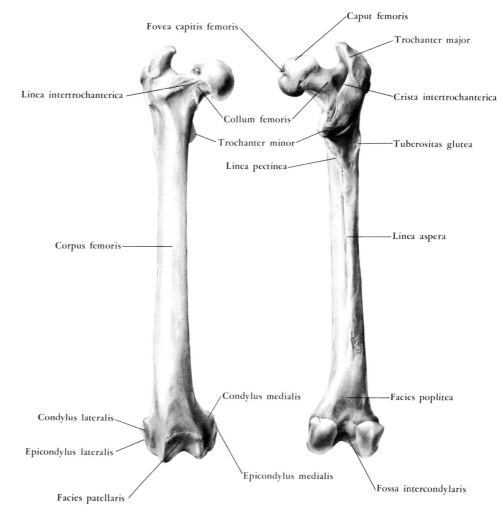

Papio

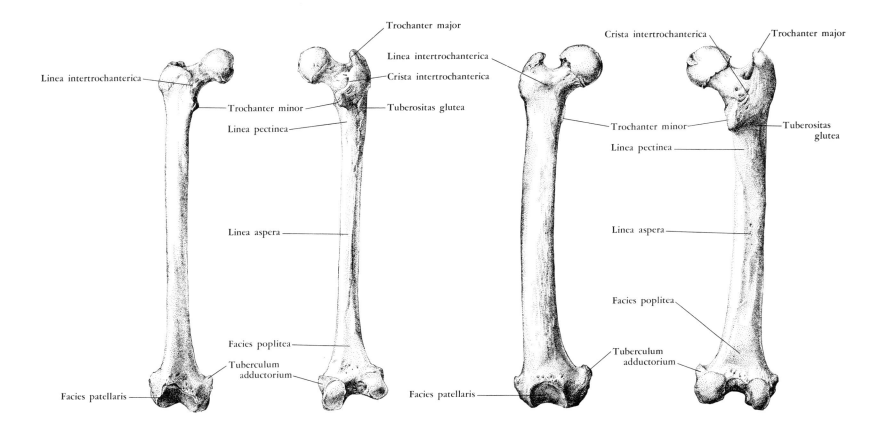

Linea intertrochanterica

Trochanter minor

Linea pectinea

Linea aspera

Facies poplitea

Tuberculum adductorium

Facies patellaris

Trochanter major

Linea intertrochanterica

Crista intertrochanterica

Tuberositas glutea

Crista intertrochanterica

Trochanter major

Trochanter minor

Tuberositas glutea

Linea pectinea

Linea aspera

Facies poplitea

Tuberculum adductorium

Facies patellaris

Homo

Pan

PLATE 24

Right Tibia

The body of the tibia is prismatic throughout its proximal half, becoming more tubular at the distal end of the bone. The anterior margin is prominent in all three primates and can be followed from the lateral border of the tuberosity distally to the anterior margin of the medial malleolus. The proximal portion of the tibia in *Papio* is more compressed mediolaterally than in the other two primates. Indeed, either side of the tibial tuberosity the body of the tibia is concave in a proximodistal direction, resulting in the high relief of this process. This portion of the tibia is much fuller in *Pan* and *Homo*.

The medial condyle is more extensive than the lateral, especially in *Homo*. The articular surfaces of the condyles are as follows. In *Homo* the medial surface is oval and broadly concave, while the articular surface of the lateral condyle is more circular and almost flat. In *Pan* the surface of the medial condyle is similar to that in *Homo,* whereas the surface of the lateral condyle is convex in its anteroposterior direction. In *Papio* the surface of the lateral condyle is similar to that in *Pan,* but the surface of the medial condyle is different from that in the other two primates, being convex rather than concave in its anteroposterior direction. The intercondylar eminence is similarly disposed in the three forms, although the intercondylar tubercles are more prolonged in *Homo*.

The most prominent feature on the distal portion of the tibia is the medial malleolus. It is very elongated in *Papio* and curves laterally near its tip to produce a deep sulcus. The medial malleolus is long in *Pan;* however, the process is normally straight and the groove is absent. In *Homo* the malleolus is thick and broad and its long axis is inclined medially.

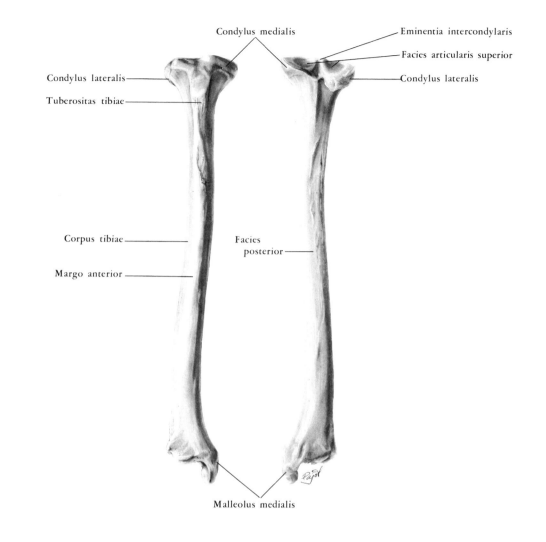

Papio

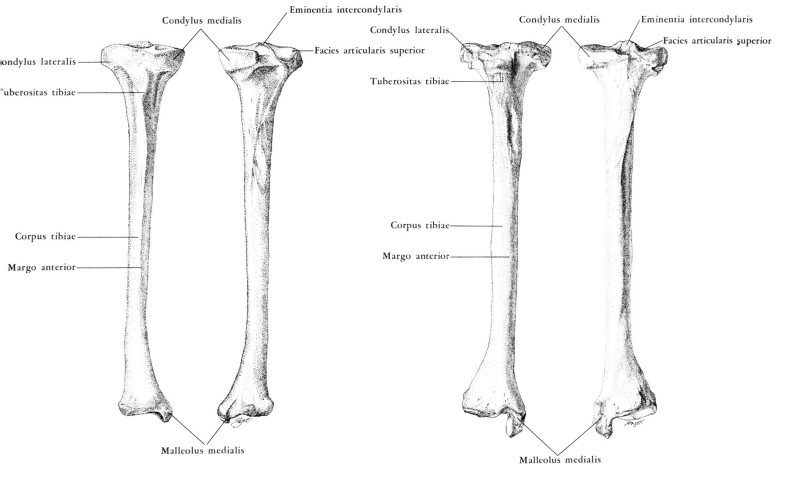

Condylus medialis

Eminentia intercondylaris

ondylus lateralis

Facies articularis superior

uberositas tibiae

Corpus tibiae

Margo anterior

Malleolus medialis

Homo

Condylus medialis

Condylus lateralis

Eminentia intercondylaris

Facies articularis superior

Tuberositas tibiae

Corpus tibiae

Margo anterior

Malleolus medialis

Pan

PLATE 25

Right Fibula

The majority of primates have a mobile fibula (Barnett and Napier 1952), that is, both the proximal and distal tibiofibular articulations are synovial, permitting some degree of rotation during ankle joint movement. Thus, all three fibulas present rather conspicuous articular facets. Proximally, there is a somewhat circular articular surface of the head for articulation with the lateral condyle of the tibia. Distally, the medial malleolar articular surface articulates with the fibular notch of the tibia.

The proximal end of each fibula bears a somewhat rounded head, although it is much compressed transversely in *Papio*. The distal end displays a rather flattened, pyramidal extension from the body, the lateral malleolus. It is short, blunt, and has no definite apex in *Papio*. The lateral malleoli are proportionately larger in *Homo* and *Pan* and each presents a rather sharp, pointed apex. The medial surface of each fibula is indented by the lateral malleolar fossa, which is more deeply excavated in *Pan* and *Homo* than in *Papio*.

The most prominent feature of the shaft is the interosseous margin. In *Pan* and *Homo* it is elevated in a keellike fashion along the anterior margin of the fibula coursing from the head distally to near the lateral malleolus. It affords attachment to the interosseous membrane. In *Papio* the margin is less distinct, especially along the distal half of the shaft.

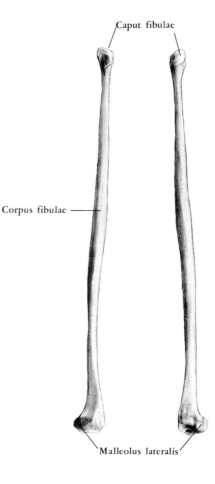

Caput fibulae

Corpus fibulae

Malleolus lateralis

Papio

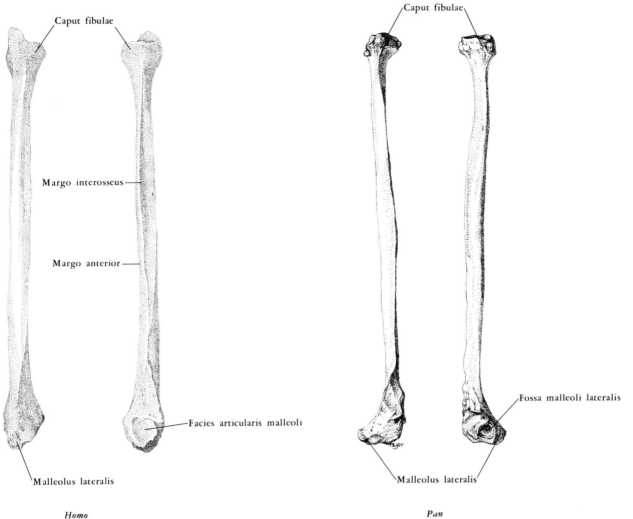

Caput fibulae

Caput fibulae

Margo interosseus

Margo anterior

Facies articularis malleoli

Fossa malleoli lateralis

Malleolus lateralis

Malleolus lateralis

Homo

Pan

PLATE 26

Right Dorsal Foot

The tarsal bones are grouped into a proximal row—calcaneus and talus—and a distal row—medial, intermediate, and lateral cuneiform bones, and the cuboid. Positioned between these two rows on the medial side is the navicular. When compared with the carpal bones, the tarsal bones are larger and show greater diversity of size. These differences are correlated, at least in part, with the function of weight bearing, especially in *Homo*.

Individually, the tarsal bones present some interesting osteologic differences among the three genera. In *Papio* and *Pan* the axis of the neck of the talus forms an angle of 20° or more with that of the articular surface for the tibia; in *Homo* this angle is always much less than 20°. The difference in the angle is correlated with the position of the hallux, being abducted in *Papio* and *Pan* and adducted in *Homo*. The articular surface for the tibia extends some distance onto the dorsal surface of the neck in *Papio* (Hill 1970), but not in *Pan* or *Homo*. The calcaneus extends posteriorly into the tuberosity, which in *Homo* projects inferiorly and posteriorly to form the heel. This posterior extension of the calcaneus is much more constricted in *Pan*, and especially in *Papio*.

The remaining tarsal bones are morphologically more similar in the three forms, except for size and proportion differences. In the latter category, note the conspicuous anteroposterior shortening of the proximal and intermediate tarsal bones in *Pan*. Le Gros Clark (1960) has attributed this to the forwardly displaced center of gravity in the Great Apes.

The metatarsals are long, cylindrical bones with enlarged proximal and distal ends. In *Papio* the third metatarsal is the longest, corresponding with the functional axis of the foot, while in *Pan* and *Homo* this axis lies between the first and second digits. Indeed, it has shifted almost to the hallux in *Homo*. Consequently, the second metatarsal bone is the longest of the series.

The hallux is approximated to the other digits only in *Homo*. It is a long, robust digit which, on occasion, may be the longest. The length of man's great toe is apparently the result of the reduction of digits II-V rather than hypertrophy of the hallux (Schultz 1936).

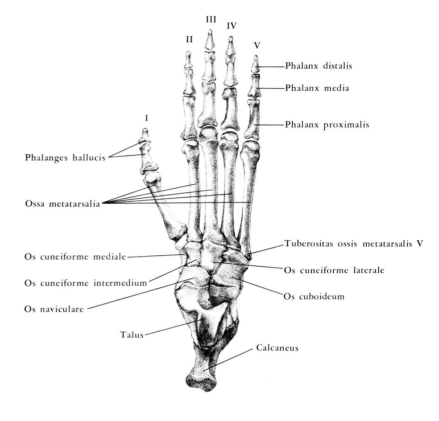

Papio

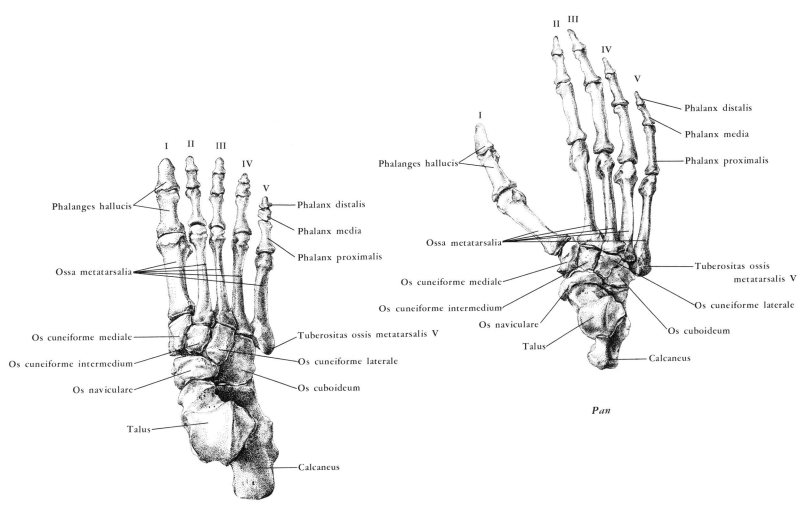

Phalanges hallucis

I II III

IV

V

Phalanx distalis

Phalanx media

Phalanx proximalis

Ossa metatarsalia

Os cuneiforme mediale

Os cuneiforme intermedium

Os naviculare

Talus

Tuberositas ossis metatarsalis V

Os cuneiforme laterale

Os cuboideum

Calcaneus

Homo

II III

IV

V

Phalanx distalis

Phalanx media

Phalanx proximalis

I

Phalanges hallucis

Ossa metatarsalia

Os cuneiforme mediale

Os cuneiforme intermedium

Os naviculare

Talus

Tuberositas ossis
metatarsalis V

Os cuneiforme laterale

Os cuboideum

Calcaneus

Pan

PLATE 27

Right Ventral Foot

The calcaneus of *Papio* displays little curvature along
its lateral border, whereas the medial surface is strongly
concave. The sustentaculum tali is prominent in the three
forms and presents a more attenuated projection in
Papio. The constricted calcaneal tuberosity of *Papio* was
noted earlier.

The navicular and cuboid bones have well-developed
tuberosities, which are readily observed in this view. Of the
three cuneiforms, the middle is the smallest; indeed, in
Papio its distal portion is so narrow that it is virtually
obscured by the medial and lateral cuneiforms.

The metatarsal bones are long in *Papio*, particularly
when compared with the short phalanges. This formation
reflects the cursorial gait of quadrupedal *Papio*. In walking,
these primates use the distal heads of the metatarsal
bones as the fulcrum for pushing off of the ground. Their
locomotion pattern, therefore, is classified as metatarsi-
fulcrumating, and a phylogenetic consequence of this
gait has been an increase in the length of the metatarsal
bones (Morton 1935; Le Gros Clark 1960). The third
metatarsal is the longest of the series. Observe the large
tuberosity of the fifth metatarsal of *Homo* pointing proximal
on the lateral side of its base.

Note the ten sesamoid bones in *Papio*. This animal
usually has ten, two at each metatarsophalangeal joint.
In *Pan* and *Homo* there are two, both located at the
metatarsophalangeal junction of the hallux.

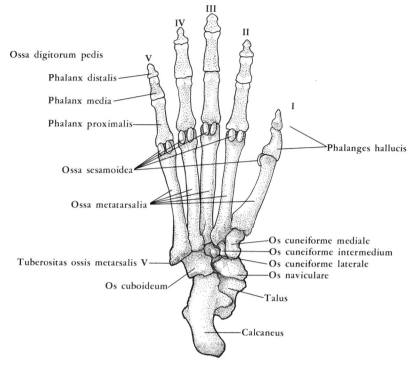

Papio

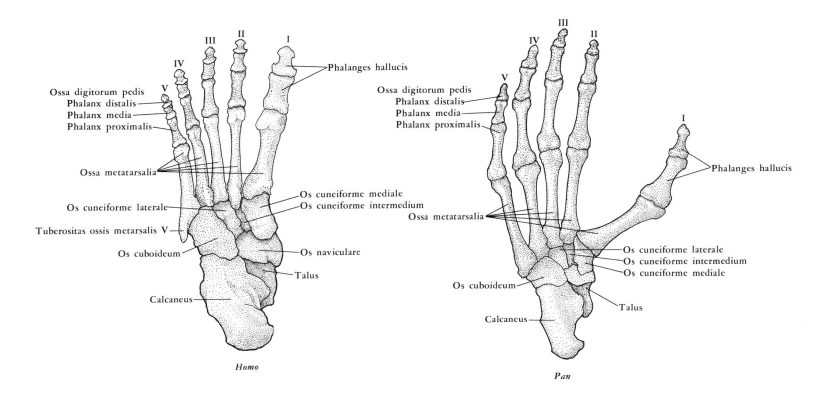

Ossa digitorum pedis
Phalanx distalis
Phalanx media
Phalanx proximalis

Ossa metatarsalia

Os cuneiforme laterale

Tuberositas ossis metarsalis V

Os cuboideum

Calcaneus

Phalanges hallucis

Os cuneiforme mediale
Os cuneiforme intermedium

Os naviculare

Talus

Homo

Ossa digitorum pedis
Phalanx distalis
Phalanx media
Phalanx proximalis

Ossa metatarsalia

Os cuboideum

Calcaneus

Phalanges hallucis

Os cuneiforme laterale
Os cuneiforme intermedium
Os cuneiforme mediale

Talus

Pan

Part 2

HEAD AND NECK

PLATE 28

Distribution of External Carotid Artery

The common carotid artery normally remains unbranched as it ascends through the neck in most primates. In anthropoid apes, especially *Pan,* it frequently gives off branches to the thyroid gland when there is no thyroid branch from the subclavian (Sonntag 1924). In *Papio* the common carotid bifurcates at the cranial border of the hyoid bone deep to the posterior belly of the digastric muscle and the twelfth nerve, whereas in *Pan* and *Homo* the division occurs more caudally in the carotid triangle. Unlike *Homo,* the external carotid in *Papio* is larger at the level of bifurcation than the internal carotid (McCoy, Swindler, and Albers 1967).

The linguofacial trunk appears consistently in *Papio* and is the general rule in *Pan* (McCoy, Swindler, and Albers 1967; Sonntag 1924). In *Homo* these vessels arise independently from the external carotid as the lingual and facial arteries. The superior thyroid, the first branch of the external carotid in *Homo,* arises from the common linguofacial trunk in *Papio* and *Pan.* As noted earlier, the superior thyroid may arise from the common carotid in *Pan.* In *Papio,* McCoy, Swindler, and Albers (1967) found the superior thyroid arising from the linguofacial trunk in 71 percent of their *Papio* sample.

One of the smaller branches of the common carotid, the ascending pharyngeal, arises from the superomedial side of the external carotid in all three primates. It is not shown here, but passes cranially and superficially over the surface of the longus colli muscle on its way to the base of the skull.

A common trunk for the occipital and posterior auricular arteries occurs more often in *Papio* and *Pan.* In the former, McCoy, Swindler, and Albers (1967) found it in 66 percent of twenty-seven *Papio* dissections. In *Homo* the occipital and posterior auricular arteries arise separately from the posterior border of the external carotid.

The superficial temporal and transverse facial arteries arise as a common stem in the majority of *Papio* specimens. This is often the condition in *Pan,* whereas in *Homo* the transverse facial arises from the superficial temporal, which is the smaller of the two terminal branches of the external carotid. The other, much larger terminal branch is the maxillary artery, which is usually interpreted as the continuation of the external carotid in *Papio* (McCoy, Swindler, and Albers 1967; Platzer 1960; Hill 1970).

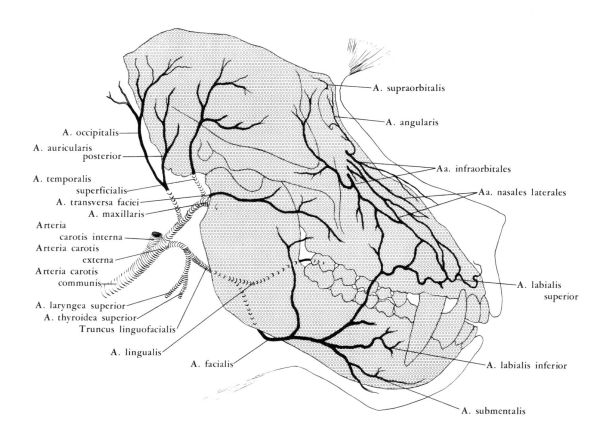

Papio

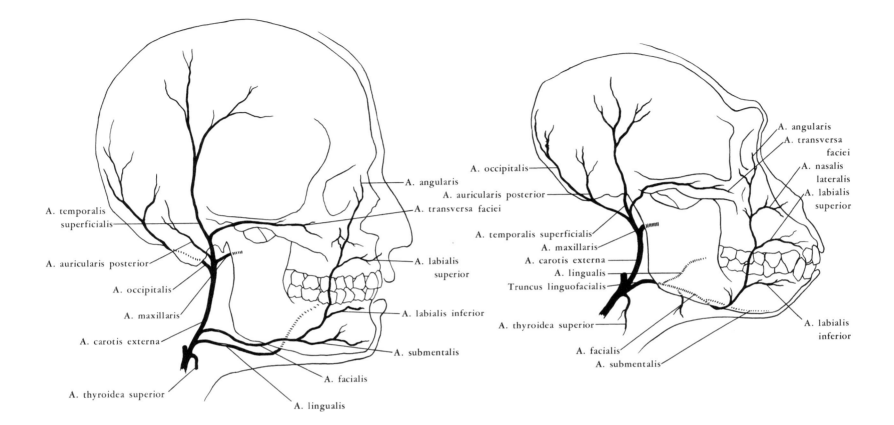

A. temporalis
superficialis

A. auricularis posterior

A. occipitalis

A. maxillaris

A. carotis externa

A. thyroidea superior

A. angularis

A. auricularis posterior

A. transversa faciei

A. labialis
superior

A. labialis inferior

A. submentalis

A. facialis

A. lingualis

A. occipitalis

A. temporalis superficialis

A. maxillaris

A. carotis externa

A. lingualis

Truncus linguofacialis

A. thyroidea superior

A. facialis

A. submentalis

A. angularis

A. transversa
faciei

A. nasalis
lateralis

A. labialis
superior

A. labialis
inferior

Homo

Pan

PLATE 29

Superficial Veins of Face and Neck

As in other regions of the body, the veins of the face and neck are divisible into superficial and deep systems. The superficial veins of the face are tributaries of the internal and external jugular veins of the neck, while the deep veins of the face are tributaries of the internal jugular only. Both systems anastomose freely with each other, creating extremely diverse drainage patterns. Variability is the rule rather than the exception.

The facial vein is the continuation of the angular and returns blood from the most distal part of the face or snout of *Papio*. There are numerous external nasal veins which form a complicated drainage pattern along the long snout of *Papio*. These ultimately drain into the facial, which in turn is a tributary of the external jugular. In *Pan* and *Homo* the tortuous course of the facial vein terminates more frequently in the internal jugular vein. Throughout its course there are rich connections with the deep veins of the face.

The retromandibular vein is normally formed by the union of the superficial temporal and maxillary veins. In addition, in *Papio* a large vessel leaves a foramen in the lateral part of the petrosquamous fissure to drain into the retromandibular vein. This is a rather constant vessel in the cercopithecids and is named the petrosquamous vein (Weinstein and Hedges 1962). The retromandibular becomes the external jugular vein.

The external jugular is formed by the junction of the posterior auricular and retromandibular veins in *Homo*. It is a tributary of the large subclavian vein. In *Papio* and other cercopithecids the external jugular is frequently divided into two vessels. One appears to be the continuation of the facial and pursues a superficial course through the neck passing ventral to the clavicle. The other is a continuation of the external jugular and passes dorsal to the clavicle. If present, the two vessels unite at a point caudal to the clavicle to join the subclavian vein or internal jugular (McCoy 1964).

The internal jugular vein commences at the jugular bulb and passes through the neck collecting blood from the brain, face, and neck. It is a direct tributary of the brachiocephalic vein.

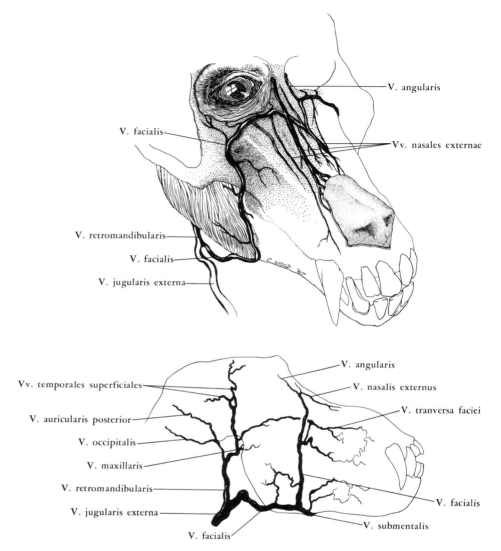

Papio

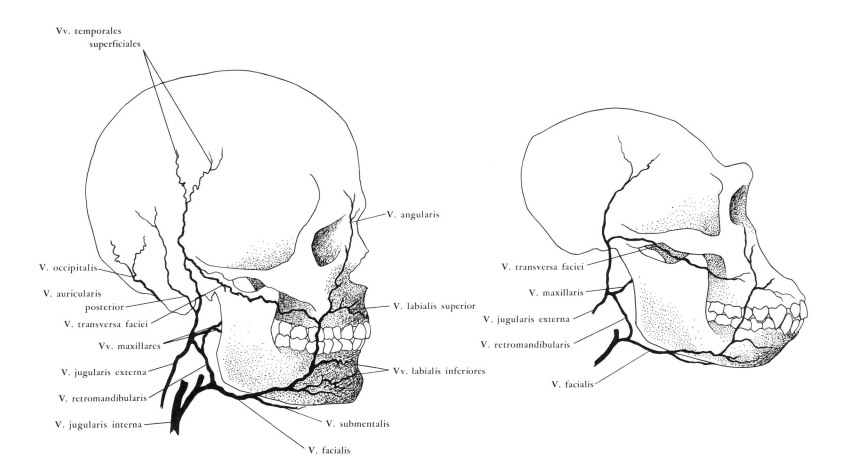

Vv. temporales
superficiales

V. angularis

V. occipitalis

V. auricularis
posterior

V. transversa faciei

Vv. maxillares

V. jugularis externa

V. retromandibularis

V. jugularis interna

V. labialis superior

Vv. labialis inferiores

V. submentalis

V. facialis

V. transversa faciei

V. maxillaris

V. jugularis externa

V. retromandibularis

V. facialis

Homo

Pan

PLATE 30

Facial Branches
of Trigeminal Nerve

The trigeminal nerve has sensory and motor roots. The ganglion associated with the sensory root is the semilunar ganglion, which lies in a pocket of dura mater on the medial surface of the petrous portion of the temporal bone (see also Plate 47). Three large nerves spring from the ganglion: the ophthalmic, maxillary, and mandibular. Of these, only the mandibular division is associated with the motor root. The general pattern of trigeminal distribution is similar in the three primates if one allows for certain minor variations in the details of the peripheral branches (Ashton and Oxnard 1958; Bowden, Mahran, and Godding 1960; Gasser and Hendrickx 1969).

The ophthalmic division separates into its three terminal branches—frontal, lacrimal and nasociliary—just before it enters the superior orbital fissure. Smaller branches of each of these three nerves reach the skin of the face. The frontal appears as the supraorbital and supratrochlear nerves, and supplies integument at the lateral corner of the eye and over the zygomatic process of the frontal bone. The nasociliary is distributed to the skin as the infratrochlear and external nasal twigs. Note that the latter nerve is a branch of the anterior ethmoidal, a terminal branch of the nasociliary which is seen in Plate 42.

The maxillary division leaves the middle cranial fossa via the foramen rotundum and enters the pterygopalatine fossa. From here it passes into the infraorbital sulcus and canal as the infraorbital nerve on its way to the skin of the midface. While still within the pterygopalatine fossa the parent trunk gives off the zygomatic nerve, which in turn gives rise to the zygomaticofacial and zygomaticotemporal rami. These nerves innervate skin around the lateral side of the orbit and the temporal region. In *Papio* the infraorbital nerve divides into nasal and labial parts (the labial separates into two twigs) while still within the infraorbital sulcus, while in *Homo* this division occurs after egress from infraorbital foramen (Ashton and Oxnard 1958). These authors also describe a divided canal in *Pan.* One thus expects to find multiple infraorbital foramina, usually three in *Papio* and two in *Pan,* more frequently than in *Homo,* where a single external opening is the rule. In all three primates there is a prominent communication between the infraorbital branches and branches of the facial nerve (Gasser and Hendrickx 1969).

The mandibular division is the largest and, along with the motor root, leaves the cranial cavity through the foramen ovale. Of the numerous branches of this nerve, only three reach to the skin: the buccal, auriculotemporal, and mental. The buccal and auriculotemporal nerves run similar courses and are distributed in like manner in these animals. The mental nerve is similarly disposed, except for the number of fascicles emerging from the mandible. In *Papio* there are usually three or four mental foramina, whereas in *Pan* and *Homo* the number is more often one.

Note that all of the terminal sensory branches of the trigeminal nerve intermingle freely with the terminal motor fibers of the facial nerve. The connections are established early in the embryonic history of the animals and remain an intricate part of their definitive distribution (ibid.).

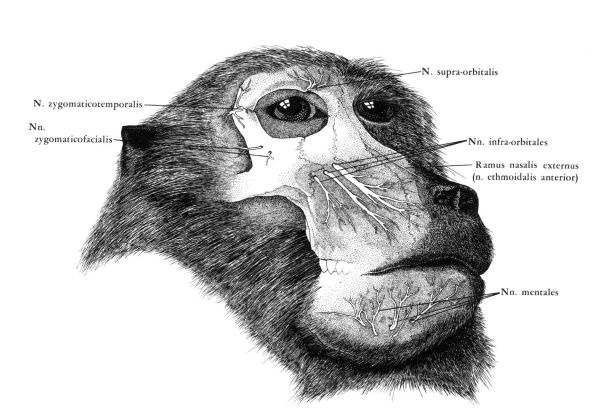

N. supra-orbitalis

N. zygomaticotemporalis

Nn. zygomaticofacialis

Nn. infra-orbitales

Ramus nasalis externus (n. ethmoidalis anterior)

Nn. mentales

Papio

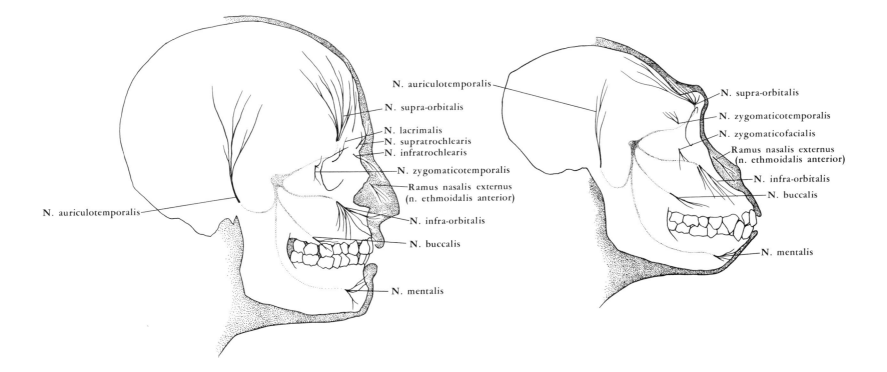

N. auriculotemporalis

N. supra-orbitalis

N. lacrimalis
N. supratrochlearis
N. infratrochlearis

N. zygomaticotemporalis

Ramus nasalis externus
(n. ethmoidalis anterior)

N. infra-orbitalis

N. buccalis

N. mentalis

N. auriculotemporalis

N. supra-orbitalis

N. zygomaticotemporalis

N. zygomaticofacialis

Ramus nasalis externus
(n. ethmoidalis anterior)

N. infra-orbitalis

N. buccalis

N. mentalis

Homo

Pan

PLATE 31

Muscles of Facial Expression

The muscles of facial expression are subdivided into cervical, oral, mental, nasal, orbital, auricular, and cranial parts. All are innervated by the facial nerve. These muscles have been investigated extensively and the reader is referred to the following authorities for the details of differentiation as exhibited by the living primates: Ruge 1887, Lightoller 1928, and Huber 1931.

The facial muscles have, for the most part, both osseous and cutaneous attachments, and are composed of fibers organized into thin sheets. The degree of differentiation varies greatly between species, as well as among individuals of the same species. The complexity of the facial muscles in *Homo* is associated with the function of emotional expression which is so characteristic of the group (Huber 1931).

A rather extensive muscle in *Papio*, the platysma, is much less developed in *Pan* and *Homo*. In fact, it has lost much of its nuchal-noto portion in *Pan,* and all of it in *Homo,* which possesses a tracheloplatysma only. Note that in *Papio* the cranial part of notoplatysma is often composed of two strata, a superficial and a deep.

The occipitofrontalis muscle consists of two frontal and two occipital bellies. Between these lies the galea aponeurotica, to which they attach. It is quite extensive in *Homo* and much reduced in *Papio* (Lightoller 1928). The chief function of these muscles is to elevate the brows, a use which *Papio* often employs.

The extrinsic and intrinsic ear muscles are well developed in *Papio.* The former are composed of a superior and a posterior sheet which together are responsible for the majority of ear movements. These muscles express a great deal of individual variation in *Homo* and *Pan.* The most constant of them in these forms is the superior auricular. The intrinsic muscles of the primate ear are thoroughly described by Huber (1931).

The disposition of the oral muscles is less complicated in *Papio* because there is less differentiation into separate muscles. Thus, the powerful zygomatic muscle mass is in broad connection with the orbicularis oculi and displays little, if any, differentiation into the major and minor heads of *Homo* and *Pan.* Hill (1970), however, described these two heads in *Papio cynocephalus.* The nasolabialis muscle is present in *Papio* and, according to Huber (1931), this sheet differentiates into the procerus and quadratus labii inferioris muscle of *Homo.*

The risorius is absent in *Papio,* and Huber (1931) has stated that it is a characteristic human structure. On the other hand, Sonntag (1924) shows it in *Pan* (Fig. 27A, p. 162), but does not mention it in the text. We were unable to define it in *Pan.*

The buccal pouch of *Papio* is a herniation of the strong, coarse fibers of the buccinator muscle through or into the platysma. Often the platysma is split into upper and lower portions.

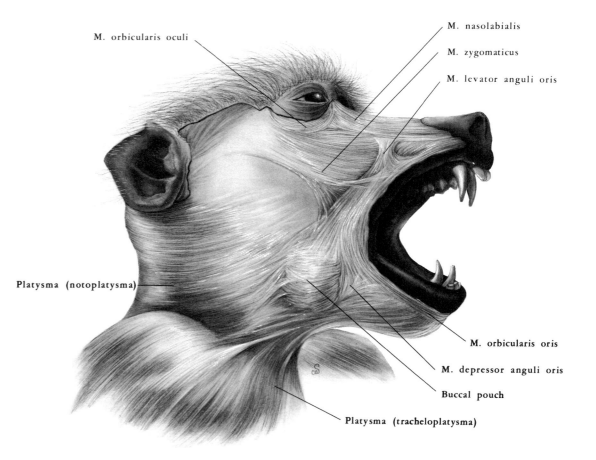

M. orbicularis oculi

M. nasolabialis

M. zygomaticus

M. levator anguli oris

Platysma (notoplatysma)

M. orbicularis oris

M. depressor anguli oris

Buccal pouch

Platysma (tracheloplatysma)

Papio

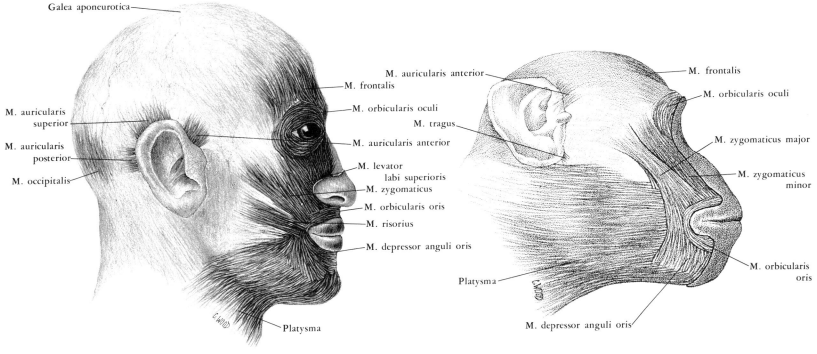

Galea aponeurotica

M. auricularis
superior

M. auricularis
posterior

M. occipitalis

M. auricularis anterior

M. frontalis

M. orbicularis oculi

M. auricularis anterior

M. levator
labi superioris

M. zygomaticus

M. orbicularis oris

M. risorius

M. depressor anguli oris

Platysma

Homo

M. auricularis anterior

M. tragus

Platysma

M. depressor anguli oris

Pan

M. frontalis

M. orbicularis oculi

M. zygomaticus major

M. zygomaticus
minor

M. orbicularis
oris

PLATE 32

Parotid Gland and Facial Nerve

The parotid gland is the largest of the salivary glands. Lying caudal and ventral to the external ear, it extends from the zygomatic arch to the angle of the mandible. In *Papio* the gland frequently extends some distance caudal to the angle of the mandible where it contacts the cephalic pole of the submandibular gland. An accessory parotid gland is present in approximately 20 percent of humans and has been reported in *Papio* (Blount and Lachman 1966; Hill 1970). When present, the accessory gland is separated from the parotid, being attached to the parotid duct as it passes across the surface of the masseter muscle.

The parotid gland is divisible into superficial and deep portions which are connected by an isthmus. The branches of the facial nerve lie between them and radiate out from beneath the ventral border of the gland.

The parotid duct emerges from the ventral border of the gland and courses across the masseter muscle. As it passes over the ventral border of the muscle, it pierces the buccinator muscle to enter the vestibule opposite the permanent maxillary second molar. The duct is accompanied by the transverse facial artery cranially and a branch of the facial nerve caudally.

The parotid gland is covered by a sheath of the cervical fascia, which is rather tough and strong enough to resist considerable tension. Within the substance of the gland a constant relation exists regarding several important structures. The most superficial structures are the nerves; the veins are on an intermediate plane; and the arteries occupy the deepest stratum. This arrangement is similar in all three primates.

The facial nerve emerges from the stylomastoid foramen and curves ventrally where it divides into its two main parts, the larger temporofacial and the smaller cervicofacial divisions. The ramifications of these major divisions are subject to much variation; but even so, a general pattern of distribution usually emerges for these three primates. The temporofacial part is responsible for supplying branches to the temporal, zygomatic, and buccal regions of the face; while the cervicofacial sends branches to the mandibular and cervical areas.

Note the auriculotemporal nerve (V3) emerging from the cranial border of the parotid gland. It communicates with the otic ganglion and is thereby responsible for conveying the postganglionic (secretory) fibers from the ninth nerve to the parotid gland.

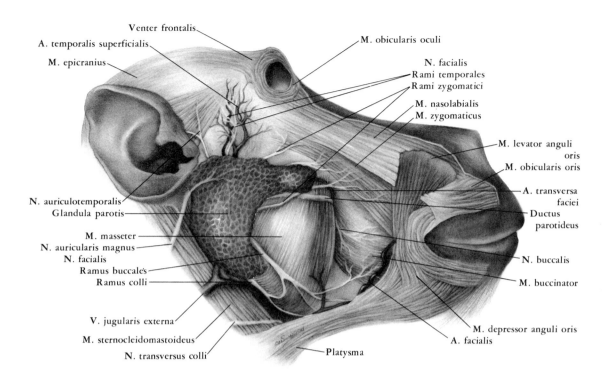

Papio

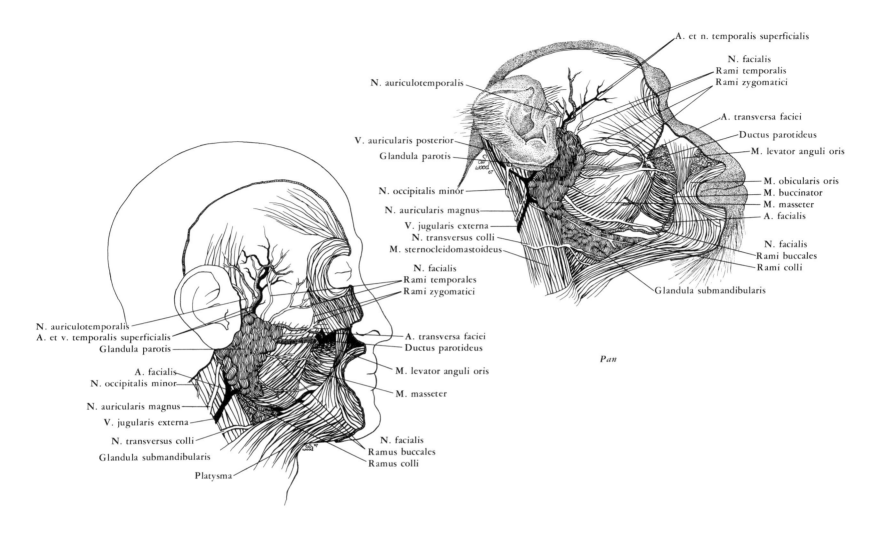

A. et n. temporalis superficialis

N. facialis
Rami temporalis
Rami zygomatici

A. transversa faciei

Ductus parotideus

M. levator anguli oris

M. obicularis oris
M. buccinator
M. masseter
A. facialis

N. facialis
Rami buccales
Rami colli

N. auriculotemporalis

V. auricularis posterior
Glandula parotis

N. occipitalis minor
N. auricularis magnus
V. jugularis externa
N. transversus colli
M. sternocleidomastoideus

Glandula submandibularis

Pan

N. facialis
Rami temporales
Rami zygomatici

N. auriculotemporalis
A. et v. temporalis superficialis
Glandula parotis

A. transversa faciei
Ductus parotideus

A. facialis
N. occipitalis minor

M. levator anguli oris

N. auricularis magnus
V. jugularis externa
N. transversus colli
Glandula submandibularis

M. masseter

N. facialis
Ramus buccales
Ramus colli

Platysma

Homo

PLATE 33

Muscles of Mastication

The craniomandibular musculature is represented by four muscles: the temporal, masseter, and medial and lateral pterygoids.

The temporalis is a powerful structure in the three primates. In *Papio* in particular, it varies in strength and size according to the age and sex of the animal. In adult males it usually reaches to the median line where along the posterior surface of the parietal bone it attaches to a low sagittal crest. In *Pan* the muscle usually attaches to a well-developed sagittal crest in the adult male. Only in *Papio* is the muscle divisible into superficial and deep portions. The former occupies much of the temporal fossa from the frontal bone to the occipital bone. The majority of the fibers attach to the coronoid process and anterior border of the ascending mandibular ramus. The deep stratum arises from the inferior portion of the temporal fossa and passes to the medial side of the coronoid process. Some of the deep fibers join the tendon of insertion of the superficial portion and together they attach to an elongated tubercle on the posterior part of the oblique line of the mandible.

The masseter can be divided in its posterior portion into superficial and deep strata. In *Pan* there frequently is an aponeurotic sheet separating the two parts and giving origin to fibers of both laminae (Sonntag 1924). The superficial portion arises from the inner side and lower border of the zygomatic arch and passes to the lower border of the mandible. The deep head leaves the posterior part of the arch, and occasionally fibers arise from the anterior aspect of the temporomandibular ligament in *Papio*. This has been reported for *Macaca mulatta* (Schwartz and Huelke 1963). The fleshy fibers of the deep head attach along the lateral aspect of the mandibular ramus.

The medial pterygoid originates from the pterygoid fossa and adjacent bones to pass to the medial side of the mandibular angle. The direction of its fibers is nearly parallel to those of the superficial head of the masseter.

The fourth muscle of mastication, the lateral pterygoid, is the smallest member of the group. It arises as two heads, one from the greater wing of the sphenoid and infra-temporal crest, the other from the lateral pterygoid plate. They converge posteriorly to attach to the pterygoid fossa of the mandible, capsule, and articular disc of the joint. It is interesting to note that the evolutionary alterations in fiber orientation of the lateral pterygoid from a more sagittal direction in the lower primates to a much greater angle with the sagittal plane in *Homo* may be one of many phenomena which have contributed to the development of the chin (DuBrul and Sicher 1954).

These four muscles are derived embryologically from the mandibular arch and are innervated by the mandibular nerve (V3).

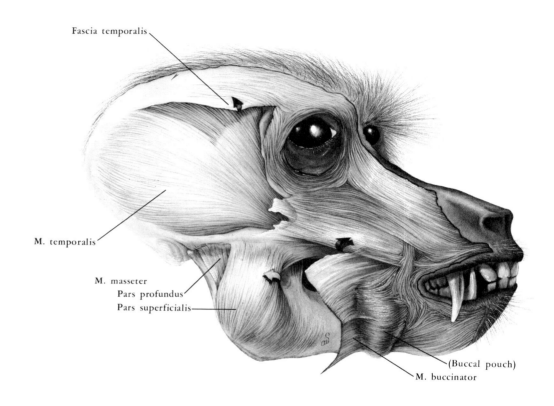

Fascia temporalis

M. temporalis

M. masseter
Pars profundus
Pars superficialis

(Buccal pouch)
M. buccinator

Papio

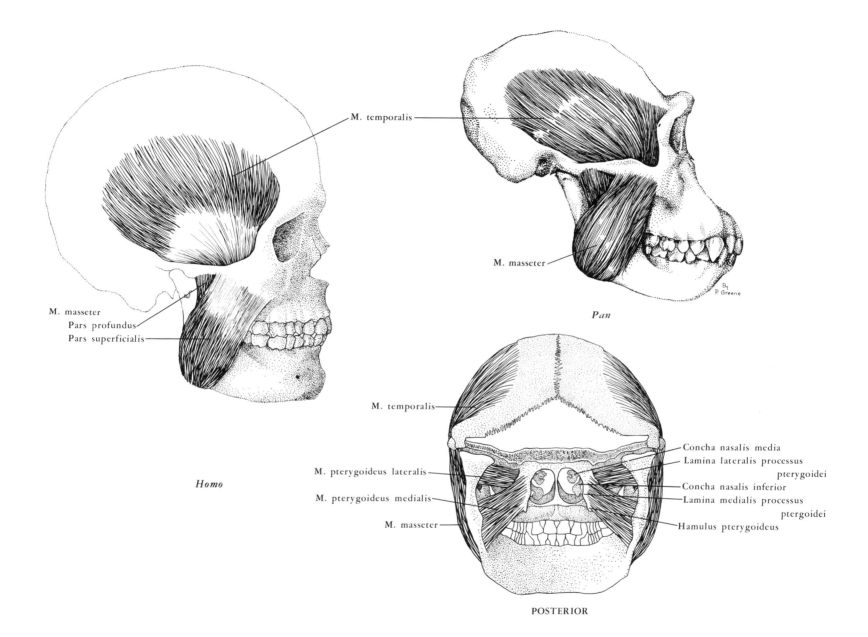

M. temporalis

M. temporalis

M. masseter
Pars profundus
Pars superficialis

M. masseter

Pan

Homo

By
P. Greene

M. temporalis

Concha nasalis media
Lamina lateralis processus
pterygoidei
M. pterygoideus lateralis
Concha nasalis inferior
M. pterygoideus medialis
Lamina medialis processus
ptergoidei
M. masseter
Hamulus pterygoideus

POSTERIOR

PLATE 34

Infratemporal Fossa I

A superficial dissection of the infratemporal fossa reveals no major differences among the three primates.

In *Papio* the external carotid artery curves sharply anteriorly after emerging from between the stylohyoid and posterior belly of the digastric muscle. This sharp angulation normally occurs after the vessel gives rise to the occipitoauricular stem and before the common trunk of the transverse facial and superficial temporal arteries (McCoy, Swindler, and Albers 1967). Hereafter, the major vessel is the maxillary artery as it passes through the pterygoid region on its way to the palatine fossa, where it becomes the infraorbital artery. Its major branches are shown here and in the following plate. Their general disposition is similar in the three primates as they arise from the customary three parts of the maxillary artery. For the most part, these branches are found accompanying the branches of the trigeminal nerve (V3).

The facial nerve is shown just after its exit from the stylomastoid foramen. In this position, it lies superficial to the posterior belly of the digastric muscle, the styloid process, and the external carotid artery. The small motor twigs to the posterior belly of the digastric and the stylohyoid muscles are visible in *Papio*. Also, note the separation of the facial nerve into its two major parts, temporofacial and cervicofacial.

Several branches of the mandibular nerve (V3) are shown passing from beneath the lateral pterygoid muscle. One of these, the auriculotemporal, is quite small and can be observed passing between the sphenomandibular ligament and the temporomandibular joint. Note the communication between this nerve and the facial nerve. This anastomosis was found in all species studied by Bowden, Mahran, and Godding (1960). The lingual and inferior alveolar nerves are large rami issuing from beneath the caudal border of the lateral pterygoid muscle. Note the small mylohyoid nerve running alongside the posterior border of the inferior alveolar nerve. This nerve produces the mylohyoid groove on the medial side of the mandibular ramus (Plate 37). The groove contains the nerve and its accompanying vessels. The topographic relation between the groove and the mandibular foramen has been studied by numerous students of the primates. An excellent summary and analysis of the phylogenetic significance of the groove-foramen relation is presented by Straus (1962).

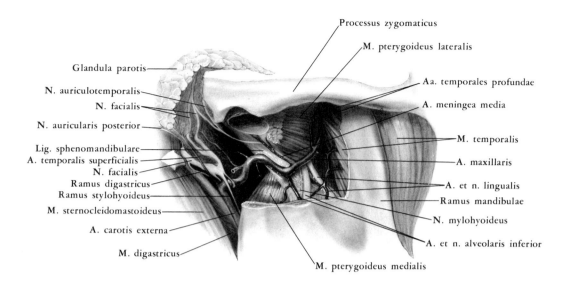

Papio

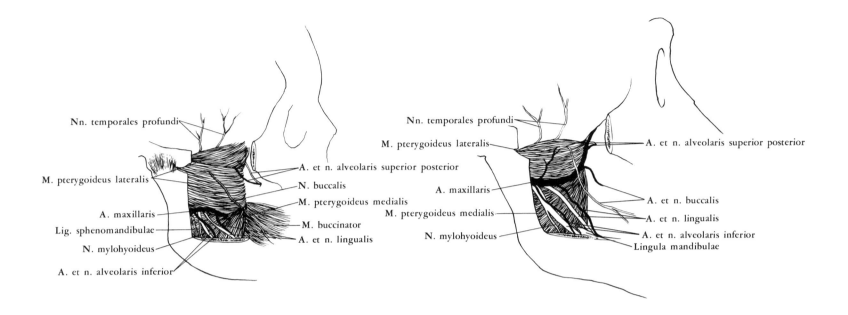

Nn. temporales profundi

M. pterygoideus lateralis

A. maxillaris

Lig. sphenomandibulae

N. mylohyoideus

A. et n. alveolaris inferior

A. et n. alveolaris superior posterior

N. buccalis

M. pterygoideus medialis

M. buccinator

A. et n. lingualis

Homo

Nn. temporales profundi

M. pterygoideus lateralis

A. maxillaris

M. pterygoideus medialis

N. mylohyoideus

A. et n. alveolaris superior posterior

A. et n. buccalis

A. et n. lingualis

A. et n. alveolaris inferior

Lingula mandibulae

Pan

PLATE 35

Infratemporal Fossa II

The mandibular division (V3) is the main nerve associated with the masticatory space. It enters the region through the foramen ovale where it divides into a smaller anterior trunk and a larger posterior trunk.

The anterior division penetrates the lateral pterygoid plate via the pterygoalar foramen in *Papio*. The latter opening is rarely present in *Pan* and *Homo;* indeed, its occurrence in *Homo* is reported to be less than 8 percent (Chouke 1946; Priman and Etter 1959). Upon entering the infratemporal fossa the anterior trunk divides into its terminal branches. The largest branch is the buccinator nerve which travels in a ventrocaudal direction from the pterygoalar foramen to the lateral surface of the buccinator muscle. It supplies sensory fibers to the mucosa of the buccal pouch in *Papio*.

The large posterior division is composed mainly of sensory fibers from the lingual, mandibular, and mental regions. It exits through the foramen ovale and passes along the medial surface of the lateral pterygoid plate. The auriculotemporal nerve originates from the posterior division at the caudal border of the pterygoalar plate, and passes medial to the neck of the condyle (Plate 36). In *Papio* the auriculotemporal nerve is rarely pierced by the middle meningeal artery whereas in *Pan* and *Homo* the artery normally passes through the nerve. In *Macaca mulatta* a splitting of the nerve is reported as a rare variation (Schwartz and Huelke 1963; McCoy 1964). It should be noted that the pterygospinous ligament is more often ossified in *Papio* than in either *Pan* or *Homo* (Priman and Etter 1959; McCoy 1964). When this ossification occurs, the auriculotemporal nerve immediately enters the foramen produced by the pterygospinous bar and is thereby shielded by bone from the middle meningeal artery.

The course of the lingual, inferior alveolar and mylohyoid nerves is similar in the three primates. Note the chorda tympani nerve entering the lingual nerve at an acute angle just caudal to the lateral pterygoid plate.

The maxillary artery usually gives rise to about eight to ten branches before exiting the masticatory space by way of the pterygopalatine fossa. As mentioned previously, the artery for descriptive purposes is divided into three parts, each part having a different relation to the lateral pterygoid muscle. The branching pattern and general areas of distribution are similar in the three animals when one allows for a few interspecific differences in the number of branches. Thus, in *Papio* the middle meningeal and tympanic arteries enjoy a common trunk of origin, whereas in *Pan* and *Homo* these arteries are usually separate. Also, the former artery enters the middle cranial fossa by way of the foramen ovale in *Papio,* rather than via the foramen spinosum as in *Pan* and *Homo*.

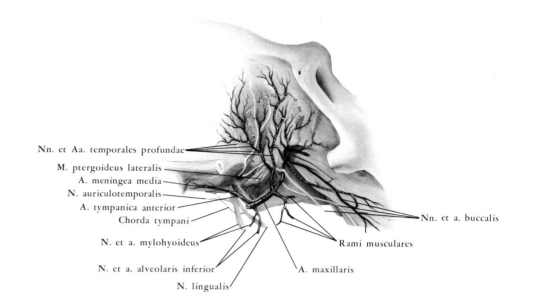

Nn. et Aa. temporales profundae

M. ptergoideus lateralis

A. meningea media

N. auriculotemporalis

A. tympanica anterior

Chorda tympani

N. et a. mylohyoideus

N. et a. alveolaris inferior

N. lingualis

Nn. et a. buccalis

Rami musculares

A. maxillaris

Papio

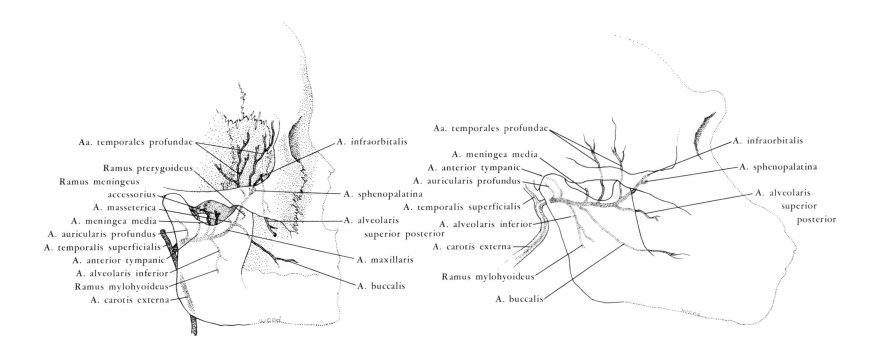

Aa. temporales profundae
A. infraorbitalis
Ramus pterygoideus
Ramus meningeus accessorius
A. sphenopalatina
A. masseterica
A. meningea media
A. alveolaris superior posterior
A. auricularis profundus
A. temporalis superficialis
A. anterior tympanic
A. alveolaris inferior
A. maxillaris
Ramus mylohyoideus
A. carotis externa
A. buccalis

Homo

Aa. temporales profundae
A. infraorbitalis
A. meningea media
A. sphenopalatina
A. anterior tympanic
A. auricularis profundus
A. alveolaris superior posterior
A. temporalis superficialis
A. alveolaris inferior
A. carotis externa
Ramus mylohyoideus
A. buccalis

Pan

PLATE 36

Infratemporal Fossa III

The infratemporal fossa is an irregularly shaped region situated medial and caudal to the zygomatic arch. Laterally it is guarded by the ramus of the mandible.

The glenoid cavity is noticeably shallow in *Papio* when compared with *Pan* and *Homo,* particularly with the latter. The postglenoid process is a well-formed, vertically projecting bar of bone in *Papio.* There is minimum development of this structure in *Homo,* while in *Pan* it occupies an intermediate position. Anteriorly, the articular surface continues onto the articular eminence. The eminence is quite distinct in *Homo* and is strongly convex in an anteroposterior direction. It is much less pronounced in *Pan* and *Papio.*

The pterygopalatine fissure is nothing more than a narrow slit in *Papio,* while in *Pan* and *Homo* the separation is much more spacious. In addition, the pyramidal process of the palatine bone is noticeably insinuated between the maxillary tuberosity and the lateral pterygoid plate in *Pan* and *Papio.* Note the position of the pterygoalar foramen on the posterolateral surface of the lateral pterygoid plate in *Papio.* The posterior extension of the lateral pterygoid plate effectively protects the foramen ovale from being entered from the lateral side.

The pterion region is of some phylogenetic interest, especially in view of the labors of Wood Jones (1948). This author believed that the type of articulation between the four bones making up this area of the skull reflected specialized characters useful in taxonomic designations. He entertained the thesis that the alisphenoid articulating with the parietal, as in *Homo,* was a primitive condition, whereas the temporofrontal pterion is a rarity in *Homo* and represents an osseous specialization in Old World monkeys and anthropoid apes. Such features as these were used by Wood Jones to support his contention of the early division of the hominids from the catarrhine stem prior to the separation of the ancestral stocks of the existing anthropoid apes.

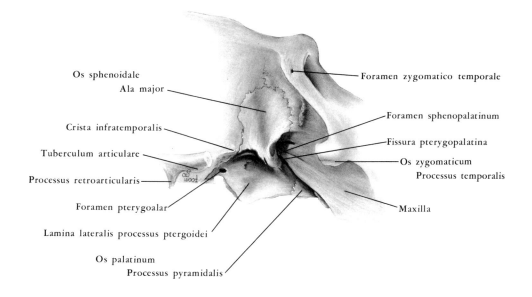

Os sphenoidale
Ala major
Crista infratemporalis
Tuberculum articulare
Processus retroarticularis
Foramen pterygoalar
Lamina lateralis processus ptergoidei
Os palatinum
Processus pyramidalis

Foramen zygomatico temporale
Foramen sphenopalatinum
Fissura pterygopalatina
Os zygomaticum
Processus temporalis
Maxilla

Papio

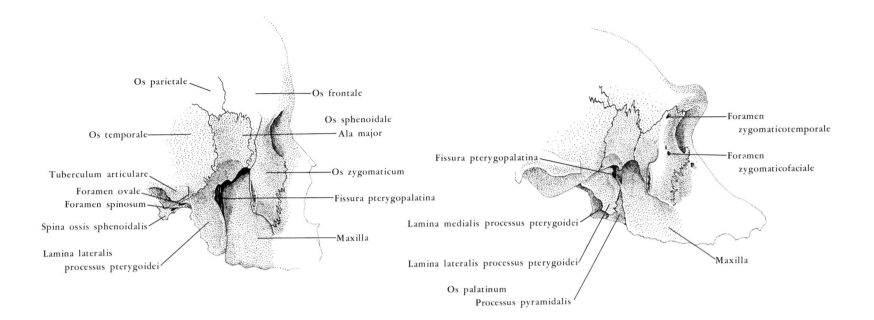

Os parietale

Os frontale

Os temporale

Os sphenoidale
Ala major

Tuberculum articulare

Os zygomaticum

Foramen ovale
Foramen spinosum

Fissura pterygopalatina

Spina ossis sphenoidalis

Lamina lateralis
processus pterygoidei

Maxilla

Homo

Foramen
zygomaticotemporale

Fissura pterygopalatina

Foramen
zygomaticofaciale

Lamina medialis processus pterygoidei

Lamina lateralis processus pterygoidei

Maxilla

Os palatinum
Processus pyramidalis

Pan

PLATE 37

Muscles of Floor of Mouth

There are four muscles connecting the hyoid bone with the skull. They lie external to the tongue musculature and are responsible for elevating the hyoid and larynx. In addition, three of them—the mylohyoid, the geniohyoid, and the anterior belly of the digastric—depress the mandible. The stylohyoid and digastric muscles are depicted in Plate 50.

The mylohyoid muscle is suspended from the medial aspect (mylohyoid line) of the body of the mandible. A median fibrous raphe serves as the area of insertion for many of the muscle fibers. The raphe passes from the hyoid to the mandible. In this position, the mylohyoid forms a muscular support for the tongue. The muscle, as well as the anterior belly of the digastric, are derived from the first (mandibular) branchial arch and, therefore, are innervated by the trigeminal (V3), via the mylohyoid nerve.

The geniohyoid muscle lies subjacent to the mylohyoid and runs from the mental depression on the medial aspect of the mandible to the corpus of the hyoid. The muscle is frequently fused with the muscles of the tongue and quite often with its companion of the opposite side. This is true in all three primates. Note that the geniohyoid is phylogenetically a muscle of the infrahyoid groups and is innervated by the first cervical nerve via the hypoglossal nerve (Howell and Straus 1933b).

The genioglossus is shown cut near its mandibular attachment in *Pan* and *Homo*. The genioglossus is a major extrinsic muscle of the tongue, composing a large part of the body of that organ (Plate 38).

The mylohyoid groove is shown. In *Homo* the type "1" sulcus is present; according to Straus (1962), this type was found in 94.1 percent of the sample studied by him. On the other hand, *Pan* displays a type "3" which these forms normally exhibit. *Papio*—and indeed the majority of Old World monkeys—is characterized by type "1." Such investigations are valuable; in the present instance, Straus's study clearly indicated the limited taxonomic and phylogenetic significance of this particular morphologic character.

Note that of these three groups of primates, *Homo* is normally the only one possessing a lingula.

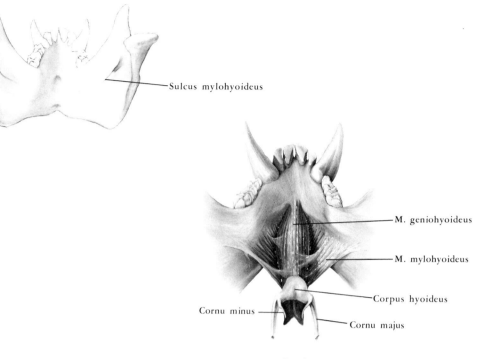

Sulcus mylohyoideus

M. geniohyoideus

M. mylohyoideus

Corpus hyoideus

Cornu minus

Cornu majus

Papio

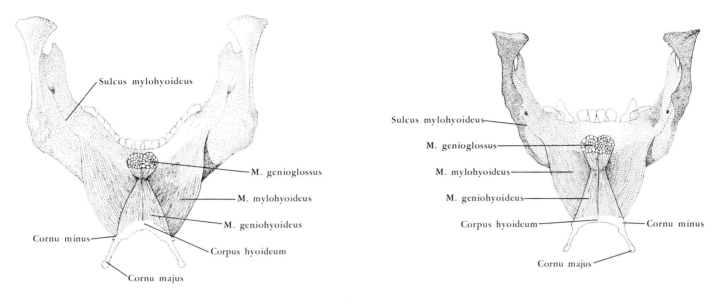

Sulcus mylohyoideus

M. genioglossus

M. mylohyoideus

M. geniohyoideus

Cornu minus

Corpus hyoideum

Cornu majus

Homo

Sulcus mylohyoideus

M. genioglossus

M. mylohyoideus

M. geniohyoideus

Corpus hyoideum

Cornu minus

Cornu majus

Pan

PLATE 38

Median Section of Tongue

The most prominent muscle from this view of the tongue and sublingual space is the genioglossus. From its mandibular attachment it passes distally into the dorsum of the tongue and to the hyoid bone. Functionally, it is considered the most important of the four extrinsic muscles of the tongue. The musculature of the tongue is supplied by the hypoglossal nerve.

The intrinsic muscles of the tongue are contained within the organ. They consist of four pairs arranged in three directions. A superior and an inferior longitudinal mass run mesiodistally; a complex of fibers passes transversely through the tongue and decussates with the vertically disposed muscle. The tongue is separated into right and left halves by the lingual septum.

The mid-sagittal section of the chin reveals several interesting morphologic differences among these animals. The angle of the chin (the relation between the front of the chin and a line drawn along the lower border of the mandible) is appreciably less in *Papio* and *Pan* than it is in *Homo*. In fact, in adult *Homo* the angle is always more than 100°, whereas in the other forms it is considerably less, particularly in Old World monkeys (Hershkovitz 1970). In a provocative article the above author clearly demonstrated that all monkeys, great apes, and man have chins. The major difference is that living hominids possess the mental protuberance which, according to Hershkovitz' argument, is a superficial feature which arose late in the evolution of the taxon. Indeed, he feels that natural selection favored the protuberance which spread rapidly through the hominids to become, ultimately, "an ornament of the chin unique to modern man."

Note the transverse shelf of bone (simian shelf) protruding distally from the symphyseal region in *Papio* and *Pan*. Mental spines are frequently absent in *Papio*, but are customarily present in *Pan* and *Homo*.

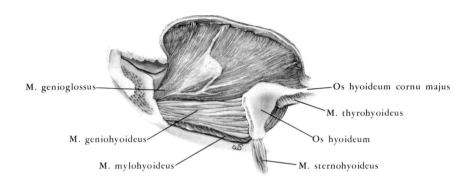

M. genioglossus — Os hyoideum cornu majus

M. geniohyoideus — M. thyrohyoideus

M. mylohyoideus — Os hyoideum

M. sternohyoideus

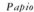

Papio

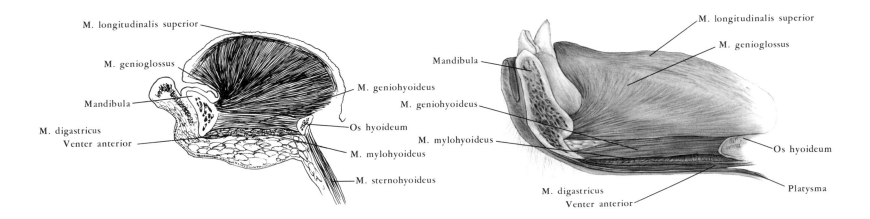

M. longitudinalis superior

M. genioglossus

Mandibula

M. digastricus
Venter anterior

M. geniohyoideus

Os hyoideum

M. mylohyoideus

M. sternohyoideus

M. longitudinalis superior

M. genioglossus

Mandibula

M. geniohyoideus

M. mylohyoideus

Os hyoideum

Platysma

M. digastricus
Venter anterior

Homo

Pan

PLATE 39

Maxillary Teeth

In *Papio* and *Pan* the outline is rectangular or
U-shaped compared with the parabolic outline in *Homo.*
This parallel-sided arrangement of the dental arches is
typical of the modern apes. Also, there is much more
sagittal elongation in the nonhuman primates. A diastema
is present between the lateral incisor and canine in *Papio*
and *Pan.* In occlusion, the mandibular canine occupies
this space while the maxillary canine resides between the
mandibular canine and third premolar.

The dental formula for the permanent teeth of the Cercopithecoidea and Hominoidea is: I, C, PM, M x 2 = 32.
The central incisors are much broader than the laterals in
the three primates. The lingual surfaces of both the central
and lateral incisors are characterized by raised enamel
marginal ridges and a concavity between. This concavity
is shaped like a sulcus in *Papio* and like a fossa in *Pan* and
Homo (Swindler, McCoy, and Hornbeck 1967). When this
lingual fossa is deep relative to elevated marginal ridges,
it is called "shovel-shaped" (Hrdlika 1920).

The canines are prominent in the males of these three
species. This is particularly true in *Papio,* where it is
hypertrophied into a powerful, projecting tooth several
times the length of the incisors. The most obvious feature
of this tooth in *Papio* is located on its mesial surface.
Here we find a deep mesial groove extending vertically
from near the tip of the crown onto the mesial surface of
the root. This groove is found on the canines of all
cercopithecoids but is absent in the hominoids.

The premolars in all three primates display two cusps,
one buccal and one lingual. In *Papio* the two cusps are
connected by an enamel ridge that effectively separates the
occlusal surface of both premolars into a small mesial
and a larger distal surface (Swindler, McCoy, and Hornbeck
1967). In all three primates, the buccal cusps are larger
than the lingual ones, and in *Papio* P⁴ is larger than P³.
In *Pan* and *Homo* these premolars are frequently equal in
size, especially in their buccal-lingual dimensions
(Schuman and Brace 1955).

The molars are approximately quadrilateral, and in
Papio they are bilophodont—that is, the mesiobuccal cusp
is connected to the mesiolingual cusp by an enamel ridge,
and the distobuccal cusp is connected by an enamel
ridge to the distolingual cusp. This dental pattern is a
specialization distinctive of the whole group of Old World
monkeys. In *Papio* the molars increase in size from M¹ to
M³, while in *Homo* it is just the opposite formula:
M¹ > M² > M³. For *Pan,* the situation is more variable, and
according to Schuman and Brace, the Liberian
chimpanzee expresses variations of both formulae in high
percentages. It is interesting to note that of all living
pongids, the chimpanzee possesses molars whose absolute
size approximates most closely those of *Homo.* This
similarity is also observed in the topographic arrangement
of the cusps, although in hominids the cusps are more
rounded and tend to be more closely aligned than in the
pongids.

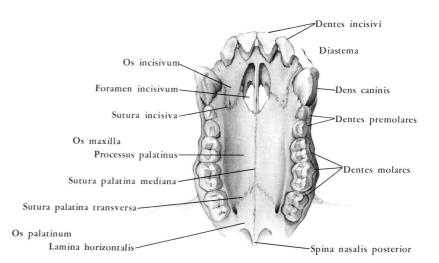

Papio

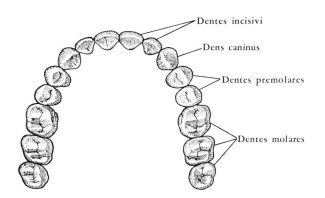

Dentes incisivi

Dens caninus

Dentes premolares

Dentes molares

Homo

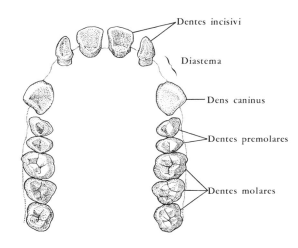

Dentes incisivi

Diastema

Dens caninus

Dentes premolares

Dentes molares

Pan

PLATE 40

Mandibular Teeth

The outline of the mandibular dental arch corresponds with the general shape of the maxillary arch, which is U-shaped in *Papio* and *Pan,* parabolic in *Homo.* A diastema is usually located between the canine and third premolar in *Papio* and *Pan.*

The central incisors are larger than the lateral ones in *Papio,* with the reverse ratio in *Pan* and *Homo.* In all three primates the four incisors form a chisel-shaped arrangement across the mesial end of the arch.

The morphologic configuration of the canine is quite different among these three primates. In *Papio* the crowns are twisted or curved labially and slightly distally from robust bases. At the same time, they are much larger in males than females. In *Pan* and *Homo* there is much less sexual dimorphism; indeed, the dimensional ranges overlap. Also, there is a tendency for interspecific overlap in the mesiodistal diameter (Schuman and Brace 1955).

The dental morphology of the premolars is characterized as heteromorphic in *Papio* and *Pan* and homomorphic in *Homo*—that is, in *Papio* and *Pan* the third premolar (sectorial) is enlarged and compressed literally to form a cutting platform for the upper canine and does not in any way resemble the fourth premolar. In *Homo* these two teeth have the same general appearance. The unicuspid sectorial third premolar is characteristic of all known Miocene, Pliocene, and living pongids (Le Gros Clark 1960). The fourth premolar is typically bicuspid in these primates, although there is a definite tendency toward multicusps (Ludwig 1957; Hornbeck and Swindler 1967).

The molars of *Papio* are bilophodont; each has four cusps, except the third, which has a fifth cusp, the hypoconulid. The lingual cusps are higher than the buccal ones and these four major cusps are separated by deep mesiodistal and buccolingual developmental grooves. In *Pan* and *Homo* the bilophodont specialization is absent, and all molars typically possess the hypoconulid, although its reduction or complete absence is common in both groups, particularly in *Homo.*

The occlusal patterns of the molars in *Pan* and *Homo* are of some interest because of their evolutionary significance. A particular arrangement between the cusps and sulci in Dryopithecine fossil pongids was first noted by Gregory (1916). This Y5 pattern (so named by Hellman in 1928) is found in all Dryopithecus molars, and it or some modification can be observed in the molars of all subsequent fossil and living hominoids. The Y5 configuration is shown in the insert. Note that in the Y5 pattern the hypoconid is between the two buccal sulci, and the single lingual fissure separates the metaconid from the entoconid. In this manner, the metaconid is always in contact with the hypoconid. These two ingredients are essential to the Y5 pattern and should not be confused with other occlusal configurations (Robinson and Allin 1966).

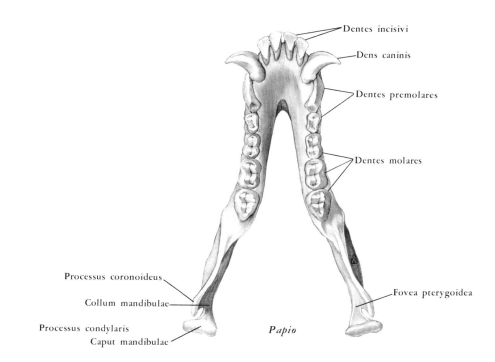

Papio

Dentes incisivi
Dens caninis
Dentes premolares
Dentes molares
Processus coronoideus
Collum mandibulae
Fovea pterygoidea
Processus condylaris
Caput mandibulae

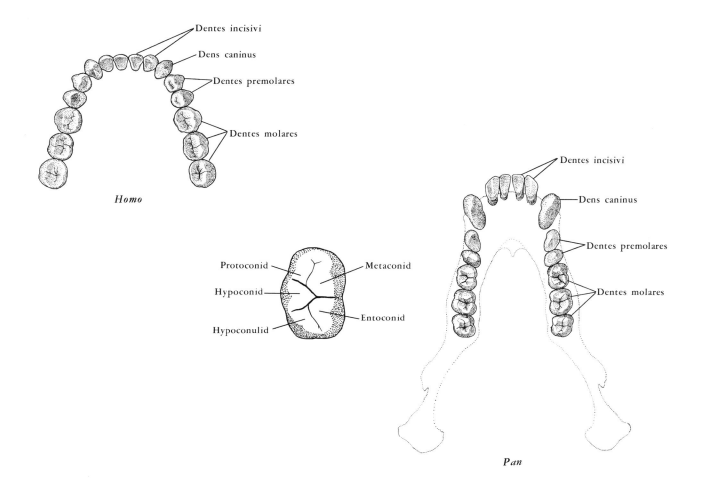

Dentes incisivi

Dens caninus

Dentes premolares

Dentes molares

Homo

Protoconid

Hypoconid

Hypoconulid

Metaconid

Entoconid

Dentes incisivi

Dens caninus

Dentes premolares

Dentes molares

Pan

PLATE 41

Orbital Cavity I

The bony orbit is lined with dense orbital periosteum, the periorbita. Distally it is continuous with the dura mater at the optic foramen and superior orbital fissure. The contents of the orbit are bound together and supported by the orbital fascia.

In *Pan* and *Homo* there are seven voluntary muscles within the orbital cavity; six attach to the eyeball and one elevates the upper eyelid. In *Papio* there is an additional ocular muscle, the accessory lateral rectus. These muscles are discussed in the following plate.

The lacrimal gland, ducts, and sac are collectively referred to as the lacrimal apparatus. The gland lies in a shallow fossa in the most craniolateral part of the orbit. The tears are conveyed by a series of ducts to the conjunctival sac. From here the fluid is conducted into the lacrimal sac and then into the nasolacrimal duct, which drains to the nose and there opens into the inferior nasal meatus. The blood supply to the gland is brought by the lacrimal artery and the infraorbital branch of the maxillary artery. The gland is innervated (sensory) by the lacrimal nerve and by autonomic motor (secretory) fibers from the facial nerve. The latter fibers represent parasympathetic, postganglionic fibers from the pterygopalatine ganglion. They pass from the ganglion to the maxillary nerve and then to its zygomatic branch. From here the fibers communicate with the lacrimal nerve, which carries them to their destination, the lacrimal gland.

The intracranial part of the optic nerve is shown at the optic chiasma. There is a partial decussation of the fibers at the chiasma; indeed, a trend is noted in the increase in the uncrossed retinal projections from prosimians to anthropoid apes to hominids (Campbell 1969). In *Homo* nearly 50 percent of the fibers remain uncrossed (Campbell 1966).

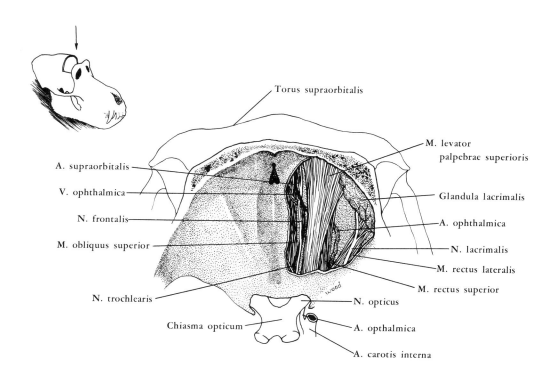

Papio

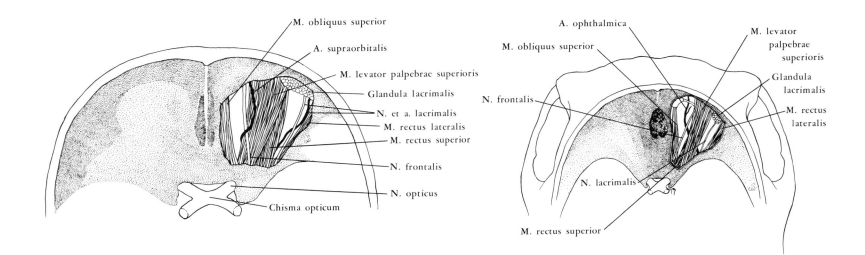

M. obliquus superior

A. supraorbitalis

M. levator palpebrae superioris

Glandula lacrimalis

N. et a. lacrimalis

M. rectus lateralis

M. rectus superior

N. frontalis

N. opticus

Chisma opticum

Homo

A. ophthalmica

M. obliquus superior

M. levator palpebrae superioris

Glandula lacrimalis

N. frontalis

M. rectus lateralis

N. lacrimalis

M. rectus superior

Pan

PLATE 42

Orbital Cavity II

The extra ocular muscles are clearly shown in *Papio*. All
of these bulbar muscles, except the inferior oblique, arise
from the distal part of the orbit, from a fibrous ring
surrounding the optic canal and the superomedial part of
the superior orbital fissure. The inferior oblique originates
from the medial margin of the orbital floor. The four recti
muscles attach to the sclera of the eyeball somewhat
anterior to its equator, while the two oblique muscles attach
just posterior to the equator. Note that these muscles are
arranged in opposite pairs, that is, superior and inferior
recti, medial and lateral recti, and so forth.

The elevator of the lid, the levator palpebrae superior
muscle, is the only bulbar muscle not attaching to the
eyeball. Instead, it attaches fanwise to the superior
palpebral cartilage of the eyelid.

The accessory lateral rectus, present in *Papio* and other
cercopithecoids, lies medial to the lateral rectus and
attaches distal to the equator of the eyeball (Wojtowicz,
Sadowski, and Kurek 1969). It is normally absent in
Pan and *Homo*.

The innervation of these muscles in the three primates
is as follows: the lateral and accessory rectus by the
abducent nerve; the superior oblique by the trochlear
nerve; and all of the other extra ocular muscles by the
oculomotor nerve. These three nerves, in addition to the
ophthalmic division of the trigeminal, enter the orbit through
the superior orbital fissure.

The ophthalmic nerve separates into three terminal
branches: frontal, nasociliary, and lacrimal. All three are
sensory and pass through the orbital cavity before exiting
onto the face.

The oculomotor nerve contains primarily somatic motor
and general visceral efferent fibers. The latter are
associated functionally with the ciliary ganglion, which is
situated in the distal part of the orbit between the optic
nerve and the lateral rectus muscle. In *Papio* it lies deep to
the accessory lateral rectus. Numerous short ciliary nerves
emerge from the ganglion and pass to the eyeball. These
nerves carry postganglionic parasympathetic fibers to the
ciliary muscle and to the sphincter muscle of the iris.
In addition, they contain postganglionic sympathetic fibers
from the superior cervical ganglion, which supplies the
dilator muscle of the iris.

The ophthalmic artery arises from the internal carotid
as it leaves the cavernous sinus. It then winds around the
anterior clinoid process under the optic chiasma or nerve
to enter the optic canal. As the artery enters the orbit, it
is firmly adherent to the optic sheath covering the nerve.
Several of the many branches of the ophthalmic are shown
here. For the most part, these arteries are similarly
disposed in the three primates. A detailed study of the
vascular pattern of the orbit in the rhesus monkey was
conducted by Hayreh (1964).

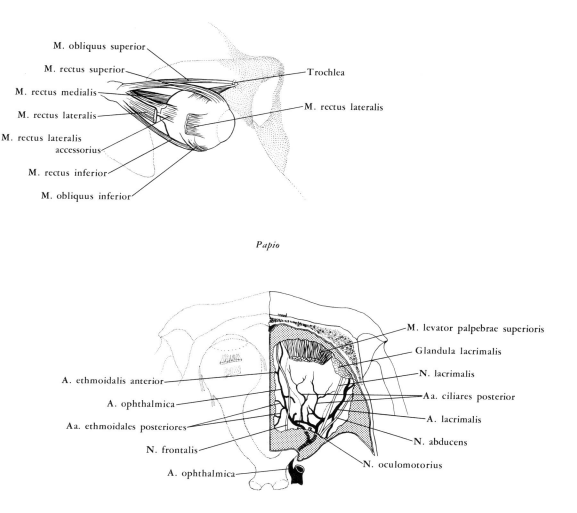

Papio

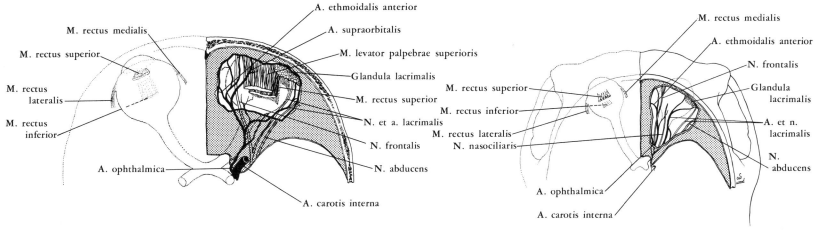

M. rectus medialis

M. rectus superior

M. rectus
lateralis

M. rectus
inferior

A. ophthalmica

A. ethmoidalis anterior

A. supraorbitalis

M. levator palpebrae superioris

Glandula lacrimalis

M. rectus superior

N. et a. lacrimalis

N. frontalis

N. abducens

A. carotis interna

Homo

M. rectus medialis

A. ethmoidalis anterior

N. frontalis

Glandula
lacrimalis

A. et n.
lacrimalis

N.
abducens

M. rectus superior

M. rectus inferior

M. rectus lateralis

N. nasociliaris

A. ophthalmica

A. carotis interna

Pan

PLATE 43

Median Sagittal Section of Head

This view of the head displays the interrelationships of several different anatomical regions—namely, the mouth, nasal cavity, pharynx, larynx, and brain. These regions are considered in detail elsewhere and only a few brief comments are presented here.

The ostium of the auditory tube is protected by the torus tubarius, which is quite large in *Pan*. The auditory tube is positioned between the middle ear and the nasopharynx.

The laryngeal ventricle is observed in *Pan* and *Homo*. The laryngeal sacs of *Pan* and *Papio* represent evaginations from this region of the larynx (see Plate 58).

The simian shelf of *Pan* and *Papio* is noted projecting posteriorly from the midline of the mandible. The geniohyoid muscle attaches to this bony ledge.

Clearly shown in this view is an important difference among the three primates, the degree of kyphosis, which is the angle between the presellary skull base and the postsellary skull base. In *Homo* the kyphosis is located in the basisphenoid, while in nonhuman primates it is situated in the presphenoid (Hofer 1969). The width of the angle is wider in *Homo* than it is in *Papio* or *Pan*, although the location of the vertex in *Pan* closely approaches its position in *Homo* (ibid.). The larger angle in *Homo* may be the reflection of the greater development of the frontal lobes of the brain as well as the establishment of erect bipedal locomotion.

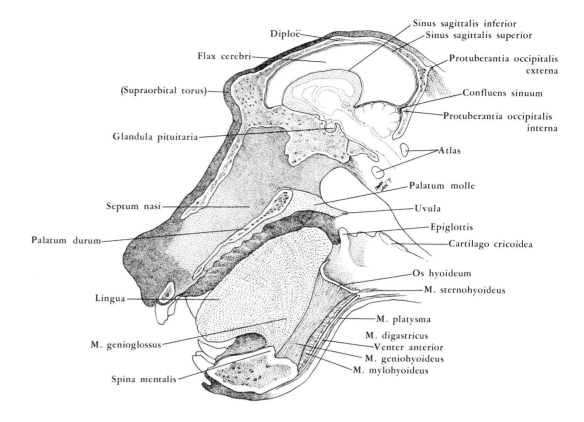

Papio

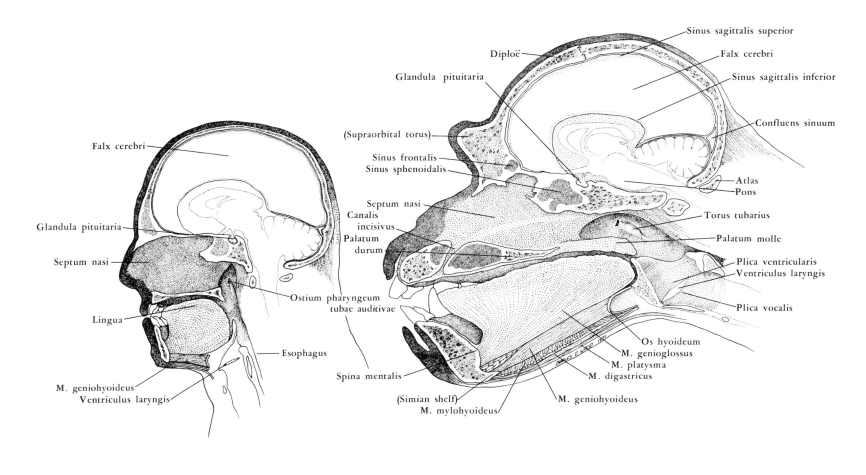

Sinus sagittalis superior

Diploë

Falx cerebri

Glandula pituitaria

Sinus sagittalis inferior

Confluens sinuum

(Supraorbital torus)

Sinus frontalis
Sinus sphenoidalis

Atlas
Pons

Septum nasi

Torus tubarius

Canalis
incisivus

Palatum molle

Palatum
durum

Plica ventricularis
Ventriculus laryngis

Plica vocalis

Os hyoideum

M. genioglossus

M. platysma

M. digastricus

Spina mentalis

(Simian shelf)
M. mylohyoideus

M. geniohyoideus

Falx cerebri

Glandula pituitaria

Septum nasi

Ostium pharyngeum
tubae auditivae

Lingua

Esophagus

M. geniohyoideus
Ventriculus laryngis

Homo

Pan

PLATE 44

Lateral Brain

The great deal of attention accorded the primate brain
through the years has resulted in an extensive amount of
literature. We would be remiss if we failed to mention the
classic works of Elliot Smith (1902, 1903), Brodman (1909),
Tilney (1928), Ariëns Kappers, Huber, and Crosby (1936),
Connolly (1950), and Crosby, Humphrey, and Lauer (1962).

The cerebral hemispheres are incompletely separated
from each other by the longitudinal fissure, and the corpus
callosum forms a bond of union between the two
hemispheres (Plate 45). The cerebral cortex spreads over
the surface of the hemisphere, and its area is increased
by the presence of gyri separated by sulci. There is a
general increase in the complexity of the fissural pattern
as one passes from prosimians to monkeys, thence to apes
and finally *Homo* (Connolly 1936). The rhinencephalon
is phylogenetically the oldest part of the cortex and is
designated as the archipallium. The newer nonolfactory
cortex is much larger and is called the neopallium. In *Homo*
the neopallium has attained its maximum development
among the primates (Elliot Smith 1902).

The cortex is demarcated by several important sulci
into the frontal, parietal, temporal, and occipital lobes. The
frontal and parietal lobes are separated by the central
sulcus, the parietal and occipital by the parieto-occipital
sulcus, and the parietal and frontal from the temporal by
the deep lateral cerebral fissure. According to Sonntag
(1924), *Homo* is the only primate possessing a complete
lateral fissure consisting of anterior horizontal, anterior
ascending, and posterior rami. The major difference is the
poorly constructed anterior limbs in the other primates,
which often results in exposure of the insula.

In *Papio* the lateral cerebral fissure normally does not
meet the superior temporal sulcus (Connolly 1936); rather,
they remain separate, running parallel courses along the
lateral surface of the temporal lobe. In *Pan* and *Homo* the
most distal ends of these grooves often join on the lateral
surface of the parietal lobe. The central sulcus, well
developed in these primates, separates the cerebral cortex
into the motor area anteriorly and the sensory area
posteriorly.

The occipital pole is incised horizontally by the lateral
calcarine sulcus in *Papio* and *Pan,* but only rarely in *Homo*.
This sulcus is frequently Y-shaped, as shown here in
Pan and *Papio,* although its dorsal ramus is often separated
in *Pan* (Connolly 1936). Such changes are the result of
the expansion of the parietal cortex displacing the visual
area to the medial side of the cerebrum in *Homo*. Also, the
lunate sulcus (simian sulcus), which sweeps so
pronouncedly across the occipital lobe in nonhuman
primates, is absent or identified with difficulty in *Homo*.

The cerebellum is divisible into three main lobes—
anterior, middle, and posterior—and these are similarly
disposed in the three primates. In *Papio* the floccular lobes
are relatively large and the petrosal lobe projects from the
anterolateral margin of the paraflocculus.

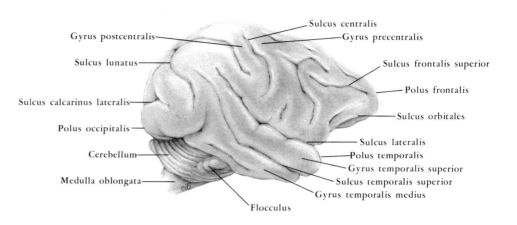

Papio

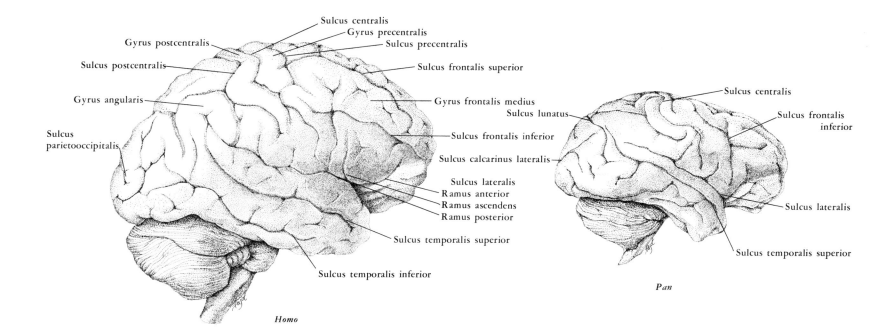

Sulcus centralis
Gyrus precentralis
Sulcus precentralis
Gyrus postcentralis
Sulcus frontalis superior
Sulcus postcentralis
Gyrus angularis
Gyrus frontalis medius
Sulcus parietooccipitalis
Sulcus frontalis inferior
Sulcus calcarinus lateralis
Sulcus lateralis
Ramus anterior
Ramus ascendens
Ramus posterior
Sulcus temporalis superior
Sulcus temporalis inferior

Homo

Sulcus centralis
Sulcus lunatus
Sulcus frontalis inferior
Sulcus lateralis
Sulcus temporalis superior

Pan

PLATE 45

Medial Brain

The brain of *Papio* is large when compared with that of other cercopithecoids. Its brain-weight/body-weight ratio agrees with that for the larger macaques (Hill 1970). According to the same author, the relative sizes of the cerebral hemispheres, pons, cerebellum, and medulla are similar to the values for *Homo*.

The medial surface of the hemisphere is perpendicular and flattened and lies parallel to the longitudinal fissure. The two hemispheres are connected by the corpus callosum. If one gently separates the two hemispheres from above, the dorsal surface of the corpus callosum is exposed. The topographical relations of most of the structures labeled in this view are similar when the size differential is considered.

The configuration of the convolutions as seen here and in the preceding plate shows a general increase in complexity from *Papio* to *Homo*. Indeed, as Connolly noted years ago (1950), there is a relation between the degree of fissuration and the size of the brain, and both of these factors are related to body weight. Of all anthropoid apes, the convolutional pattern of the gorilla's brain most closely resembles *Homo* (Sonntag 1924; Connolly 1936). The major difference from *Papio* to *Homo* is the development of secondary and tertiary sulci which adds greater details of fissuration. The folding of the cerebral cortex in the adult brain of *Homo* results in a surface area of approximately 2,300 square centimeters, of which about one-third is exposed and two-thirds lie hidden in the walls and floors of the sulci and fissure (Voneida 1966).

The largest brain in anthropoid apes occurs in the male gorilla, where a cranial capacity of 650 cc. has been reported (Hill 1953). However, the range for the species, including both sexes, is 380-590 cc. The brain of *Pan* is slightly smaller, running from about 320 to 480 cc., with an average of 410 cc. On the other hand, the cranial capacity of *Homo* ranges from less than 900 cc. to approximately 2,250 cc. (Le Gros Clark 1960). According to most authorities, the anatomical differences between the brain of pongids and hominids appear to be quantitative— for example, cell densities—rather than qualitative. For as Le Gros Clark (1960) stated, "there is no known neomorphic element" that distinguishes the one from the other (p. 262).

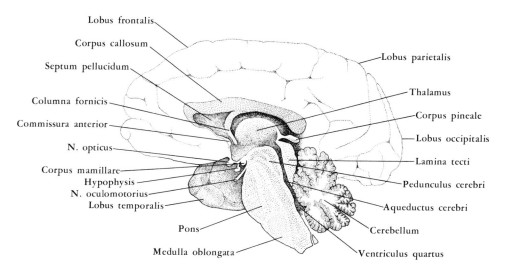

Papio

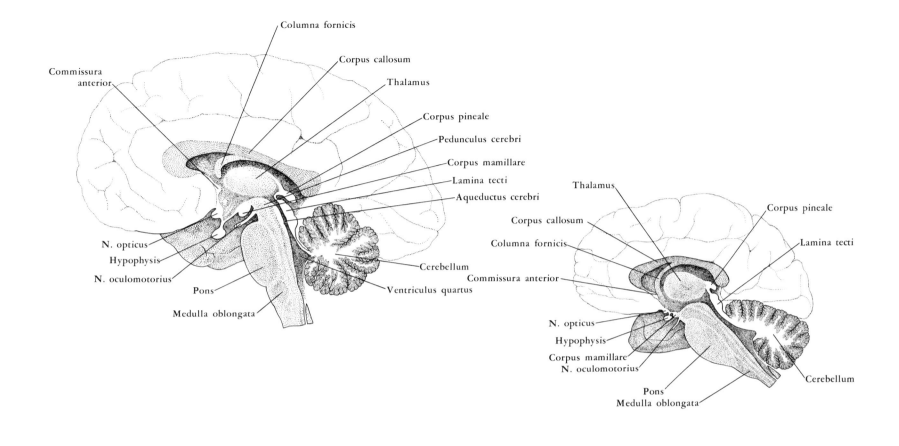

Columna fornicis

Corpus callosum

Thalamus

Commissura
anterior

Corpus pineale

Pedunculus cerebri

Corpus mamillare

Lamina tecti

Aqueductus cerebri

N. opticus

Hypophysis

N. oculomotorius

Pons

Medulla oblongata

Cerebellum

Ventriculus quartus

Homo

Thalamus

Corpus pineale

Corpus callosum

Columna fornicis

Lamina tecti

Commissura anterior

N. opticus

Hypophysis

Corpus mamillare

N. oculomotorius

Cerebellum

Pons

Medulla oblongata

Pan

PLATE 46

Ventral Brain I: Arteries

The arteries at the base of the brain display the familiar polygon known as the cerebral arterial circle. It is formed anteriorly on each side by the anterior cerebral arteries from the internal carotids. The two arteries are connected by the anterior communicating artery. Posteriorly, the posterior cerebral arteries from the basilar are united on either side with the internal carotid via the posterior communicating arteries.

A modification of this basic pattern occurs rather frequently among the Cercopithecidae. In these monkeys, the anterior cerebrals of each side unite as they enter the longitudinal cerebral fissure to form the common anterior cerebral artery. *Papio* exhibits this common artery, as did *Macaca cyclopsis* (Sakuma 1961). In *Macaca mulatta* it occurred in 96 percent of specimens (Kassell and Langfitt 1965). Both investigations reported the presence of an anterior communicating vessel connecting the anterior cerebrals just proximal to their union. This communication has not been reported in *Papio*. Kassell and Langfitt also reported an artery joining each internal carotid at the level of the hypophysis. This was not mentioned by Sakuma, nor is it present in *Papio*.

The common anterior cerebral is present in *Pan;* however, it is variable among the Pongidae (Watts 1933, 1934; Hindze 1930). In *Homo,* Alpers, Berry, and Paddison (1959) found it in only 2 percent of their cases.

Separate origins for the anterior and posterior inferior cerebellar arteries are not observed in *Papio;* rather, there is a common trunk from the basilar artery, which runs ventrolateral to the radix of the abducent nerve before bifurcating. Sakuma (1961) reported separate origins for these arteries in *Macaca cyclopsis;* however, they both arose from the basilar and, in addition, the anterior inferior cerebellar ran deep to the stem of the abducent nerve. In *Homo* and *Pan,* the anterior and posterior inferior cerebellar arteries normally arise from the basilar and vertebral arteries, respectively. Also, the anterior vessel generally passes ventral to the abducent radix.

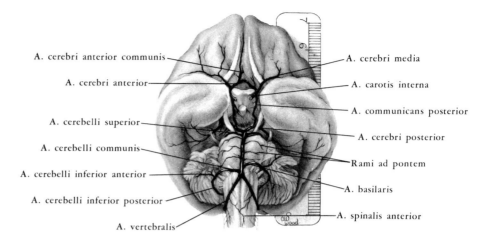

A. cerebri anterior communis
A. cerebri anterior
A. cerebelli superior
A. cerebelli communis
A. cerebelli inferior anterior
A. cerebelli inferior posterior
A. vertebralis
A. cerebri media
A. carotis interna
A. communicans posterior
A. cerebri posterior
Rami ad pontem
A. basilaris
A. spinalis anterior

Papio

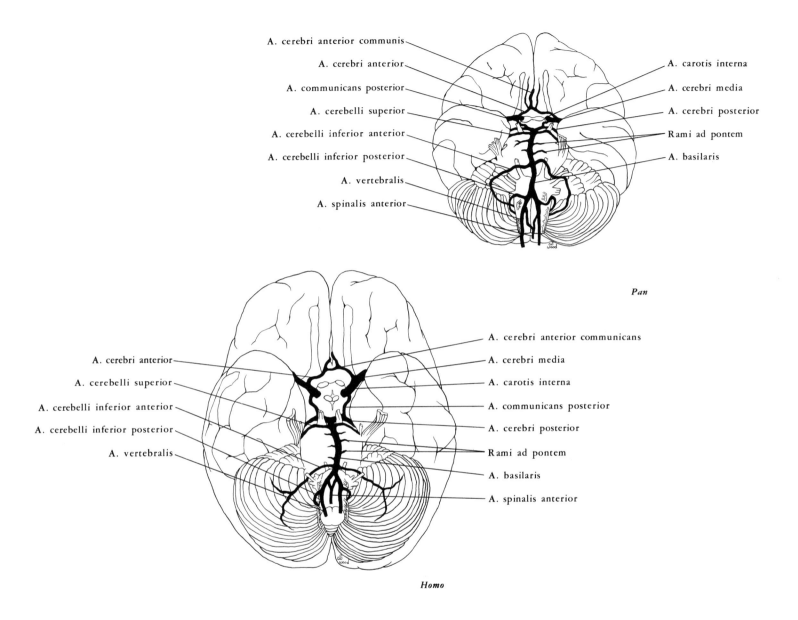

A. cerebri anterior communis

A. cerebri anterior

A. communicans posterior

A. cerebelli superior

A. cerebelli inferior anterior

A. cerebelli inferior posterior

A. vertebralis

A. spinalis anterior

A. carotis interna

A. cerebri media

A. cerebri posterior

Rami ad pontem

A. basilaris

Pan

A. cerebri anterior

A. cerebelli superior

A. cerebelli inferior anterior

A. cerebelli inferior posterior

A. vertebralis

A. cerebri anterior communicans

A. cerebri media

A. carotis interna

A. communicans posterior

A. cerebri posterior

Rami ad pontem

A. basilaris

A. spinalis anterior

Homo

PLATE 47

Ventral Brain II: Nerves

At the rostral end of the brain the olfactory tract and bulb pass along the orbital surface of the frontal lobe. The fila of the olfactory nerve originate from the bulb and pass to the olfactory epithelium of the nasal fossa.

The optic nerve, actually a fiber tract of the brain, arises from the optic chiasma. The fibers from the medial or nasal half of each retina cross in the optic chiasma.

The oculomotor nerve is large: originating from the oculomotor sulcus on the medial surface of the cerebral peduncle, it occupies a large portion of the interpeduncular fossa. Note that the oculomotor nerve lies between the superior cerebellar and posterior cerebral arteries.

The small trochlear nerve is seen peeping out from beneath the lateral border of the pons. Actually, its superficial origin lies deeper from the dorsal surface of the anterior medullary velum.

The large trigeminal nerve arises from the lateral aspect of the middle of the pons. It has two roots, the portio major or sensory root and the portio minor or motor root. The semilunar ganglion is associated with the sensory root, while the motor root crosses the deep surface of the ganglion to pass out the foramen ovale with the mandibular division. Particularly in *Papio,* the maxillary trunk is the largest of the three divisions of the trigeminal. This division of the trigeminal is correlated with the extremely long snout in these animals (Hill 1970).

The small abducent nerve arises from the posterior border of the pons just rostral to the pyramid.

The facial and acoustic nerves arise very close together from the lateral border and caudal part of the pons. Note the proximity of these nerves to the flocculus. The acoustic trunk consists of two parts, the vestibular and cochlear nerves.

The glossopharyngeal, vagus, and accessory nerves are lined up as a series of filaments from the posterior lateral sulcus of the medulla oblongata. The ninth nerve occupies the rostral end of the series, the tenth nerve is in the middle, while the eleventh nerve lies caudal to both. Indeed, the accessory also arises from the lateral aspect of the cranial four to six cervical segments of the spinal cord.

The hypoglossal is the last cranial nerve. Its superficial origin is from the anterior lateral sulcus of the medulla oblongata between the olive and the pyramid.

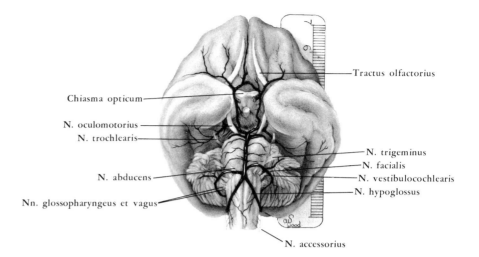

Chiasma opticum

N. oculomotorius

N. trochlearis

N. abducens

Nn. glossopharyngeus et vagus

Tractus olfactorius

N. trigeminus

N. facialis

N. vestibulocochlearis

N. hypoglossus

N. accessorius

Papio

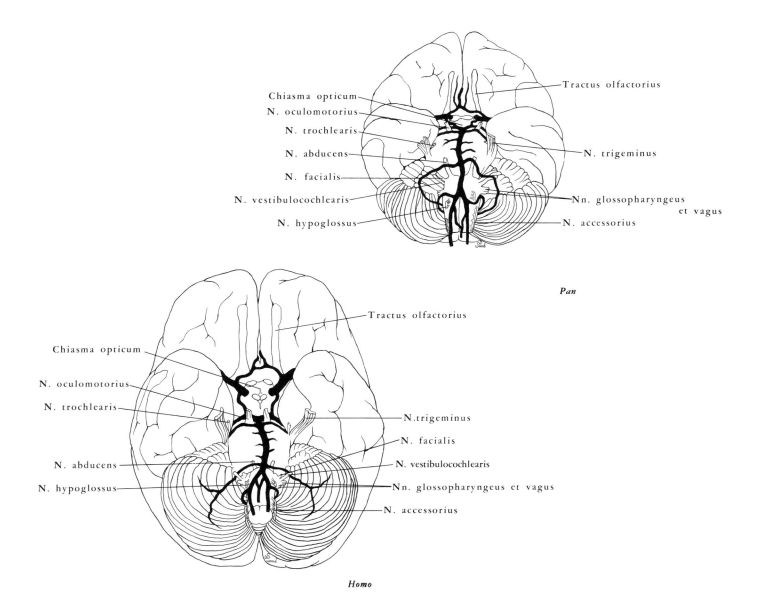

Chiasma opticum
N. oculomotorius
N. trochlearis
N. abducens
N. facialis
N. vestibulocochlearis
N. hypoglossus

Tractus olfactorius

N. trigeminus

Nn. glossopharyngeus et vagus

N. accessorius

Pan

Tractus olfactorius

Chiasma opticum
N. oculomotorius
N. trochlearis
N. abducens
N. hypoglossus

N. trigeminus

N. facialis

N. vestibulocochlearis

Nn. glossopharyngeus et vagus

N. accessorius

Homo

PLATE 48

Interior of Skull: Cranial Nerves

The olfactory tract and bulb occupy the trough between the cribriform plate and the convex orbital plate of the frontal bone. The orbital plate is much more convex in *Papio* than in the other forms. The filaments making up the olfactory nerve pass through foramina in the cribriform plate to terminate in the bulb. In *Homo* and *Pan* there are as many as twenty filaments from each side, whereas in *Papio* this number is greatly reduced; in fact, Hill (1970) reported a single, thick trunk in *Papio*.

The optic nerve enters the middle cranial fossa by traversing the optic canal. The third, fourth, and sixth nerves are shown lying just medial to the semilunar ganglion on the left side. Actually, at this point the three nerves are about to enter the walls of the cavernous sinus. They pass through the sinus to enter the orbit via the superior orbital fissure. In their course they are joined by the ophthalmic nerve (V1). Note the third, fourth, and sixth nerves piercing the dura just distolateral to the dorsum sellae.

The large trigeminal is seen separating into its three divisions on the left side. The ophthalmic was considered above. The maxillary division passes into the pterygopalatine fossa via the foramen rotundum. The mandibular nerve exits the middle cranial fossa by the foramen ovale. In *Papio* this foramen is merely a separation between the sphenoid and the rostral part of the petrous temporal; in *Pan* it is within the temporal bone, while in *Homo* it is located entirely within the sphenoid bone.

The seventh and eighth nerves lie in the posterior cranial fossa and leave it through the internal acoustic meatus. The eighth nerve passes to the vestibular and cochlear mechanisms of the ear. The seventh nerve enters the facial canal and follows this route to the stylomastoid foramen, where it emerges from the temporal bone.

The ninth, tenth, and eleventh nerves exit the posterior cranial fossa through the jugular foramen. In *Pan* and *Homo* the glossopharyngeal presents the superior and inferior ganglia as it enters the foramen, whereas in *Papio* there is usually only the inferior (Hill 1970). Note the spinal portion of the accessory in *Papio*. The spinal part unites with the cranial fibers after it enters the posterior cranial fossa through the foramen magnum.

The twelfth nerve is shown piercing the dura to enter the hypoglossal canal (anterior condylar foramen).

The greater and lesser petrosal nerves are shown on the left side of *Papio*. The greater petrosal arises from the facial nerve. For the connections of the intraosseous part of the seventh nerve in *Papio,* see Vidic´ 1970. The nerve leaves the geniculate ganglion and travels through the facial hiatus, which opens as a small slit on the upper surface of the petrous temporal. From here it passes to the pterygopalatine ganglion. Sympathetic fibers (deep petrosal) join the nerve just before it enters the pterygoid canal, where it becomes the nerve of the pterygoid canal.

The small petrosal, a branch of the ninth nerve, enters the middle cranial fossa just medial to the greater petrosal. It runs anteriorly to pass through the foramen ovale in *Papio* and terminates in the otic ganglion.

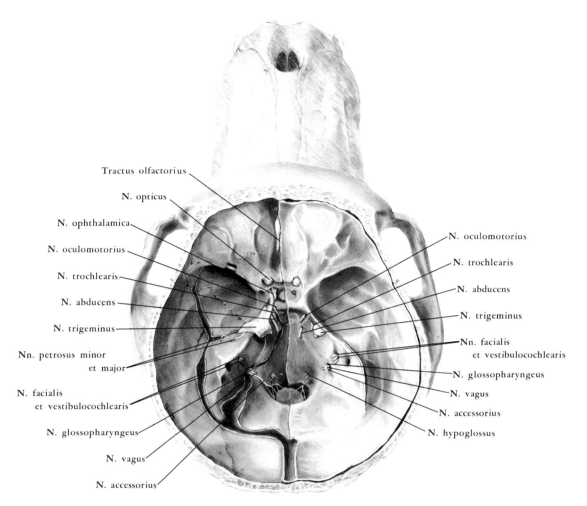

Tractus olfactorius

N. opticus

N. ophthalamica

N. oculomotorius

N. trochlearis

N. abducens

N. trigeminus

Nn. petrosus minor et major

N. facialis et vestibulocochlearis

N. glossopharyngeus

N. vagus

N. accessorius

N. oculomotorius

N. trochlearis

N. abducens

N. trigeminus

Nn. facialis et vestibulocochlearis

N. glossopharyngeus

N. vagus

N. accessorius

N. hypoglossus

Papio

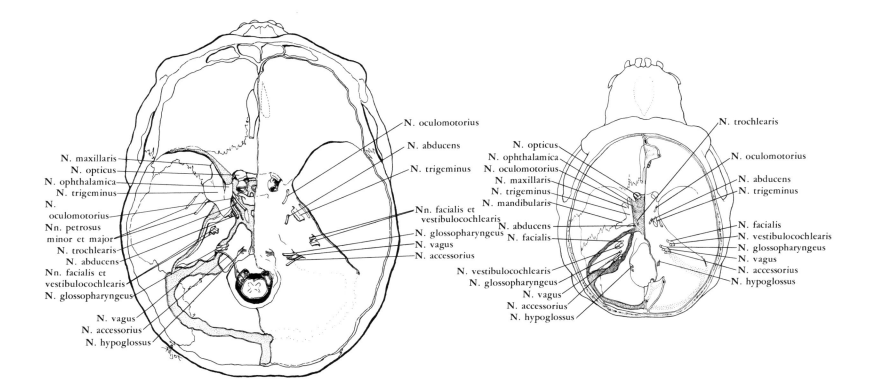

N. oculomotorius

N. abducens

N. trigeminus

N. maxillaris
N. opticus
N. ophthalamica
N. trigeminus
N.
oculomotorius
Nn. petrosus
minor et major
N. trochlearis
N. abducens
Nn. facialis et
vestibulocochlearis
N. glossopharyngeus

Nn. facialis et
vestibulocochlearis
N. glossopharyngeus
N. vagus
N. accessorius

N. vagus
N. accessorius
N. hypoglossus

Homo

N. trochlearis

N. opticus
N. ophthalamica
N. oculomotorius
N. maxillaris
N. trigeminus
N. mandibularis

N. oculomotorius

N. abducens
N. trigeminus

N. abducens
N. facialis

N. facialis
N. vestibulocochlearis
N. glossopharyngeus
N. vagus
N. accessorius
N. hypoglossus

N. vestibulocochlearis
N. glossopharyngeus
N. vagus
N. accessorius
N. hypoglossus

Pan

PLATE 49

Interior of Skull: Dural Sinuses

The dural sinuses are endothelially lined blood channels situated between the meningeal and periosteal layers of the dura mater. The sinuses are divided into paired and unpaired systems. In general the disposition of the sinuses is similar among the three species, particularly between *Pan* and *Homo*. In *Papio* certain differences warrant discussion.

The unpaired midline sinuses—superior sagittal, inferior sagittal, and straight—are essentially the same in the three animals. The occipital sinus is present in *Papio* and the other species, although it was reported absent in *Macaca mulatta* by Weinstein and Hedges (1962). They also noted that the basilar plexus was either absent or insignificantly developed in this monkey. This venous plexus is present in *Papio,* extending from the cavernous sinus to the inferior petrosal sinus. Its communications with the marginal sinus and the internal vertebral venous plexus are poorly formed, if they exist at all.

In *Pan* and *Homo* the superior petrosal sinus connects the cavernous sinus to the transverse sinus. In *Papio* the former receives blood from the middle cerebral vein and does not communicate with the cavernous sinus. This arrangement was also reported in *Macaca mulatta* (Weinstein and Hedges 1962). The confluence of middle cerebral vein and superior petrosal sinus occurs in the attached margin of the tentorium cerebelli just cranial to the internal acoustic meatus. The superior petrosal sinus ends in the transverse sinus. Note the subarcute fossa in *Papio.* This deep depression in the medial wall of the petrous bone houses the floccular lobe of the cerebellum.

In *Papio* the cavernous sinus communicates mainly with the ophthalmic vein anteriorly and the inferior petrosal sinus posteriorly. The internal carotid artery passes through the sinus upon leaving the carotid canal. Its course in the sinus in *Papio* is much less tortuous, and certainly it fails to make the strong sigmoid curve characteristic of *Pan* and *Homo.*

The petrosquamous sinus is prominent in *Papio* and other cercopithecoids, but is only occasionally present in *Homo* (ibid.). It was not present in our sample of *Pan.* The sinus opens into the transverse sinus posteriorly, and anteriorly it passes from the middle cranial fossa through the petrosquamous foramen located just lateral to the internal acoustic meatus. A number of cerebral veins empty into it before it passes into the retromandibular vein.

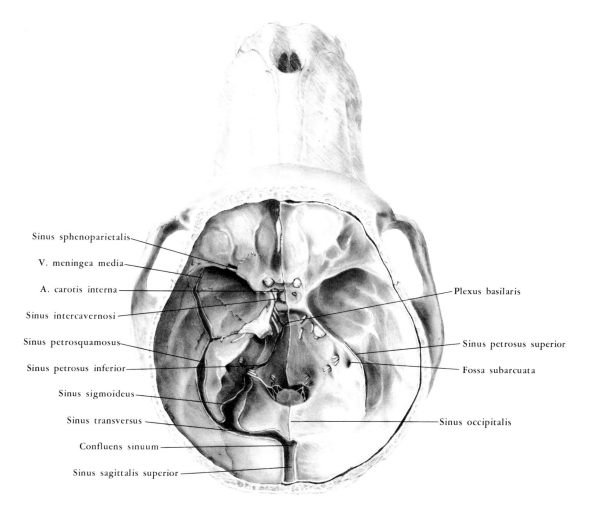

Sinus sphenoparietalis
V. meningea media
A. carotis interna
Sinus intercavernosi
Sinus petrosquamosus
Sinus petrosus inferior
Sinus sigmoideus
Sinus transversus
Confluens sinuum
Sinus sagittalis superior
Plexus basilaris
Sinus petrosus superior
Fossa subarcuata
Sinus occipitalis

Papio

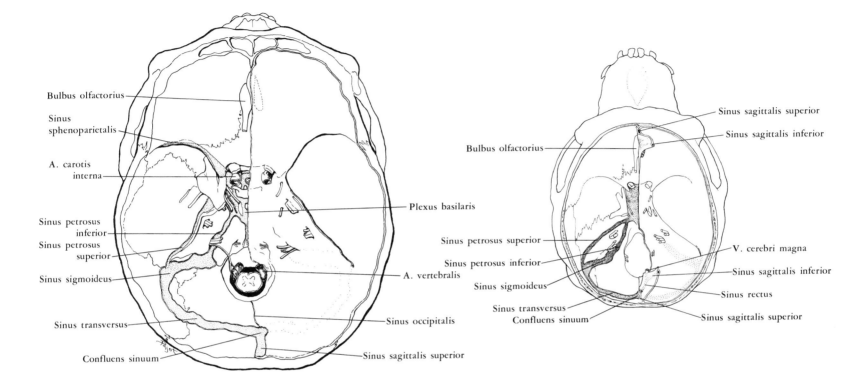

Bulbus olfactorius

Sinus sphenoparietalis

A. carotis interna

Sinus petrosus inferior

Sinus petrosus superior

Sinus sigmoideus

Sinus transversus

Confluens sinuum

Plexus basilaris

A. vertebralis

Sinus occipitalis

Sinus sagittalis superior

Homo

Bulbus olfactorius

Sinus sagittalis superior

Sinus sagittalis inferior

Sinus petrosus superior

Sinus petrosus inferior

Sinus sigmoideus

Sinus transversus

Confluens sinuum

V. cerebri magna

Sinus sagittalis inferior

Sinus rectus

Sinus sagittalis superior

Pan

PLATE 50

Ventral Neck I

Several different groups of muscles are depicted in this view of the ventral neck. The most superficial layer is the platysma, which was encountered previously. In *Papio* the cervical portion of the platysma is well developed, and there is usually a great deal of interlacing of fibers below the chin. The degree of decussation displays marked individual variability among *Papio,* as well as in *Homo* (Loth 1949).

Of the deeper muscles, the digastric warrants special attention. The muscle possesses two posterior bellies in all three primates. These bellies arise medial to the mastoid processes and gradually narrow to become tendons. In *Homo* this intermediate tendon is united to the hyoid bone by an aponeurotic expansion from its caudal border, and the two anterior bellies converge on the anterior ends of the tendons. The anterior bellies remain widely separated, and the mylohyoid muscle is exposed between them. A much different arrangement obtains in *Papio.* The tendons become continuous anterior to the hyoid, forming a fibrous arcade to which attach the muscle fibers of the anterior belly. Since these fibers are continuous across the midline, the result is a single anterior belly termed "the digastric sling" by Schwartz and Huelke (1963). In *Pan* both arrangements occur with about equal frequency, while in *Pongo* only the posterior belly is present and it runs to the mandibular angle (Sonntag 1924).

The submandibular gland is seen lying on the superficial surface of the anterior belly of the digastric. It is a lobulated structure divisible into two or three parts. The gland is enclosed in a connective tissue capsule. In addition, there are often accessory glands present along the sub-mandibular duct. In *Papio* the submandibular and sublingual glands are usually completely separated, a situation which also exists in *Macaca mulatta* (Leppi 1967; Celemencki and Zajac 1968). In all three animals, the free border of the mylohyoid muscle grooves the anterior surface of the gland.

Note the air sac in *Pan* lying between the two sternohyoid muscles. Discussion of this interesting structure is delayed until later (Plate 58).

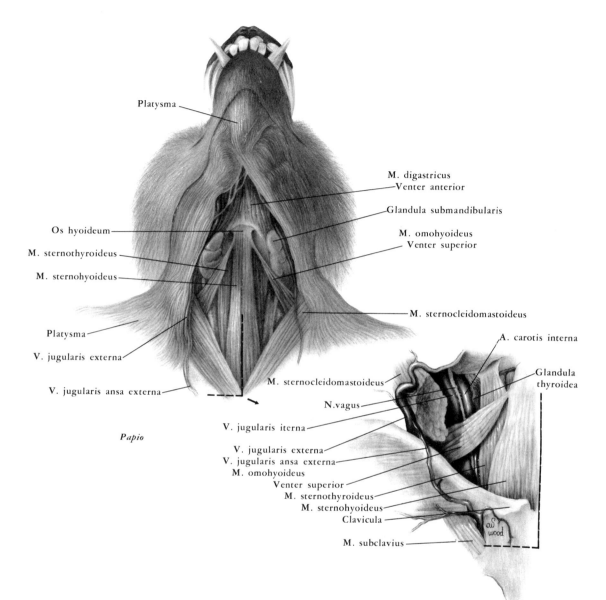

Platysma

M. digastricus
Venter anterior

Glandula submandibularis

Os hyoideum

M. omohyoideus
Venter superior

M. sternothyroideus

M. sternohyoideus

M. sternocleidomastoideus

Platysma

A. carotis interna

V. jugularis externa

Glandula thyroidea

V. jugularis ansa externa

M. sternocleidomastoideus

N.vagus

V. jugularis iterna

Papio

V. jugularis externa
V. jugularis ansa externa
M. omohyoideus
Venter superior
M. sternothyroideus
M. sternohyoideus
Clavicula

M. subclavius

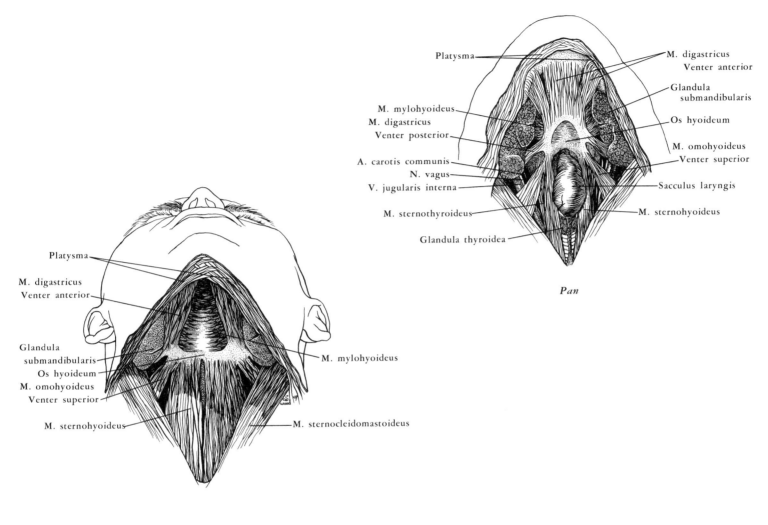

Platysma

M. digastricus
Venter anterior

M. mylohyoideus
M. digastricus
Venter posterior

A. carotis communis
N. vagus
V. jugularis interna

M. sternothyroideus

Glandula thyroidea

M. digastricus
Venter anterior

Glandula
submandibularis

Os hyoideum

M. omohyoideus
Venter superior

Sacculus laryngis

M. sternohyoideus

Pan

Platysma

M. digastricus
Venter anterior

Glandula
submandibularis
Os hyoideum
M. omohyoideus
Venter superior

M. sternohyoideus

M. mylohyoideus

M. sternocleidomastoideus

Homo

PLATE 51

Ventral Neck II

Two muscles of mastication are shown in *Papio,* the masseter and the temporalis. The former is laminated into superficial and deep parts, of which the superficial portion is seen attaching along the lower border of the mandible. The powerful temporalis attaches to the coronoid process and the anterior border of the ascending ramus of the mandible.

The fleshy mylohyoid has a median raphe in *Papio* and *Homo,* but it is absent in *Pan* (Sonntag 1924). The remainder of the muscles have been discussed earlier.

The thyroid gland is shown in *Pan and Homo.* In these forms the gland consists of two lateral lobes on either side of the trachea and an interconnecting isthmus lying ventral to the trachea. In *Pan* the isthmus is frequently wanting, and in *Papio* it is absent in the majority of animals. Occasionally a pyramidal lobe is present in *Homo;* however, this cranial extension of the thyroid gland has not been reported in *Papio* or *Pan* (Hill 1970; Sonntag 1924). In general, many variations can be anticipated regarding the form of the gland in these animals. An interesting anomaly is a persistent thyroglossal duct passing from the thyroid gland to the foramen caecum at the base of the tongue. The duct may persist in part or in its entirety, and Batson (1946) found thyroglossal remains in over half of the human cadavers he studied. Parathyroid glands are present on the dorsal surface of the thyroid gland. In *Papio* these are more often embedded in the substance of the gland. In *Homo* there are usually superior and inferior glands, although their number and locations are variable.

The common carotid artery, internal jugular vein, and vagus nerve are shown in their characteristic arrangement. Their topography—vein lateral, artery medial, and nerve between—is a constant and stable relation through this region of the neck in all three animals. Note the phrenic nerve lying on the superficial surface of the anterior scalene muscle in *Papio.* As in the case of the carotid sheath and its contents mentioned above, this arrangement is the same in these three primates.

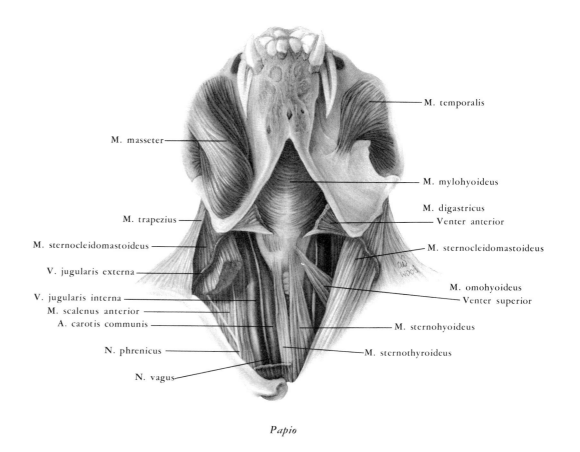

M. temporalis

M. masseter

M. mylohyoideus

M. digastricus
Venter anterior

M. trapezius

M. sternocleidomastoideus

M. sternocleidomastoideus

V. jugularis externa

V. jugularis interna
M. scalenus anterior
A. carotis communis

M. omohyoideus
Venter superior

M. sternohyoideus

N. phrenicus

M. sternothyroideus

N. vagus

Papio

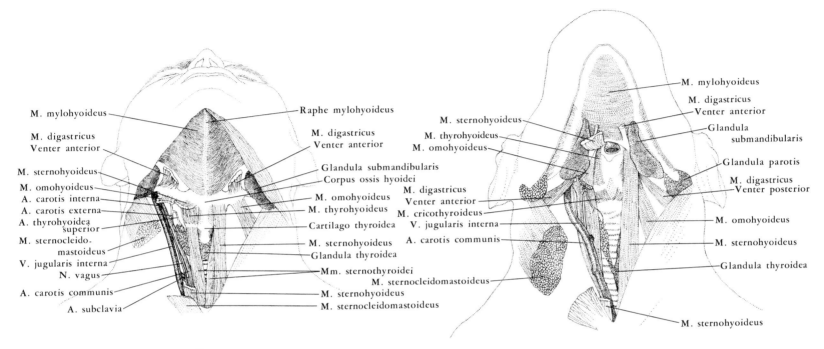

M. mylohyoideus

Raphe mylohyoideus

M. digastricus
Venter anterior

M. digastricus
Venter anterior

Glandula submandibularis
Corpus ossis hyoidei

M. sternohyoideus

M. omohyoideus
A. carotis interna
A. carotis externa
A. thyrohyoidea superior

M. omohyoideus
M. thyrohyoideus
Cartilago thyroidea

M. sternocleido-mastoideus
V. jugularis interna
N. vagus
A. carotis communis
A. subclavia

M. sternohyoideus
Glandula thyroidea
Mm. sternothyroidei
M. sternohyoideus
M. sternocleidomastoideus

Homo

M. sternohyoideus
M. thyrohyoideus
M. omohyoideus

M. digastricus
Venter anterior
M. cricothyroideus
V. jugularis interna
A. carotis communis

M. mylohyoideus
M. digastricus
Venter anterior
Glandula submandibularis

Glandula parotis

M. digastricus
Venter posterior

M. omohyoideus

M. sternohyoideus

Glandula thyroidea

M. sternohyoideus

Pan

PLATE 52

Root of Neck

The anatomical structures at the root of the neck are closely packed and intimate. Here we see the large brachiocephalic trunk issuing from the arch of the aorta. Near the cranial border of the right sternoclavicular joint it bifurcates into the right common carotid and the right subclavian arteries. The former ascends into the neck within the carotid sheath; the latter passes deep to the anterior scalene muscle and continues laterally where, as it runs across the first rib, it becomes the axillary artery. This most medial portion of the subclavian usually gives rise to three separate arteries: the vertebral, internal thoracic, and thyrocervical trunk. In *Papio* the thyrocervical trunk and internal thoracic arteries frequently share a common origin. In *Papio* and *Homo* the inferior thyroid artery usually arises from the thyrocervical trunk; in *Pan* the artery frequently appears as a branch of the common carotid. The costocervical artery commonly arises from the subclavian as it passes from beneath the anterior scalene muscle. The origin of this artery from the left subclavian is usually from the first portion of the artery.

Observe the vagus nerve crossing superficially to the subclavian artery where it gives off its recurrent laryngeal branch. The latter quickly assumes the groove between the trachea and the esophagus to ascend into the neck. On the left, the recurrent laryngeal loops around the aortic arch.

Note the sympathetic trunk passing through the neck deep to the carotid sheath. There are typically three cervical ganglia present in the three animals. Also, there is noticeable anastomosing between the cardiac branches of the cervical sympathetic chain and the vagus (Zuckerman 1938).

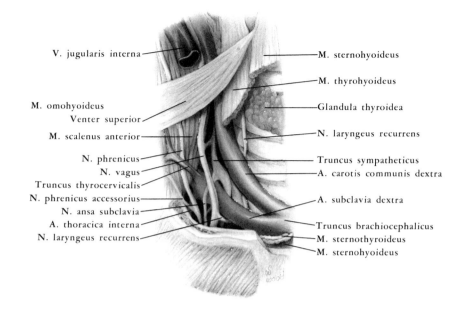

Papio

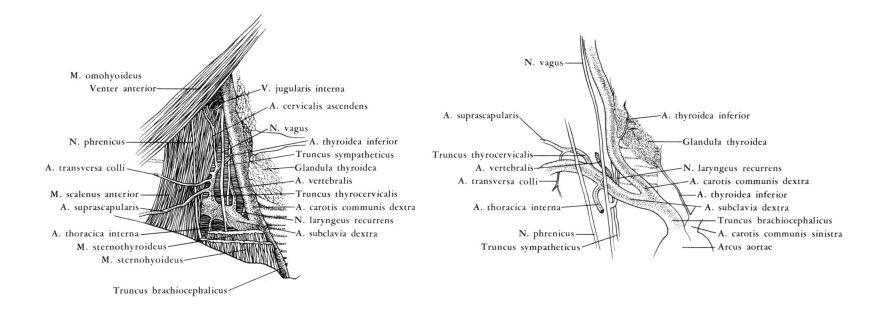

M. omohyoideus
Venter anterior
V. jugularis interna
A. cervicalis ascendens
N. vagus
N. phrenicus
A. thyroidea inferior
Truncus sympatheticus
Glandula thyroidea
A. transversa colli
A. vertebralis
Truncus thyrocervicalis
M. scalenus anterior
A. carotis communis dextra
A. suprascapularis
N. laryngeus recurrens
A. thoracica interna
A. subclavia dextra
M. sternothyroideus
M. sternohyoideus

Truncus brachiocephalicus

Homo

N. vagus
A. suprascapularis
A. thyroidea inferior
Truncus thyrocervicalis
Glandula thyroidea
A. vertebralis
N. laryngeus recurrens
A. transversa colli
A. carotis communis dextra
A. thyroidea inferior
A. thoracica interna
A. subclavia dextra
Truncus brachiocephalicus
N. phrenicus
A. carotis communis sinistra
Truncus sympatheticus
Arcus aortae

Pan

PLATE 53

Lateral Neck I

The facial nerve has just issued through the stylomastoid foramen. In *Homo,* note the protection offered the nerve by the well-developed mastoid process.

The glossopharyngeal and vagus nerves enter the region via the jugular foramen. The former, destined for the tongue and cranial portion of the pharynx, is a mixed nerve carrying both motor and sensory fibers. Some of the sensory fibers are special visceral afferent and carry the sensation of taste from the posterior one-third of the tongue. Observe the nerve curving anteriorly through the deep lateral neck to pass subjacent to the hyoglossus muscle. This is a constant arrangement in the three animals.

The vagus has the greatest distribution of any of the cranial nerves. Here we see the superior laryngeal arising from the vagus and passing caudoventrally toward the larynx. It divides almost immediately into the internal and external rami. The internal nerve pierces the thyrohyoid membrane and is sensory from the laryngeal mucosa as far caudally as the true vocal cords. The external branch innervates the cricothyroid muscle. The recurrent laryngeal of the vagus supplies the other muscles of the larynx.

The hypoglossal nerve is somatic motor to the tongue. It swings anteriorly through the neck deep to the digastric and stylohyoid tendons and on to the lateral surface of the hyoglossus muscle, then disappears between the mylohyoid and genioglossus muscles.

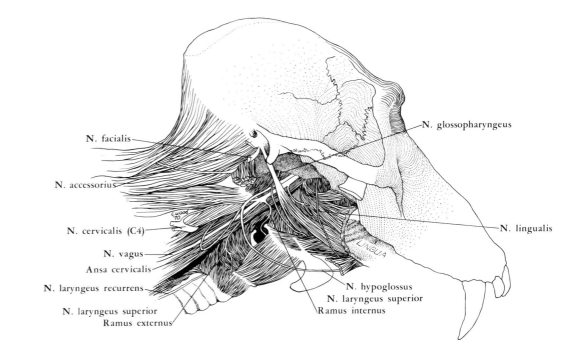

Papio

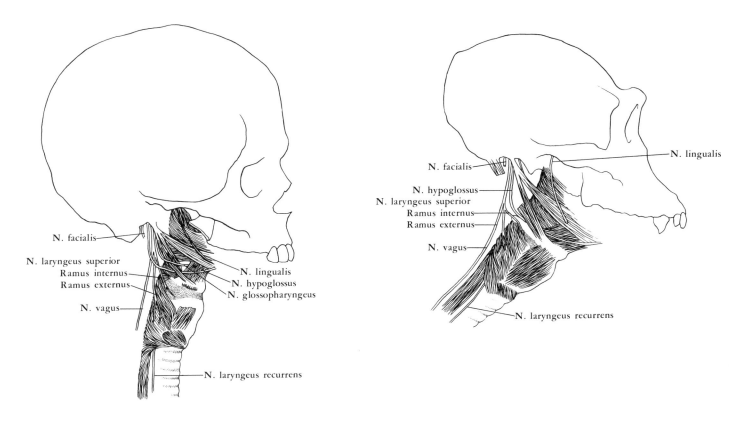

N. facialis

N. laryngeus superior
Ramus internus
Ramus externus

N. vagus

N. lingualis
N. hypoglossus
N. glossopharyngeus

N. laryngeus recurrens

Homo

N. facialis

N. lingualis

N. hypoglossus
N. laryngeus superior
Ramus internus
Ramus externus

N. vagus

N. laryngeus recurrens

Pan

PLATE 54

Lateral Neck II

The muscles shown in this plate represent several different morphological and functional groups. The levator veli palatini and tensor veli palatini are muscles of the soft palate. The former is composed of parallel fibers running from the region of the petrous temporal and auditory tube to the midline of the soft palate. When the muscle contracts, it elevates the soft palate and closes the pharyngeal isthmus. The tensor passes from the spine of the sphenoid and auditory tube to attach to the aponeurosis of the soft palate. The muscle becomes tendinous as it swings around the pterygoid hamulus. It tightens the soft palate and opens the auditory tube. The palatoglossus, palatopharyngeus, and uvular are part of the soft palate musculature. The former two muscles pass from the sides of the palate to the lateral border of the tongue and lateral wall of the pharynx, respectively. The uvular muscles make up the major portion of the uvula. Note that all of these muscles are supplied by the vagus except the tensor, which is innervated by the trigeminal (V3), since it is derived embryologically from the mandibular arch.

The three muscles originating from the styloid process are the stylohyoid, styloglossus, and stylopharyngeus. They pass to the hyoid bone, tongue, and pharyngeal wall, and are innervated by the facial, hypoglossal, and glossopharyngeal nerves.

The esophagus continues from the pharynx to the stomach. It has three parts: cervical, thoracic, and abdominal. The abdominal portion is very short in *Papio*, since the esophagus enters the stomach almost immediately after passing through the diaphragm. In all three animals, the esophagus commences at the caudal border of the cricoid cartilage and in *Papio* the cervical portion deviates slightly to the right as it courses through the neck. It therefore lacks the left flexure of human anatomy. In *Papio* the total length of the esophagus ranges from 11 to 15 cm., while in *Homo* it is usually between 23 and 30 cm. long (Hill 1970; Blount and Lachman 1966).

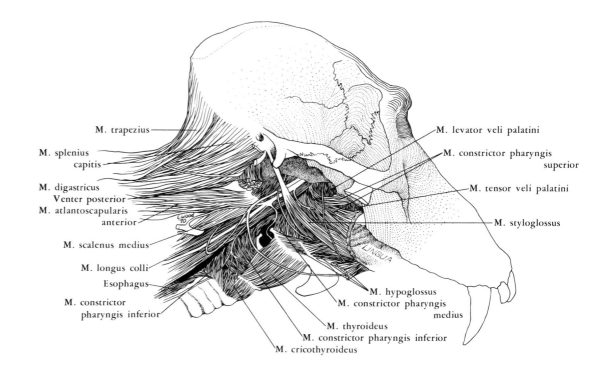

Papio

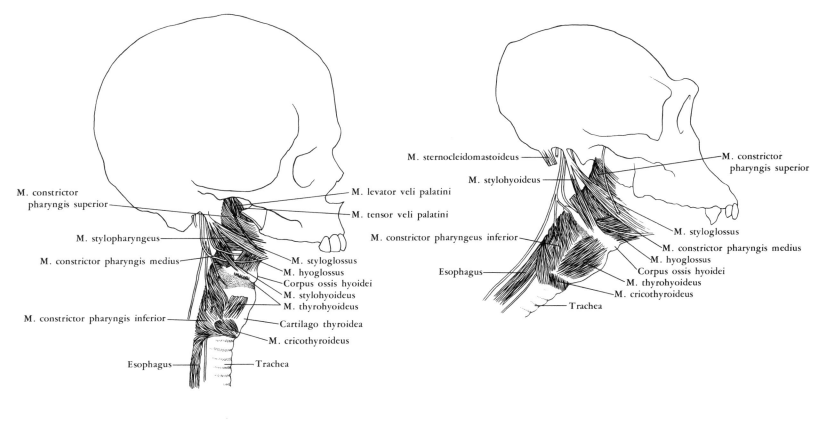

M. constrictor
pharyngis superior

M. levator veli palatini

M. tensor veli palatini

M. stylopharyngeus

M. constrictor pharyngis medius

M. styloglossus
M. hyoglossus
Corpus ossis hyoidei
M. stylohyoideus
M. thyrohyoideus

M. constrictor pharyngis inferior

Cartilago thyroidea

M. cricothyroideus

Esophagus

Trachea

Homo

M. sternocleidomastoideus

M. constrictor
pharyngis superior

M. stylohyoideus

M. constrictor pharyngeus inferior

M. styloglossus

M. constrictor pharyngis medius
M. hyoglossus
Corpus ossis hyoidei
M. thyrohyoideus
M. cricothyroideus

Esophagus

Trachea

Pan

PLATE 55

Pharyngeal Region I

The pharynx is a musculofibrous passageway extending from the base of the skull to the esophagus at the caudal border of the cricoid cartilage. Dorsally, the pharynx is in relation to the centra of the cervical vertebrae, while ventrally it communicates with the nasal, oral, and laryngeal cavities.

The muscles of the pharynx are the superior, middle, and inferior constrictors. The superior muscle drapes from its cranial attachment at the pharyngeal tubercle of the occipital bone to attach to the medial pterygoid lamina and pterygomandibular raphe. From all of these locations the muscle fibers pass to insert in the median pharyngeal raphe. The latter structure runs almost the complete length of the pharynx, affording attachment to the three constrictors. The middle and inferior constrictors attach ventrally to the hyoid bone and to the thyroid and cricoid cartilages, respectively. The three muscles constrict the pharynx and are innervated by the vagus nerve.

Several spaces are associated with the formation of the pharyngeal constrictors. These are more or less similar in the three primates, and the structures related to them are identical. Beginning cranially, the space between the free border of the superior constrictor and the skull is occupied by the pharyngobasilar fascia. Although not shown, the ascending palatine artery crosses the free border on its way to the soft palate. The glossopharyngeal nerve and stylopharyngeus muscle pass between the superior and middle constrictors. The internal laryngeal nerve and superior laryngeal artery enter the larynx between the middle and inferior constrictors. The recurrent laryngeal nerve and inferior laryngeal artery pass through the hiatus between the inferior constrictor and the esophagus.

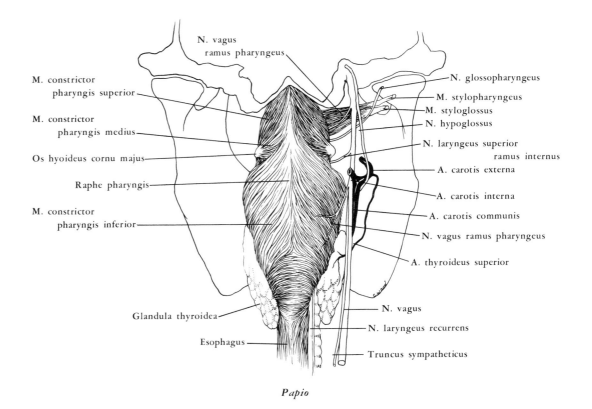

Papio

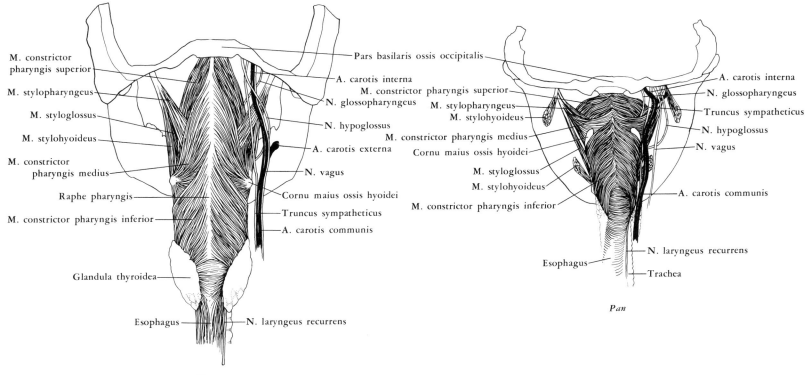

M. constrictor pharyngis superior
M. stylopharyngeus
M. styloglossus
M. stylohyoideus
M. constrictor pharyngis medius
Raphe pharyngis
M. constrictor pharyngis inferior
Glandula thyroidea
Esophagus

Pars basilaris ossis occipitalis
A. carotis interna
N. glossopharyngeus
N. hypoglossus
A. carotis externa
N. vagus
Cornu maius ossis hyoidei
Truncus sympatheticus
A. carotis communis
N. laryngeus recurrens

Homo

A. carotis interna
N. glossopharyngeus
M. constrictor pharyngis superior
Truncus sympatheticus
M. stylopharyngeus
M. stylohyoideus
N. hypoglossus
M. constrictor pharyngis medius
N. vagus
Cornu maius ossis hyoidei
M. styloglossus
M. stylohyoideus
A. carotis communis
M. constrictor pharyngis inferior
N. laryngeus recurrens
Esophagus
Trachea

Pan

PLATE 56

Pharyngeal Region II

The pharynx is divided into three parts according to its communications; thus, there is a nasal pharynx, which is respiratory, and an oral and a laryngeal pharynx, which are both respiratory and alimentary.

The nasal portion is directly dorsal to the nasal cavity and is exclusively respiratory in function. The orifice of the auditory tube occupies a part of the lateral wall of the nasal pharynx. This passageway establishes communication between the nasopharynx and the middle ear. The aggregation of lymphoid tissue in the roof and posterior wall of the nasopharynx is the pharyngeal tonsil or "adenoid."

The oral pharynx opens ventrally into the mouth. Several walls are described, one of which demands attention. The lateral wall is composed of two arches or folds of mucosa, the palatoglossal and palatopharyngeal arches. Their prominence is due to the muscles lying within the folds which, incidentally, carry the same names as the arches. The palatine tonsil resides in the fossa produced by these two pillars. Note that there are usually irregular masses of lymphoid tissue near the root of the tongue, which are collectively known as the lingual tonsil. These three areas of tonsilar tissue (lymphoid) surround the pharynx and are designated the "tonsilar ring." This ring demarcates the anterior limit of the embryonic foregut and is assumed to play a protective role as a functional part of the lymph system. The three tonsilar groups are present in these primates.

The laryngeal pharynx is the most caudal part of the pharynx and lies dorsal to the larynx. Note that the laryngeal pharynx is much wider cranially than it is caudally. The epiglottis occupies much of the cranial portion of this part of the pharynx. The superior aperture of the larynx is easily observable in *Homo*. Just caudal to this opening, note the dorsal wall of the larynx containing the arytenoid and cricoid cartilages. The aryepiglottic fold connects the arytenoid cartilage to the epiglottis.

The piriform recess lies on either side of the larynx. The internal laryngeal nerve lies just deep to the mucosa lining this depression.

The sulcus terminalis, shown on the tongue of *Homo* separates this organ into a large anterior body and a small posterior root.

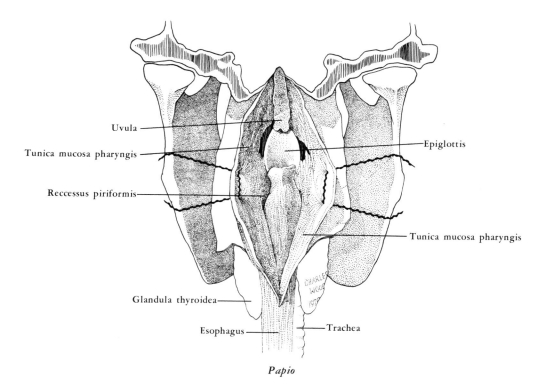

Uvula

Tunica mucosa pharyngis

Reccessus piriformis

Glandula thyroidea

Esophagus

Epiglottis

Tunica mucosa pharyngis

Trachea

Papio

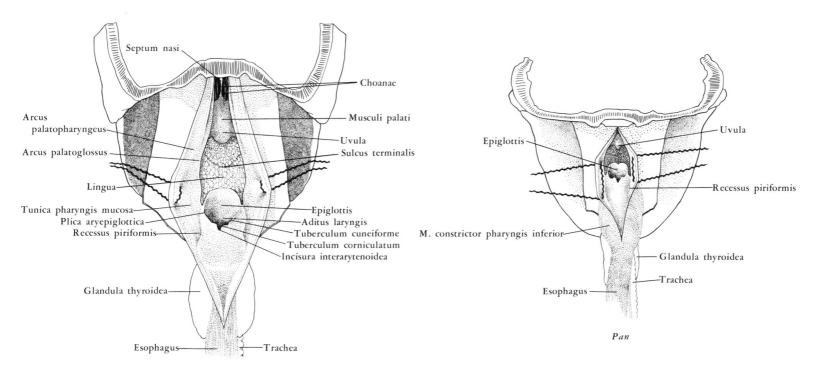

Septum nasi

Choanae

Arcus palatopharyngeus

Musculi palati

Arcus palatoglossus

Uvula

Sulcus terminalis

Lingua

Tunica pharyngis mucosa

Epiglottis

Plica aryepiglottica

Aditus laryngis

Recessus piriformis

Tuberculum cuneiforme

Tuberculum corniculatum

Incisura interarytenoidea

Glandula thyroidea

Esophagus

Trachea

Homo

Epiglottis

Uvula

Recessus piriformis

M. constrictor pharyngis inferior

Glandula thyroidea

Trachea

Esophagus

Pan

PLATE 57

Pharyngeal Region III

The larynx is made up of cartilages, elastic membranes, and intrinsic muscles. The cartilages are the thyroid, cricoid, epiglottis, and arytenoid. In addition, cuneiform and corniculate cartilages are present, although they are extremely small in *Papio* and *Pan*. The interrelationships of these various cartilages as they make up the framework of the larynx are essentially the same in the three primates. The thyroid is placed ventrally, with the epiglottis situated dorsocranially. The cricoid is positioned caudally and makes contact with the first tracheal ring. The two arytenoid cartilages sit on the cranial border of the cricoid cartilage. The arytenoids give attachment to the vocal ligaments. The cuneiform cartilages are distinct and lie within the aryepiglottic folds just anterior to the small corniculate cartilages. The latter, as mentioned above, are very minute in *Pan* and particularly in *Papio*. Indeed, they are completely absent in *Macaca mulatta* (Geist 1933).

The intrinsic muscles are responsible for modifying the size of the superior laryngeal aperture, the rima glottidis, and the amount of tension on the vocal ligaments. Two of these muscles, the cricoarytenoid and the arytenoid, are shown here. The former helps to widen the rima glottidis, thereby tensing the vocal ligaments, while the latter approximates the arytenoid cartilages, thus narrowing the rima glottidis. Both of these muscles—indeed, all of the intrinsic muscles of the larynx except the cricothyroid— are innervated by the recurrent laryngeal. The cricothyroid is supplied by the external branch of the superior laryngeal.

The cavity of the larynx is similar in the three animals. The ventricular folds, or false vocal cords, are visible on either side of the larynx. Just caudal to these, the vocal folds, or true vocal cords, project into the laryngeal cavity. Between the ventricular and vocal folds the laryngeal ventricle can be found. This is a small, lateral evagination in *Homo*, but in *Papio*, and particularly in *Pan*, this recess expands into the laryngeal air sacs (Plate 58). In *Homo* the ventricular appendix occasionally extends as far cranially as the great cornu of the hyoid bone.

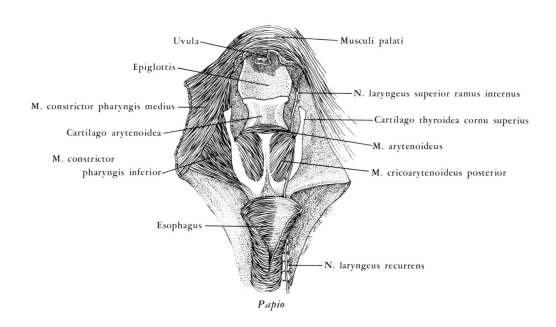

Papio

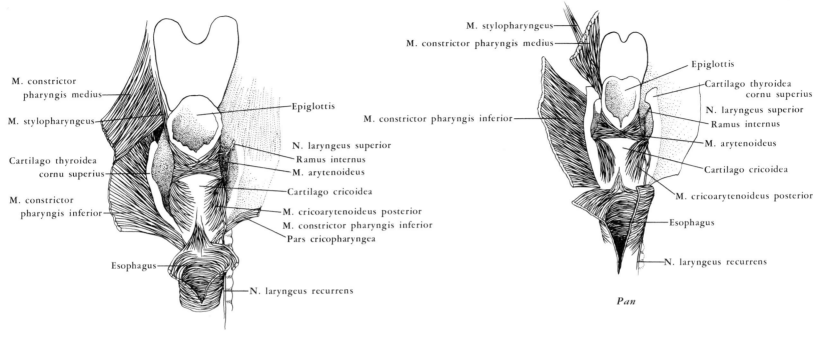

M. constrictor
pharyngis medius

M. stylopharyngeus

Cartilago thyroidea
cornu superius

M. constrictor
pharyngis inferior

Esophagus

Epiglottis

N. laryngeus superior
Ramus internus
M. arytenoideus

Cartilago cricoidea

M. cricoarytenoideus posterior
M. constrictor pharyngis inferior
Pars cricopharyngea

N. laryngeus recurrens

Homo

M. stylopharyngeus

M. constrictor pharyngis medius

M. constrictor pharyngis inferior

Epiglottis

Cartilago thyroidea
cornu superius

N. laryngeus superior
Ramus internus

M. arytenoideus

Cartilago cricoidea

M. cricoarytenoideus posterior

Esophagus

N. laryngeus recurrens

Pan

PLATE 58

Laryngeal Sac

There is no true laryngeal sac in *Homo*. A small diverticulum, the ventricular appendix, extends from the laryngeal ventricle and on rare occasions it may reach to the hyoid bone.

In *Papio* a globular midline outpocketing of the laryngeal membrane forms the median air sac. It lies in the concavity of the hyoid bone and extends caudally onto the thyrohyoid membrane. Such structures have been reported in various species of monkeys (Hilloowala 1970). In addition, *Papio* has slightly expanded laryngeal ventricles which are homologous with the ventricular appendix of *Homo*. Hilloowala correctly distinguishes between the two types, and he calls the former structure an air sac and the latter an air space. He also believes that the air sac is larger and more prominent in herbivorous animals.

In *Pan* the laryngeal space communicates with the ventricles and consists of a central and two lateral parts. The former extends to the hyoid bone cranially and to the manubrium sterni caudally. In the latter position it lies between the sternocleidomastoid muscle, and here can be found the orifices leading to the right and left lateral parts. The right and left diverticula are frequently of unequal size, as shown here. In this example, the right portion extends much more caudally beneath the pectoralis major; indeed, it nearly reaches the sixth rib. Also, there are often extensions into the axilla. The laryngeal sac receives its vascular supply and innervation from adjacent vessels and nerves.

The gorilla and orang have the most complicated system of laryngeal spaces found among the primates (Raven 1950; Sonntag 1924). In both animals the apparatus consists of numerous conjoined diverticula extending into the neck, axilla, and along the thoracic wall. They increase in size with age, and in old male orangs lateral offshoots pass around the mandible toward the ears and cheeks. The space may become infected and not infrequently the animal expires (Guilloud and McClure 1969).

To our knowledge, the function of these spaces is not completely understood. Some say they are resonating chambers which add resonance to the voice; others claim that their function is mechanical, assisting in the support of the heavy jaws. Finally, at least one student ascribes a herbivorous function to the midline variety possessed by monkeys.

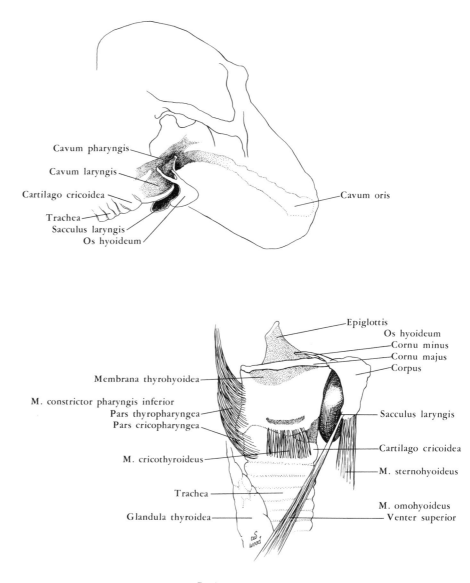

Papio

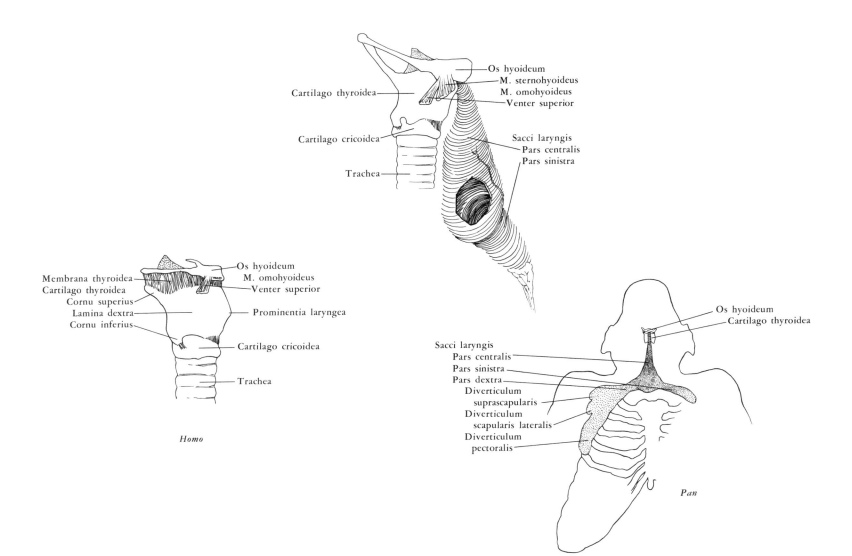

Os hyoideum
M. sternohyoideus
M. omohyoideus
Venter superior

Cartilago thyroidea

Cartilago cricoidea

Trachea

Sacci laryngis
Pars centralis
Pars sinistra

Membrana thyroidea
Cartilago thyroidea
Cornu superius
Lamina dextra
Cornu inferius

Os hyoideum
M. omohyoideus
Venter superior

Prominentia laryngea

Cartilago cricoidea

Trachea

Homo

Os hyoideum
Cartilago thyroidea

Sacci laryngis
Pars centralis
Pars sinistra
Pars dextra
Diverticulum
suprascapularis
Diverticulum
scapularis lateralis
Diverticulum
pectoralis

Pan

Part 3

SUPERIOR MEMBER

PLATE 59

Superficial Veins

The veins of the upper member are composed of the superficial and deep systems. The superficial veins are spread within the superficial fascia of the upper member. They commence in the venous plexuses of the hand. The deep veins are companions of the arteries and usually appear as venae comitantes. The two systems anastomose with each other at frequent intervals along their course.

In *Homo* two large veins, the cephalic and basilic, occupy prominent positions within the superficial fascia of the upper member. The former lies to the radial side of the limb, while the latter is located to the ulnar side of the extremity. Both veins begin in the dorsal venous network of the hand and empty into the axillary vein. Note that the basilic vein disappears into the deep brachial fascia slightly distal to mid-arm, whereas the cephalic remains superficial until it pierces the clavipectoral fascia. The median antebrachial and median cubital veins are particularly variable in the forearm of *Homo.* When present, the median cubital vein offers an excellent vessel for venipuncture.

In *Papio* and *Pan* a different superficial drainage system is presented. The major difference noted is the lack—indeed, the absence—of several superficial vessels normally found in *Homo.* In both animals the large basilic vein is entirely missing, and although the cephalic vein is present in both creatures, in *Pan* it reaches only as far as the antecubital fossa where it joins a well-marked brachial vein. Interestingly, the gorilla *(Gorilla gorilla)* is similar to *Pan* in lacking the basilic and humeral portions of the cephalic vein (Raven 1950). In *Papio* the cephalic vein is demonstrable along the radial side of the limb as far as the clavipectoral fascia. In the median cubital region several superficial vessels usually arise from the deeper system, and one of these has been here designated the median cubital of human anatomy.

The student should be continually alerted to anatomical variability and no morphological system represents this ever-present factor better than the superficial veins.

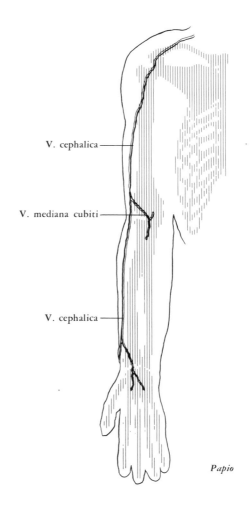

V. cephalica

V. mediana cubiti

V. cephalica

Papio

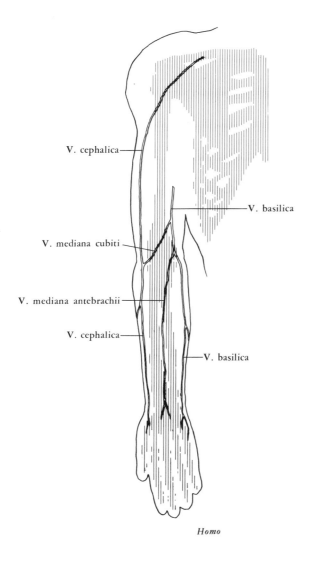

V. cephalica

V. basilica

V. mediana cubiti

V. mediana antebrachii

V. cephalica

V. basilica

Homo

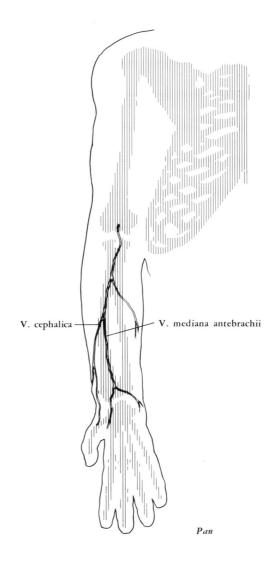

V. cephalica

V. mediana antebrachii

Pan

PLATE 60

Cutaneous Nerves

The cutaneous nerves are sensory branches arising from deeper-lying nerves. They lie within the superficial fascia and their appearance in this fascial layer, as well as their distribution, is widely variable. The most common arrangements are shown here, and one will note the general similarity in pattern among the three primates.

The cutaneous nerves of the superior member are branches of the brachial plexus, except for the supraclavicular nerves, which are cutaneous terminals from the cervical plexus. Only the lateral supraclavicular branches are shown as they pass obliquely across the acromion to supply the skin of the cranial and dorsal parts of the shoulder.

The cutaneous distribution on the ventral surface displays only a single difference. The superficial ramus of the radial nerve which makes its appearance along the extreme lateral border of the volar surface of the thumb in *Homo* and *Pan* remains entirely on the dorsal surface of the wrist and thumb in *Papio*. Other than this, the patterns are practically identical.

In *Homo* the lateral antebrachial cutaneous nerve sends a branch along the dorsal part of the radial surface of the forearm. In *Papio* and *Pan* this same area of skin is supplied by the posterior antebrachial cutaneous nerve.

The general pattern of distribution is extremely similar among the three primates, and those differences that do exist are slight and of doubtful anatomical importance.

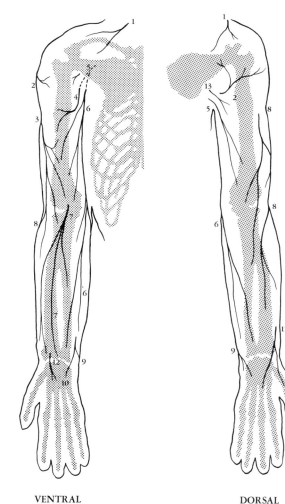

VENTRAL   DORSAL

Papio

1 Nn. supraclaviculares
2 N. cutaneus brachii lateralis superior
3 N. cutaneus brachii lateralis inferior
4 N. cutaneus brachii medialis
5 N. cutaneus brachii posterior
6 N. cutaneus antebrachii medialis
7 N. cutaneus antebrachii lateralis
8 N. cutaneus antebrachii posterior
9 Ramus dorsalis n. ulnaris
10 Ramus palmaris n. ulnaris
11 Ramus superficialis n. radialis
12 Ramus palmaris n. median
13 N. intercostobrachialis

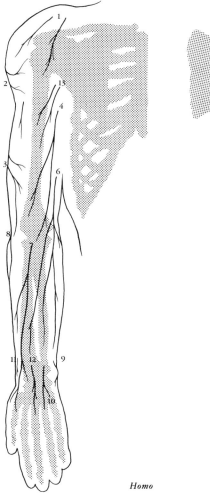
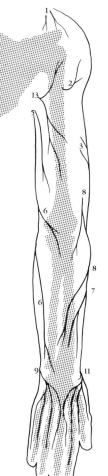
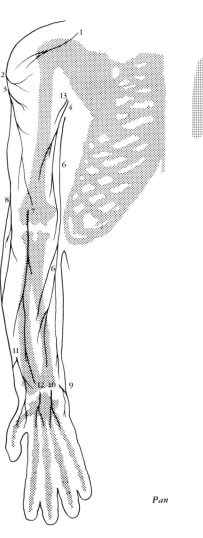

Homo

VENTRAL   DORSAL

Pan

VENTRAL   DORSAL

PLATE 61

Arterial Pattern

The plasticity of the vascular system is a well-documented fact in primate anatomy. In fact, it is virtually impossible to ascertain the normal pattern in a particular group of primates. One simply need read the excellent works of Manners-Smith on the nonhuman primates or the equally knowledgeable research of Michels on man to appreciate quickly the magnitude of this variability (Manners-Smith 1912; Michels 1955). Thus, only a general pattern, with certain major interspecific differences noted, is presented for each taxon.

The axillary artery continues directly from the subclavian into the axilla. Its first branch, the superior thoracic (Plate 66), is usually present in *Papio* and *Homo,* but is often absent in other members of the Cercopithecidae and *Pan.* The thoracoacromial artery arises next; like the superior thoracic, it is frequently absent in Old World monkeys (Manners-Smith 1912). It is normally present in *Papio,* and consistently present in *Homo* and *Pan.*

Moving laterally, the major difference encountered is the general reduction in the number of independent branches from this portion of the axillary in *Papio* and *Pan* when compared to *Homo.* In the former animals there is usually a common trunk for the subscapular, circumflex scapular, and humeral circumflex arteries. There is a tendency for the anterior humeral circumflex to be derived independently from the axillary in *Papio* and some of the mangabeys according to Manners-Smith (1912). The usual condition in *Homo* is to have three separate arteries arising from the distal part of the axillary.

The brachial artery commences at the distal border of the axilla and runs to the region of the elbow, where it bifurcates into its terminals, the radial and ulnar arteries. In *Papio* the division occurs proximal to the elbow, while in *Pan* and *Homo* it takes place at or distal to the joint. Note that the median nerve crosses the brachial artery superficially in *Papio* and *Homo,* whereas this relation is reversed in *Pan.* The largest branch of the brachial, the deep brachial, arises near the beginning of the brachial or, on occasion, directly from the axillary. The superior ulnar collateral artery is usually a branch of the deep brachial in *Papio,* but more often arises from the brachial in *Pan* and *Homo.* Collateral circulation around the elbow is carried out by a series of complex anastomosing vessels shown in the plate. Their exact origins are subject to some variation.

The radial and ulnar arteries are large vessels. The radial appears to be the continuation of the brachial, but it is usually smaller in caliber than the ulnar, especially in *Pan* and *Homo.* In *Papio,* and most other cercopithecoids, the radial is frequently the larger and more prominent vessel (Manners-Smith 1912; Lineback 1933). The interosseous arteries are similarly disposed in the three animals.

In *Papio* and other cercopithecoids there is a single volar arch which corresponds to the superficial palmar arch in *Pan* and *Homo.* The latter primates have, in addition, the deep arch shown here. The distribution of the digital arteries is similar in the three species.

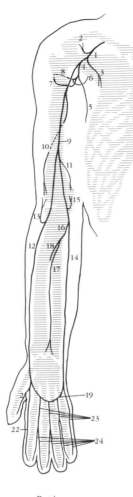

Papio

1 A. axillaris
2 A. thoraco-acromialis
3 A. thoracica lateralis
4 A. subscapularis
5 A. thoracodorsalis
6 A. circumflexa scapulae
7 A. circumflexa humeri anterior
8 A. circumflexa humeri posterior
9 A. brachialis
10 A. profunda brachii
11 A. collateralis ulnaris superior
12 A. radialis
13 A. recurrens radialis
14 A. ulnaris
15 A. recurrens ulnaris
16 A. interossea communis
17 A. interossea anterior
18 A. interossea posterior
19 Arcus palmaris superficialis
20 Arcus palmaris profundus
21 A. princeps pollicis
22 A. radialis indicis
23 Aa. digitales palmares communes
24 Aa. digitales palmares propriae

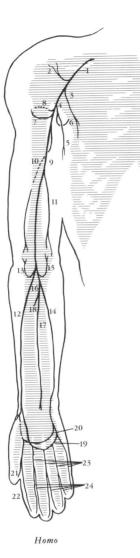

Homo

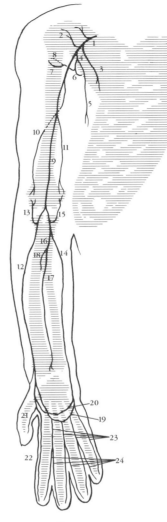

Pan

PLATE 62

Dorsal Scapular I

The muscles connecting the upper member to the vertebral column and the anterolateral thoracic walls are considered under "Back" and "Thorax," respectively. In this section, we are concerned with the muscles of the shoulder and upper limb proper.

In *Papio* the deltoid is easily separable into its component parts: clavicular, acromial, and spinal. Only the spinal portion is observable in this view. In all three animals the spinodeltoid attaches to the spine of the scapula and enjoys an extensive attachment to the fascia covering the infraspinatus muscle. The fascial connection is particularly well developed in *Papio* and *Pan*. From here the spinodeltoid converges obliquely in both lateral and ventral directions to attach to a thick intramuscular tendon, which in turn affords attachment for the muscle to the deltoid prominence on the lateral side of the shaft of the humerus. The location of this tuberosity on the humerus varies somewhat among the three animals. Its position tends to migrate distally on the humerus as one moves from quadrupedal *Papio* to brachiating *Pan* (Plate 15). The relation in *Homo* is more like *Pan*. This difference in muscle attachment is interpreted as offering the brachiators a greater mechanical advantage in lifting the humerus as they cavort through the trees.

The teres major is a rather thick, flattened muscle passing from the caudal border of the scapula laterally to attach to the proximal end of the humerus. The muscle is usually intimately united along its caudal border with the large latissimus dorsi.

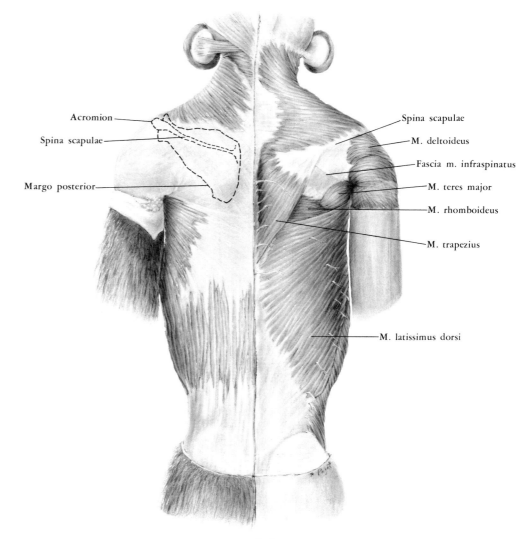

Acromion

Spina scapulae

Margo posterior

Spina scapulae

M. deltoideus

Fascia m. infraspinatus

M. teres major

M. rhomboideus

M. trapezius

M. latissimus dorsi

Papio

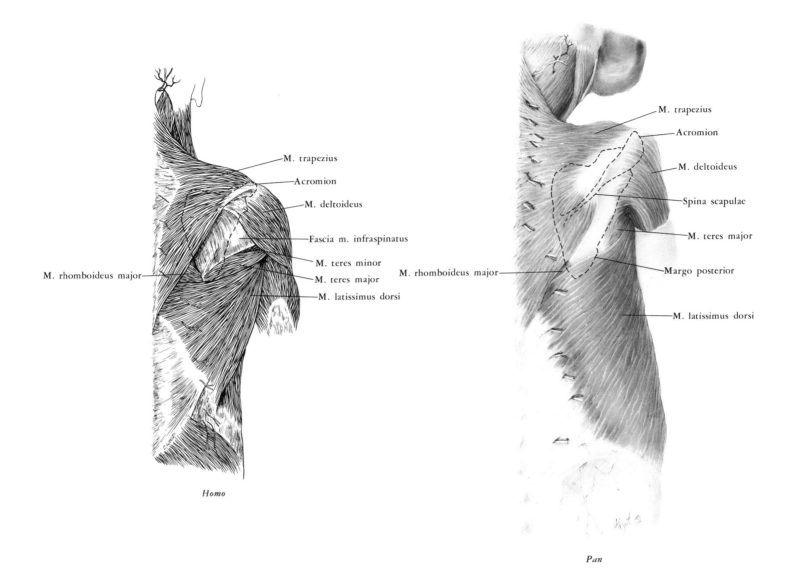

M. trapezius

Acromion

M. deltoideus

Fascia m. infraspinatus

M. teres minor

M. rhomboideus major

M. teres major

M. latissimus dorsi

Homo

M. trapezius

Acromion

M. deltoideus

Spina scapulae

M. teres major

M. rhomboideus major

Margo posterior

M. latissimus dorsi

Pan

PLATE 63

Dorsal Scapular II

The supraspinatus and infraspinatus muscles occupy most of the dorsal surface of the scapula. They pass laterally to attach to the two most proximal impressions on the greater tubercle of the humerus. The teres minor is a cylindrical muscle closely associated with the caudal portion of the infraspinatus. Indeed, in many specimens of all three species, the two muscles are extremely difficult to separate, particularly along their proximal portions. The teres minor ends at the most distal impression on the greater tubercle.

The dorsoepitrochlearis is a part of the triceps that has become secondarily attached to the latissimus dorsi. The muscle arises from the latissimus dorsi near the junction of the muscle and tendon, and accompanies the long head of the triceps to the elbow, where it passes to the medial epicondyle of the humerus. The muscle is normally absent in *Homo,* but present in prosimians, monkeys, and anthropoid apes (Howell and Straus 1933b). Sonntag (1922) refers to it as a "climbing muscle," but notes that it may be larger in certain ground-dwelling monkeys than in purely arboreal forms.

The triceps is large and easily separable into its three heads: long, lateral, and medial. Among the three primates, only the attachment of the long head is different. In *Papio* and *Pan* the long head arises from an extensive area along the axillary border of the scapula, whereas in *Homo* it is limited to the infraglenoid tubercle of the scapula. As a result of this large attachment, the triangular space of human anatomy is covered; therefore, the circumflex scapular artery does not make an appearance on the dorsal surface of the scapular muscles.

The quadrangular space is present in the three species, and in each the larger axillary nerve and posterior humeral circumflex artery swing through it to gain access to the deep surface of the deltoid. Just cranial to the teres minor, observe the suprascapular nerve and artery winding around the neck of the scapula through the greater scapular notch. While distal to the teres major, the radial nerve and deep brachial artery are observed in the triangular separation between the long and lateral heads of the triceps.

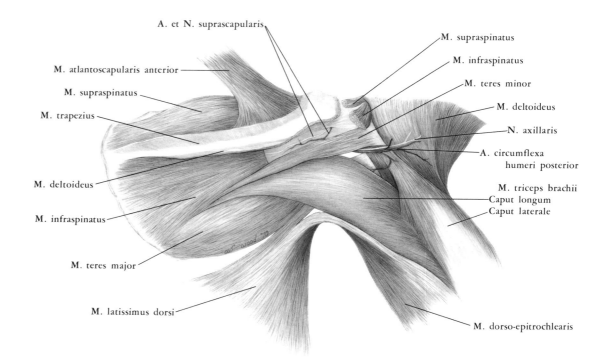

Papio

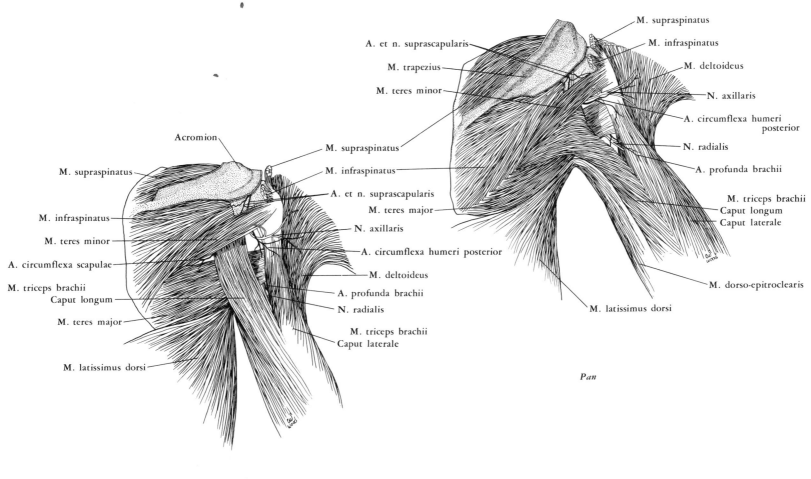

M. supraspinatus

Acromion

A. et n. suprascapularis

M. trapezius

M. teres minor

M. supraspinatus

M. infraspinatus

M. supraspinatus

M. infraspinatus

M. deltoideus

N. axillaris

A. circumflexa humeri posterior

N. radialis

A. profunda brachii

M. triceps brachii
Caput longum
Caput laterale

M. infraspinatus

M. teres minor

A. et n. suprascapularis

M. teres major

N. axillaris

A. circumflexa scapulae

A. circumflexa humeri posterior

M. triceps brachii
Caput longum

M. deltoideus

A. profunda brachii

N. radialis

M. teres major

M. triceps brachii
Caput laterale

M. dorso-epitroclearis

M. latissimus dorsi

M. latissimus dorsi

Homo

Pan

PLATE 64

Ventral Thorax

The deltoid is a coarsely fasciculated muscle composed of three parts: clavicular, acromial, and spinal. The clavicular portion has an extensive attachment to the clavicle in *Papio;* indeed, it so encroaches upon the clavicle that the pectoralis major is limited to the region of the sternoclavicular joint. In *Pan* the deltoid occupies the lateral half, and in *Homo* the lateral third of the clavicle. The acromial portion is large and easily separated from the other parts in *Papio.* In *Papio* and *Homo,* the cephalic vein intervenes between the caudal border of the deltoid and the cranial border of the pectoralis major. The absence of this vein in *Pan* may account for the frequent fusion between the deltoid and pectoralis major muscles.

The serratus anterior is a large muscular sheet positioned between the ribs and the scapula, occupying much of the lateral part of the chest. In *Papio* there may or may not be a cervical portion to the muscle. If present, it arises from the transverse processes of the caudal four or five cervical vertebrae. The cervical portion is present in *Macaca mulatta,* but Hill does not mention it in *Papio anubus* (Howell and Straus 1933b; Hill 1970). The thoracic part arises from the cranial eight to eleven ribs in all three animals. From this attachment the fibers extend dorsolaterally to insert into the length of the vertebral border of the scapula.

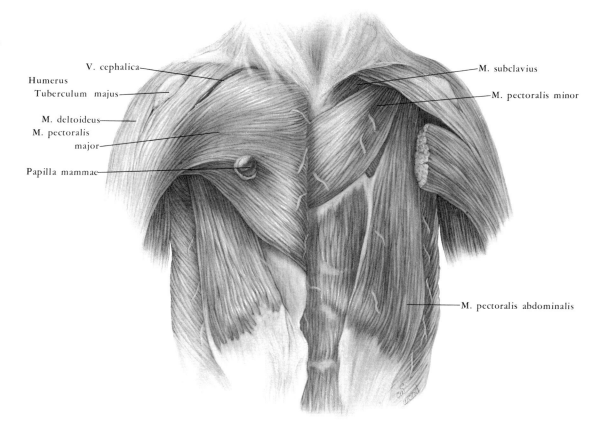

V. cephalica

Humerus
Tuberculum majus

M. deltoideus

M. pectoralis
major

Papilla mammae

M. subclavius

M. pectoralis minor

M. pectoralis abdominalis

Papio

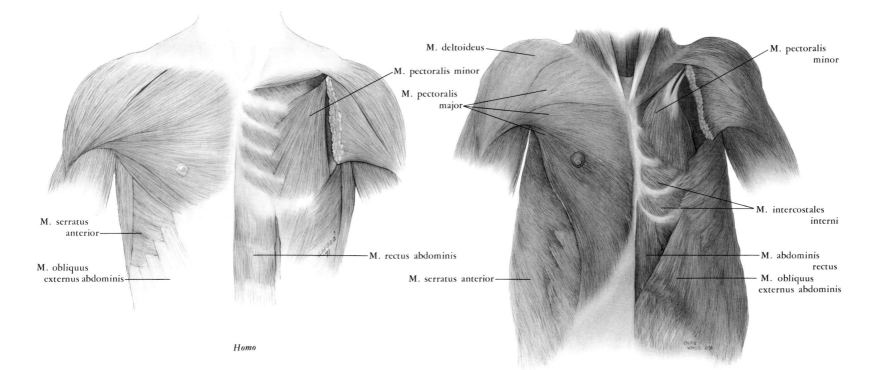

M. deltoideus

M. pectoralis minor

M. pectoralis major

M. pectoralis minor

M. intercostales interni

M. serratus anterior

M. obliquus externus abdominis

M. rectus abdominis

Homo

M. serratus anterior

M. abdominis rectus

M. obliquus externus abdominis

Pan

PLATE 65

Axillary Region I

Several important muscular relations are observed in this deep view of the posterior wall of the axilla and the proximal wall of the axilla and the proximal part of the arm.

In *Papio* the thin, narrow, tendinous branch of the panniculus carnosus is seen attaching to the humerus deep to the pectoral musculature. As noted elsewhere, this muscle is absent in *Pan* and *Homo*.

The subscapular muscle occupies the entire subscapular fossa of the scapula. From this extensive attachment it passes laterally to end as a tendon upon the lesser tubercle of the humerus. The muscle is often coarse with fibers arranged around several intramuscular septa in *Papio*. Indeed, Hill (1970) reports as many as five separate fusiform bellies present in *Papio hamadryas*.

The muscles of the brachium are the biceps, coraco-brachialis, brachialis, triceps, and dorsoepitrochlearis. The last muscle is absent in *Homo*. The biceps is a long fusiform muscle occupying the ventral surface of the arm. It arises by two heads: the long head attaches to the cranial margin of the glenoid cavity, while the short head shares a common origin with the coracobrachialis from the coracoid process. The two bellies join at various distances along the arm to continue to the proximal radius, where the muscle attaches.

The coracobrachialis possesses two parts in *Papio*: middle and deep. A third part was superficial to these, but does not appear in living primates (Howell and Straus 1933b). The deep portion is absent in *Pan* and *Homo*, who have retained only the middle part of the muscle (ibid.). The deep coracobrachialis passes from the coracoid process laterally deep to the short biceps and coracobrachialis medius to attach upon the surgical neck of the humerus. The coracobrachialis medius, or coracobrachialis in *Pan* and *Homo*, is disposed deep to the short biceps. The muscle passes from the coracoid process to the shaft of the humerus, where it attaches between the medial head of the triceps and the brachialis.

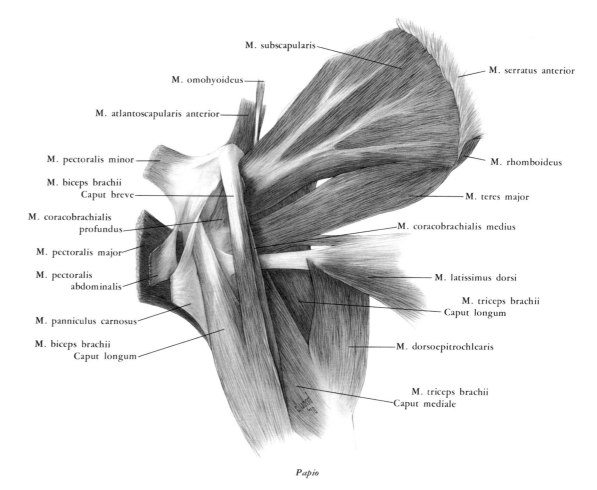

Papio

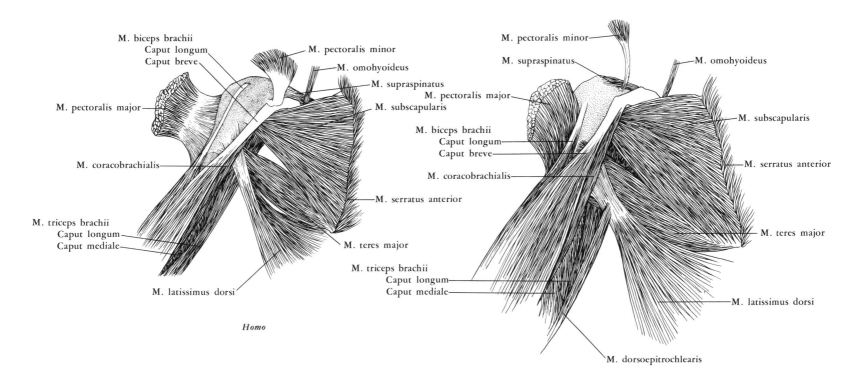

M. biceps brachii
Caput longum
Caput breve

M. pectoralis minor

M. omohyoideus

M. supraspinatus

M. pectoralis major

M. subscapularis

M. coracobrachialis

M. serratus anterior

M. triceps brachii
Caput longum
Caput mediale

M. teres major

M. latissimus dorsi

Homo

M. pectoralis minor

M. supraspinatus

M. omohyoideus

M. pectoralis major

M. subscapularis

M. biceps brachii
Caput longum
Caput breve

M. serratus anterior

M. coracobrachialis

M. teres major

M. triceps brachii
Caput longum
Caput mediale

M. latissimus dorsi

M. dorsoepitrochlearis

Pan

PLATE 66

Axillary Region II

The arrangement and interrelation of the various structures within the deep axilla is exceedingly complex mainly because there is a large number of structures coursing through a rather circumscribed pyramidal space between the medial side of the brachium and the craniolateral part of the chest. The major structures are axillary vessels and branches, brachial plexus and branches, and lymph nodes.

There is a great deal of variation associated with the branches of the axillary artery in these three primates. In general, the axillary gives rise to five or six independent trunks in *Homo,* whereas this number is reduced in *Papio* and *Pan* to two or three (Plate 61). As mentioned earlier, the most notable difference is the presence of a common humeral circumflex trunk in *Papio* and *Pan.* This is shown in the insert for *Pan.* Note that in *Papio* the anterior humeral circumflex frequently arises independently from the axillary, as shown here in the insert (Manners-Smith 1912; Hill 1970). The usual pattern in *Homo* is to have the subscapular and anterior and posterior humeral circumflex arteries arising separately from the distal portion of the axillary artery.

The subscapular artery is usually large in all three primates and gives rise to the scapular circumflex artery prior to assuming the axillary border of the subscapularis muscle. Hill (1970) described two subscapular arteries running parallel courses on the subscapular and teres major muscles.

Finally, observe that the brachial artery lies deep to the formation of the median nerve in its proximal portion in *Papio* and *Homo,* but superficial to the nerve in *Pan.* Sonntag (1924) noted a similar arrangement in *Pan.*

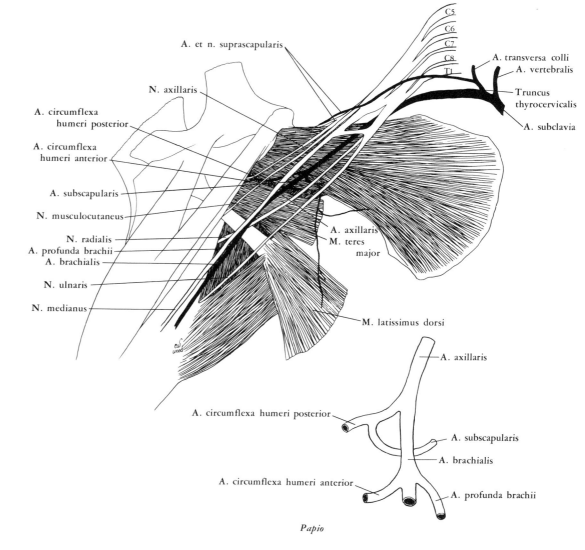

Papio

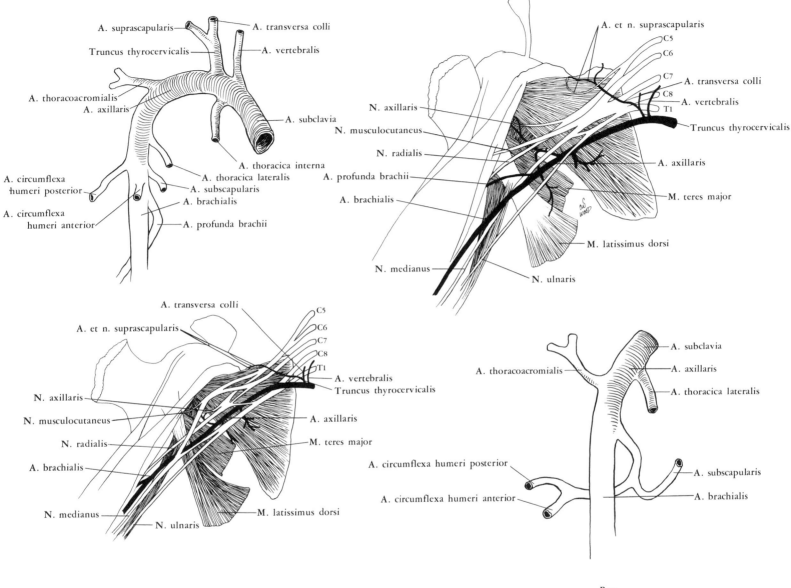

A. suprascapularis — A. transversa colli

Truncus thyrocervicalis — A. vertebralis

A. thoracoacromialis
A. axillaris — A. subclavia

A. circumflexa humeri posterior
A. circumflexa humeri anterior — A. thoracica interna
A. thoracica lateralis
A. subscapularis
A. brachialis
A. profunda brachii

A. et n. suprascapularis
C5
C6
C7
A. transversa colli
C8
A. vertebralis
T1
Truncus thyrocervicalis

N. axillaris
N. musculocutaneus
N. radialis
A. profunda brachii
A. axillaris
A. brachialis
M. teres major
N. medianus
M. latissimus dorsi
N. ulnaris

A. transversa colli
C5
C6
A. et n. suprascapularis
C7
C8
T1
A. vertebralis
Truncus thyrocervicalis
N. axillaris
N. musculocutaneus
A. axillaris
N. radialis
M. teres major
A. brachialis
N. medianus
M. latissimus dorsi
N. ulnaris

Homo

A. thoracoacromialis
A. subclavia
A. axillaris
A. thoracica lateralis

A. circumflexa humeri posterior
A. circumflexa humeri anterior
A. subscapularis
A. brachialis

Pan

PLATE 67

Brachial Plexus

The brachial plexus is formed by the ventral primary divisions of the fifth to eighth cervical nerves and the first thoracic nerve. In all three animals, the plexus often receives communicating branches from the fourth cervical and the second thoracic nerves. For excellent studies of the brachial plexus of primates, the reader is referred to Kerr 1918; Miller 1934; De Garis 1939; and Chase and De Garis 1940. The plexuses depicted here represent the normal conditions encountered, and while there are occasional variants observed in each species, the reader must be apprised of the relative stability of the basic arrangement of the plexus among the higher primates (Chase and De Garis 1940). For example, Chase and De Garis found their most prevalent type of plexus present in 82 percent of *Macaca mulatta,* and Kerr had an incidence of 93.7 percent for the most common type of *Homo.* Certain rather consistent differences between the plexuses are discussed briefly.

In *Papio* the long thoracic nerve is formed from roots C6 and C7, while in *Pan* and *Homo* it customarily arises from root C5 in addition to C6 and C7. The absence of C5 in *Papio* was also reported by Harris (1939) and Hill (1970). The number of subscapular nerves is subject to some variability. Thus, in *Papio* and *Homo* the usual number is two, whereas *Pan* frequently has as many as three to five (Sonntag 1924; Kusakabe et al. 1965). Also, in *Papio* the thoracodorsal nerve may arise from the posterior division of the lower trunk before the formation of the posterior cord (Harris 1939).

In *Papio* the medial brachial and medial antebrachial cutaneous nerves normally have a common trunk of origin from the medial cord. Indeed, Chase and De Garis (1940) proposed the term "medial cutaneous" for this common trunk in *Macaca mulatta.* In *Pan* and *Homo* these nerves usually have separate origins from the medial cord.

Note the presence of C4 in the brachial plexus of *Pan.* As mentioned above, such contributions occur in all three animals, but it appears to be a more fundamental component of the plexus in the Anthropoidea (Harris 1939; Kusakabe et al. 1965).

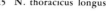

1	N. dorsalis scapulae	6	N. musculocutaneus
2	N. subclavius	7	N. axillaris
3	N. suprascapularis	8	N. radialis
4	N. subscapularis	9	N. medianus
5	N. pectoralis lateralis	10	N. ulnaris

11	N. thoracodorsalis
12	N. cutaneus antebrachii medialis
13	N. cutaneus brachii medialis
14	N. pectoralis medialis
15	N. thoracicus longus

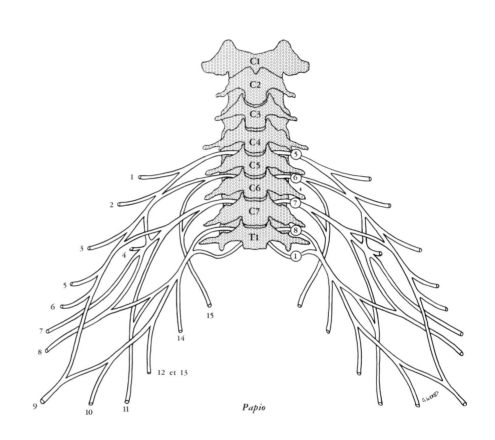

Papio

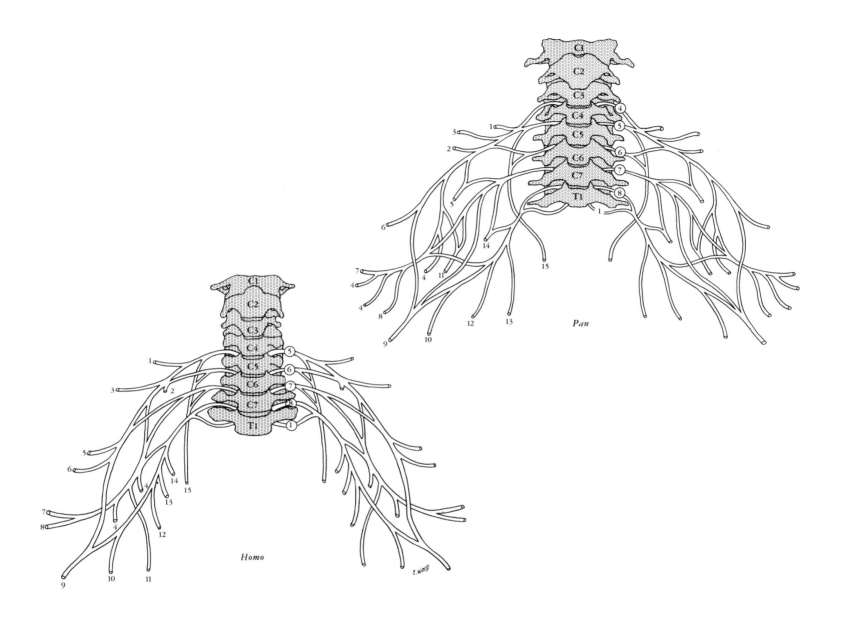

Homo

Pan

C. WOOD

PLATE 68

Medial Arm

The musculocutaneous nerve in *Papio* passes between the two portions of the coracobrachialis, whereas in *Pan* and *Homo* the nerve pierces the muscle, a condition which is usually confined to the great apes and man (Howell and Straus 1933b).

The relation of the median nerve to the brachial artery is of interest. In all three primates the median nerve lies initially on the lateral side of the brachial artery; at approximately mid-arm it passes to the medial side of the artery. In *Homo* the nerve crossed superficial to the artery in 82 percent of 307 limbs studied (Grant 1962). In *Pan* and *Papio* the artery crosses superficial to the nerve. Sonntag (1924) reported an identical condition for *Pan* and other Anthropoidea. For *Papio* the story is somewhat confusing: in all our specimens the artery crossed superficial to the nerve, but Hill (1970) reported the reverse relation in his study of *Papio*. The relation of the median nerve to the brachial artery varies because only one of the original two brachial arteries remains in the adult. If the ventral artery persists, as in *Papio* and *Pan*, then the artery crosses superficial to the nerve; if the dorsal artery remains, as in *Homo*, the condition is reversed. Of course, both types are encountered among the primates.

The superficial brachial artery warrants mentioning even though it was not encountered in our specimens (see insert). This anomalous artery arises from the axillary artery and passes superficial to the medial limb of the loop forming the median nerve, and then courses through the brachium where, near the elbow, it bifurcates into the radial and ulnar arteries. The artery has been reported in most groups of primates and the concerned reader is referred to the excellent investigations of Manners-Smith 1912; Chase and De Garis 1948; McCormack, Cauldwell, and Anson 1953.

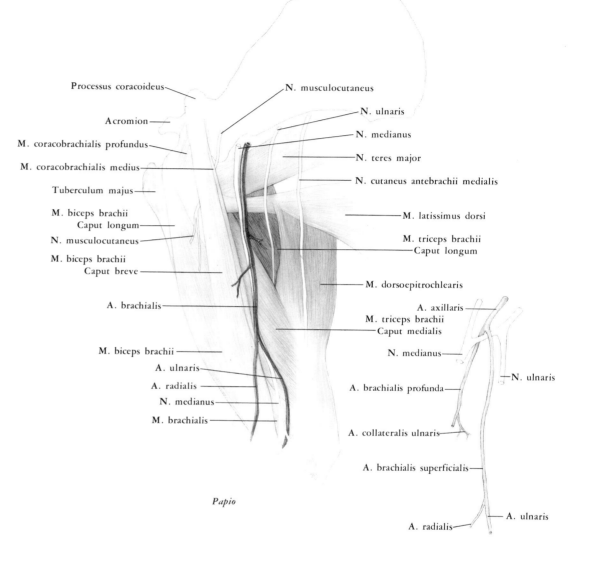

Processus coracoideus

Acromion

M. coracobrachialis profundus

M. coracobrachialis medius

Tuberculum majus

M. biceps brachii
Caput longum

N. musculocutaneus

M. biceps brachii
Caput breve

A. brachialis

M. biceps brachii

A. ulnaris

A. radialis

N. medianus

M. brachialis

N. musculocutaneus

N. ulnaris

N. medianus

N. teres major

N. cutaneus antebrachii medialis

M. latissimus dorsi

M. triceps brachii
Caput longum

M. dorsoepitrochlearis

A. axillaris

M. triceps brachii
Caput medialis

N. medianus

A. brachialis profunda

N. ulnaris

A. collateralis ulnaris

A. brachialis superficialis

A. ulnaris

A. radialis

Papio

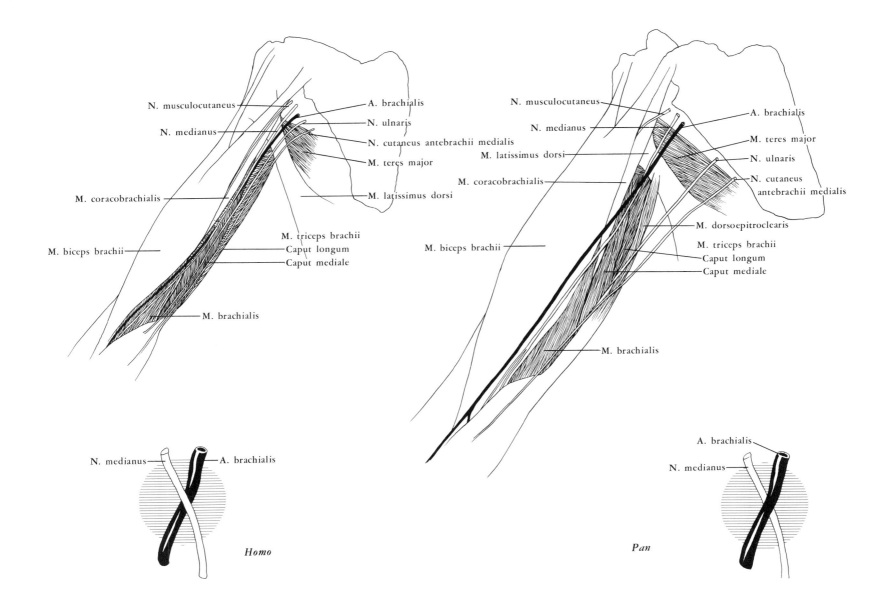

N. musculocutaneus
N. medianus
M. coracobrachialis
M. biceps brachii
M. brachialis

A. brachialis
N. ulnaris
N. cutaneus antebrachii medialis
M. teres major
M. latissimus dorsi
M. triceps brachii
Caput longum
Caput mediale

N. medianus
A. brachialis

Homo

N. musculocutaneus
N. medianus
M. latissimus dorsi
M. coracobrachialis
M. biceps brachii

A. brachialis
M. teres major
N. ulnaris
N. cutaneus antebrachii medialis
M. dorsoepitroclearis
M. triceps brachii
Caput longum
Caput mediale
M. brachialis

A. brachialis
N. medianus

Pan

PLATE 69

Lateral Arm

The powerful muscles occupying the dorsolateral surface of the arm—notably, the deltoid and triceps—are shown here.

The deltoid was discussed in Plates 62 and 64 but deserves additional comment here. It is a thick, large muscle in all three primates, and is more easily divisible into its three parts in *Papio*. In quadrupedal *Papio* the deltoid is a powerful protractor and retractor of the arm, and these potential functions are clearly suggested in this plate. As noted earlier, the humeral attachment of the muscle is more distally placed in *Pan* and *Homo*.

The long and lateral heads of the triceps are shown here. Note was made earlier of the extensive attachment of the long head to the axillary border of the scapula in *Papio*. The three parts converge about mid-shaft to form a broad tendon that continues to receive fibers from the humerus nearly as far as the olecranon fossa in *Papio*. Except for the attachment of the long head, the organization of the muscle is similar in the three primates. The brachialis muscle is seen lying subjacent to the biceps. It occupies much of the ventral surface of the humeral shaft and is a thick, powerful muscle, especially in *Papio*. Indeed, Hill (1970) found it partially divisible into a superficial and a deep lamina.

The most proximal of the forearm muscles, the brachioradialis, is clearly visible from the lateral side of the arm. Its proximal attachment to the lateral epicondyloid ridge of the humerus may extend nearly to the deltoid muscle in *Papio*. Note that the radial nerve (not visible here) courses either medial to the origin of the muscle or, on occasion, may pierce the muscle.

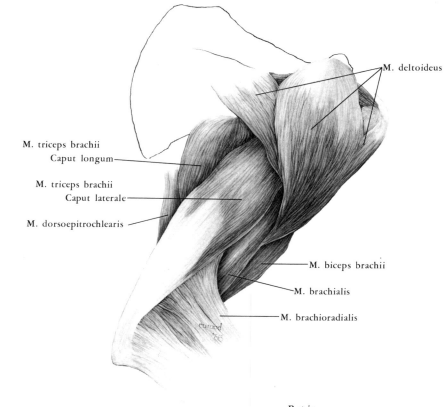

M. deltoideus

M. triceps brachii
Caput longum

M. triceps brachii
Caput laterale

M. dorsoepitrochlearis

M. biceps brachii

M. brachialis

M. brachioradialis

Papio

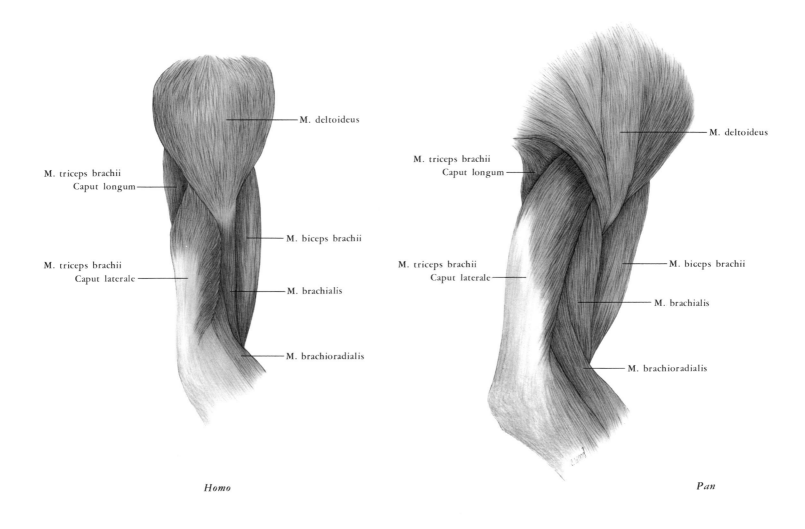

M. deltoideus

M. triceps brachii
Caput longum

M. biceps brachii

M. triceps brachii
Caput laterale

M. brachialis

M. brachioradialis

Homo

M. deltoideus

M. triceps brachii
Caput longum

M. biceps brachii

M. triceps brachii
Caput laterale

M. brachialis

M. brachioradialis

Pan

PLATE 70

Cubital Fossa

The cubital fossa is the triangular space outlined by the brachioradialis laterally and the pronator teres medially. The apex of the triangle is where the two muscles meet. Several important structures pass through the region: the brachial artery, median nerve, and the biceps tendon in *Pan* and *Homo*. The major difference in *Papio* is that the brachial artery normally divides into its terminals prior to entering the cubital fossa. Therefore, the radial artery rather than the brachial artery occupies the central position in the fossa. Also, note that in *Papio* the ulnar artery passes along the medial side of the median nerve before plunging beneath the pronator teres muscle. The recurrent branch of the radial artery sends small muscular branches into adjacent muscles as it ascends to anastomose with the deep brachial artery.

The median nerve gives off several muscular twigs to the flexor muscles as it passes through the area. On the other hand, the radial nerve divides into its superficial and deep branches in the cranial part of the fossa, just deep to the brachioradialis muscle. The superficial branch continues through the forearm under cover of the brachioradialis. The deep branch passes to the dorsum of the forearm through the supinator muscle and continues into the carpal region.

The biceps tendon is the most notable structure occupying the floor of the cubital fossa. In all three animals it is a strong, well-developed tendon as it attaches to the tuberosity of the radius. The existence of a well-formed lacertus fibrosus is present only in *Homo,* being completely absent in *Papio* and very much reduced in *Pan* and other anthropoids (Sonntag 1924).

Three of the long flexors are visible in *Papio:* pronator teres, palmaris longus, and flexor carpi radialis. Of these, only the pronator presents a major difference; in *Papio* it lacks the deep (or ulnar) head that is present in *Pan* and *Homo*. The deep head expresses some variability among the primates and, according to Sonntag (1924), it is present in *Pan* and *Pongo,* but absent in *Gorilla* and *Hylobates*. When the two heads are present, the median nerve passes between them.

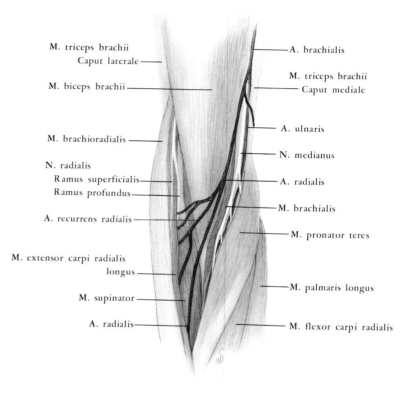

Papio

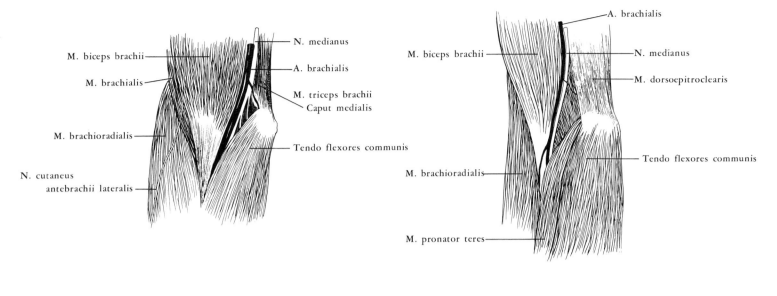

M. biceps brachii

M. brachialis

M. brachioradialis

N. cutaneus
antebrachii lateralis

N. medianus

A. brachialis

M. triceps brachii
Caput medialis

Tendo flexores communis

Homo

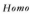

A. brachialis

M. biceps brachii

N. medianus

M. dorsoepitroclearis

Tendo flexores communis

M. brachioradialis

M. pronator teres

Pan

PLATE 71

Posterior Elbow

The muscles shown here belong to both the arm and forearm. Of the former group, the large triceps and relatively thin dorsoepitrochlearis are seen attaching to the olecranon process of the ulna in *Papio* and *Pan*. The dorsoepitrochlearis is a detached part of the triceps which has become connected with the latissimus dorsi muscle (Howell and Straus 1933b). According to these same authors, the muscle is present in all prosimians and monkeys, and often found in anthropoid apes. It is normally absent in *Homo*.

The lateral anconeus muscle represents another detached portion from the triceps complex. The muscle is simply known as the anconeus in *Pan* and *Homo*. It is a small, rather insignificant muscle in all three animals, and may on occasion be entirely absent in *Homo*. The small epitrochleoanconeus is visible in *Papio* and *Pan* as it passes between the medial epicondyle and the olecranon. It is apparently related to the flexor carpi ulnaris muscle (ibid.). Note the exposed ulnar nerve as it passes over the dorsal surface of the medial epicondyle. At this location the nerve is covered only by skin and fascia and is easily palpated as the "funny bone." The superior ulnar collateral artery is its companion through the distal half of the brachium.

The ventral and dorsal antebrachial muscles are usually divided for convenience of description into two groups, superficial and deep. These muscles are better shown in later plates and here we note only the proximal portions of the superficial layers. The flexors arise by a common tendon from the medial epicondyle of the humerus, whereas the extensors arise more individually from the lateral side of the distal humerus as well as from the lateral epicondyle.

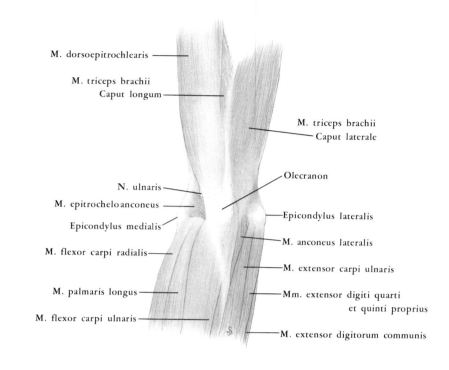

M. dorsoepitrochlearis

M. triceps brachii
Caput longum

M. triceps brachii
Caput laterale

Olecranon

N. ulnaris

M. epitrochelo anconeus

Epicondylus medialis

M. flexor carpi radialis

M. palmaris longus

M. flexor carpi ulnaris

Epicondylus lateralis

M. anconeus lateralis

M. extensor carpi ulnaris

Mm. extensor digiti quarti
et quinti proprius

M. extensor digitorum communis

Papio

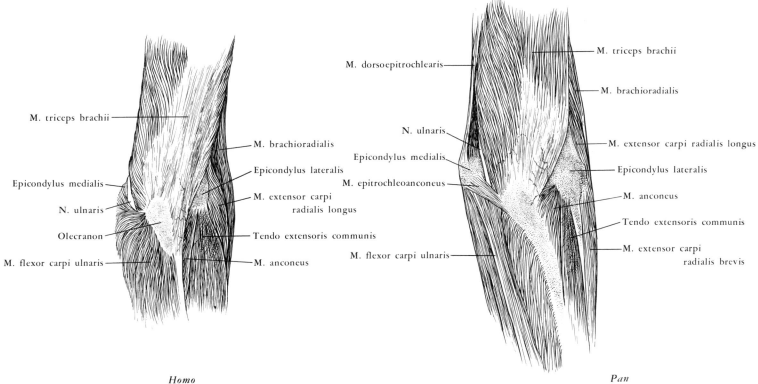

M. triceps brachii

M. brachioradialis

Epicondylus lateralis

M. extensor carpi
radialis longus

Tendo extensoris communis

M. anconeus

M. triceps brachii

Epicondylus medialis

N. ulnaris

Olecranon

M. flexor carpi ulnaris

Homo

M. dorsoepitrochlearis

N. ulnaris

Epicondylus medialis

M. epitrochleoanconeus

M. flexor carpi ulnaris

M. triceps brachii

M. brachioradialis

M. extensor carpi radialis longus

Epicondylus lateralis

M. anconeus

Tendo extensoris communis

M. extensor carpi
radialis brevis

Pan

PLATE 72

Ventral Forearm I

The superficial antebrachial muscles are shown here. They are rather massive muscles with the exception of the palmaris longus, which may be nothing more than a tendon for half of its length. It may be entirely absent in one or both forearms, especially in *Gorilla*, where Loth (1949) reported it lacking in 85 percent of his sample. In the same study he noted its absence in *Homo* ranging anywhere from 3 to 25 percent of his specimens. It was more often lacking from the right side than from the left.

The remaining muscles of the group are more or less similar with two exceptions: (1) the pronator teres has a single head of origin in *Papio*, two heads in *Pan* and *Homo;* (2) the flexor carpi radialis arises from both the humerus and much of the proximal shaft of the radius in *Pan* and the other anthropoid apes (Sonntag 1924; Howell and Straus 1933b). In *Papio* and *Homo* the flexor arises from the humerus only, although radial origins are reported as variants in *Homo*.

The large and powerful brachioradialis is observable in this view. In *Papio* it is long and narrow when compared with its counterpart in *Pan* and *Homo*. Although a flexor of the forearm, it occupies much of the radial border of the ventral surface of the forearm. In all three animals, the muscle covers much of the radial artery, which would otherwise run a superficial course through the forearm. Note the superficial branch of the radial artery arising more proximally in *Papio* and passing to the palmar surface of the hand.

At the wrist the flexor retinaculum passes superficially across the tendons of the antebrachial muscles as they course into the hand. The one exception is the palmaris longus, which lies superficial to the retinaculum and continues into the palm as the palmar aponeurosis. Note that the median nerve lies to the ulnar side of the palmaris longus tendon and is partially covered by it. Also, at the wrist the ulnar nerve is frequently seen peeking out from beneath the deep surface of the flexor carpi ulnaris.

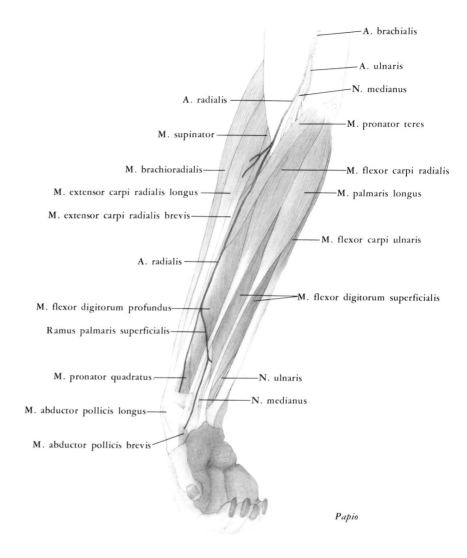

A. brachialis

A. ulnaris

N. medianus

A. radialis

M. pronator teres

M. supinator

M. brachioradialis

M. flexor carpi radialis

M. extensor carpi radialis longus

M. palmaris longus

M. extensor carpi radialis brevis

M. flexor carpi ulnaris

A. radialis

M. flexor digitorum profundus

M. flexor digitorum superficialis

Ramus palmaris superficialis

M. pronator quadratus

N. ulnaris

N. medianus

M. abductor pollicis longus

M. abductor pollicis brevis

Papio

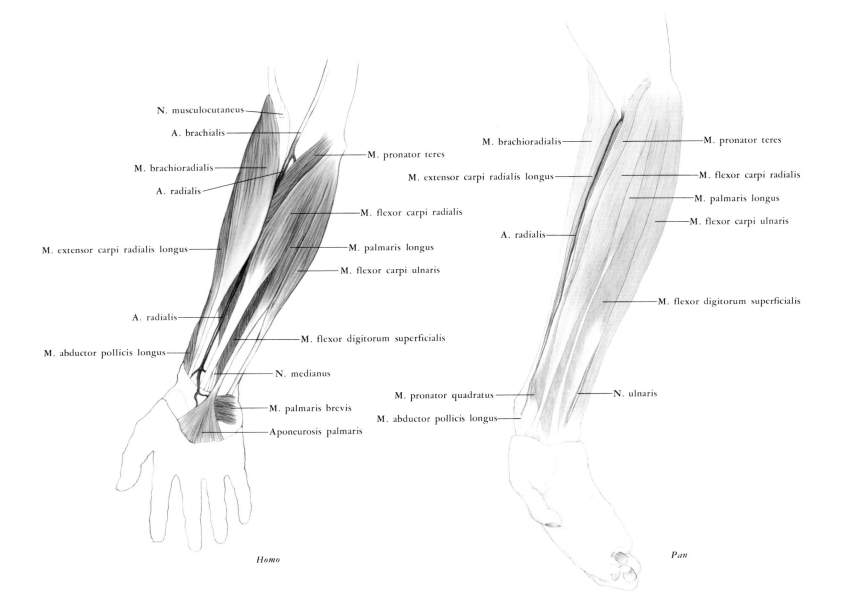

N. musculocutaneus

A. brachialis

M. brachioradialis

A. radialis

M. extensor carpi radialis longus

A. radialis

M. abductor pollicis longus

M. pronator teres

M. flexor carpi radialis

M. palmaris longus

M. flexor carpi ulnaris

M. flexor digitorum superficialis

N. medianus

M. palmaris brevis

Aponeurosis palmaris

Homo

M. brachioradialis

M. extensor carpi radialis longus

A. radialis

M. pronator quadratus

M. abductor pollicis longus

M. pronator teres

M. flexor carpi radialis

M. palmaris longus

M. flexor carpi ulnaris

M. flexor digitorum superficialis

N. ulnaris

Pan

PLATE 73

Ventral Forearm II

The deepest and largest muscle of the superficial group
of palmar antebrachial muscles is shown here.

In *Papio* the superficial flexor of the digits arises from
the medial condyle of the humerus, there being no attachments to the coronoid process of the ulna and shaft of
the radius as in *Pan* and *Homo* (Champneys 1871; Sonntag
1924). On the other hand, Hill (1970) found an ulnar
coronoid head present in *Papio hamadryas* as well as a
large number of fibers coming from the flexor profundus,
which could be interpreted as representing a radial head.
It is usually thought that the radial origin occurs only in the
anthropoid apes and man, and that the coronoid head
rarely occurs in the lower primates (Howell and Straus
1933b).

The superficial flexor, about mid-forearm, gives rise
to four tendons. In all three primates the tendons possess
the following arrangement: the tendons destined for the
third and fourth digits lie superficial to those for the second
and fifth, and all four pass deep to the palmar retinaculum
at the wrist. Note that the tendons split (shown in *Papio)*
in the region of the middle phalanges, permitting the
passage of the deep tendons (Plate 78).

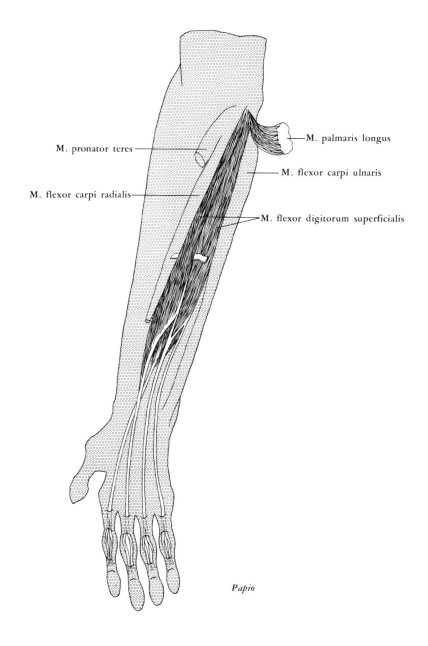

M. pronator teres

M. palmaris longus

M. flexor carpi ulnaris

M. flexor carpi radialis

M. flexor digitorum superficialis

Papio

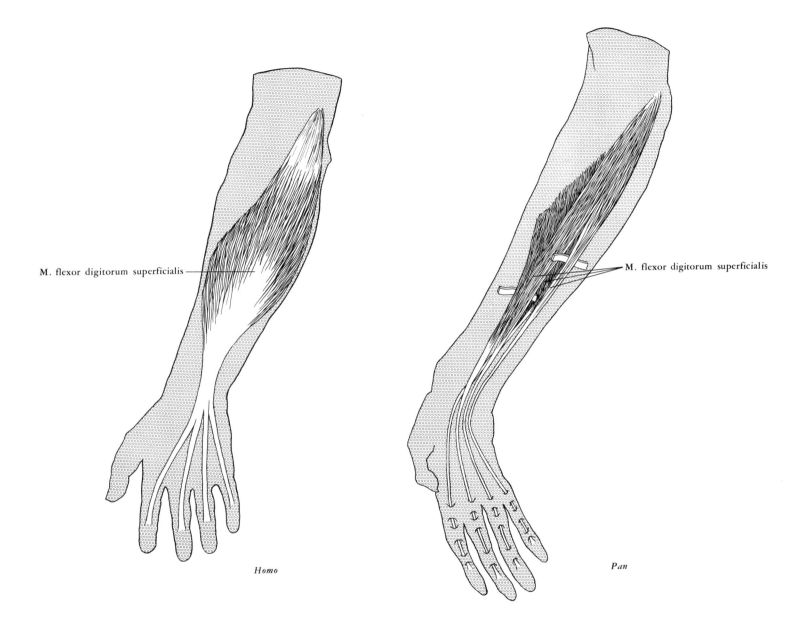

M. flexor digitorum superficialis

M. flexor digitorum superficialis

Homo

Pan

PLATE 74

Ventral Forearm III

The deepest stratum of forearm muscles and related structures is depicted here.

In *Papio* the deep flexor arises as two portions, ulnar and radial. The bellies of the two portions are separate, but the tendons come together just proximal to the wrist. Note the accessory head to the radial portion of the profundus arising from the superficial flexor. It is normally present in lower primates and not infrequent in *Homo* and *Pan* (Howell and Straus 1933b). The radial portion supplies tendons to the first, second, and third digits, while the ulnar part is responsible for the third, fourth, and fifth digits. The long flexor of the thumb is not separate in *Papio* but remains a part of the radial portion. The tendon supplying the pollex is smaller than the other tendons to the digits and separates only after the common tendon passes beneath the flexor retinaculum. At this point, the thin pollex tendon crosses obliquely the tendon of the second digit on its way to the distal phalanx of the thumb.

In *Pan* the deep flexor arises from the proximal shaft of the ulna, as it does in *Homo* according to Champneys (1871) and Sonntag (1924). These two authors differ, however, regarding the disposition of the long thumb flexor. Champneys found the muscle differentiated from the deep flexor for most of its extent—that is, having a separate radial origin—whereas Sonntag described a thin, "tendinous thread" arising from the tendon of the index finger. Our specimens displayed an intermediate condition in which a more or less separate belly was present terminating in two tendons, a large one to the index finger and a small, thin one to the thumb. The degree of differentiation is apparently quite variable among the anthropoid apes (Howell and Straus 1933b). In all three primates, the deep tendons pass through the slits of the superficial tendons.

Note that the deep flexor is innervated by the median nerve in *Papio,* while being duly supplied by the median and ulnar nerves in *Pan* and *Homo.*

Observe the common interosseous artery from the ulnar giving rise to the anterior and posterior interosseous arteries just distal to the elbow in *Papio*. These arteries supply numerous muscular branches to the deep muscles as they pass through their respective flexor and extensor compartments of the forearm.

Note the close relation between the ulnar nerve and artery as they pass through the forearm on the surface of the deep flexor. Both of these structures pass superficial to the flexor retinaculum at the wrist.

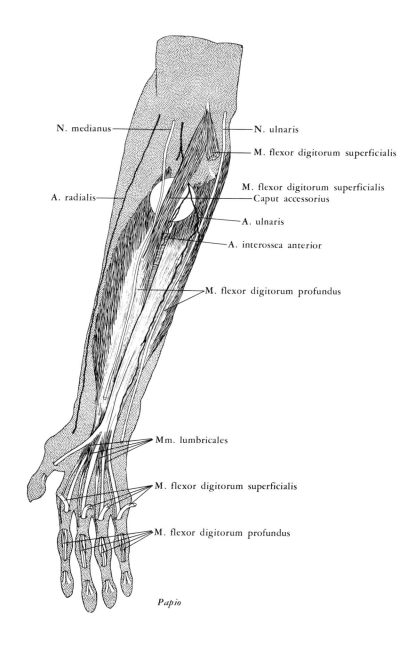

N. medianus

N. ulnaris

M. flexor digitorum superficialis

M. flexor digitorum superficialis
Caput accessorius

A. radialis

A. ulnaris

A. interossea anterior

M. flexor digitorum profundus

Mm. lumbricales

M. flexor digitorum superficialis

M. flexor digitorum profundus

Papio

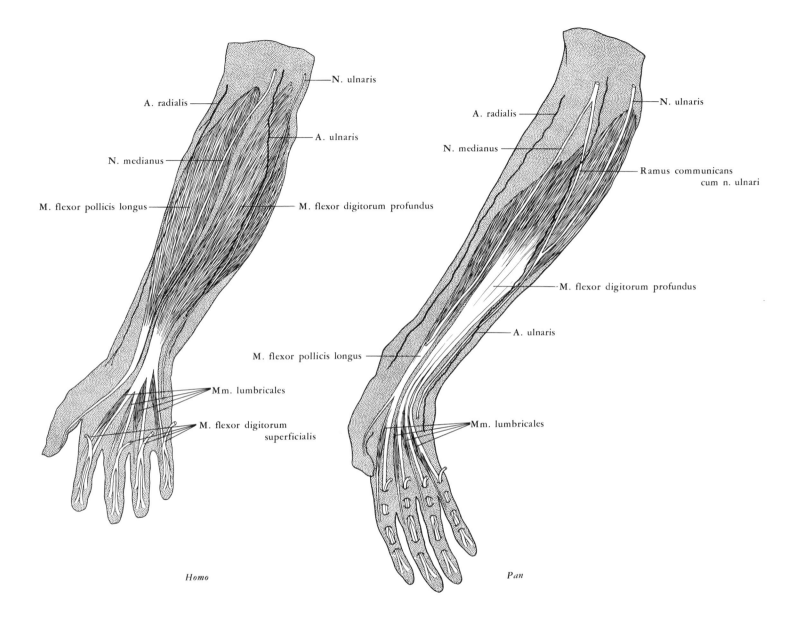

N. ulnaris

A. radialis

A. ulnaris

N. medianus

M. flexor pollicis longus

M. flexor digitorum profundus

Mm. lumbricales

M. flexor digitorum superficialis

Homo

N. ulnaris

A. radialis

N. medianus

Ramus communicans cum n. ulnari

M. flexor digitorum profundus

A. ulnaris

M. flexor pollicis longus

Mm. lumbricales

Pan

PLATE 75

Posterior Forearm

The central muscle mass of the dorsal forearm is composed of the common extensor. To either side lie the well-formed radial and ulnar extensors; the former usually consists of a long and short part, although complete differentiation into these components is often lacking in Old World monkeys (Howell and Straus 1933b; Hill 1970; Champneys 1871). The common extensor remains undivided until its tendon passes beneath the extensor retinaculum, where it splits into four digital tendons. In all three primates the muscle normally supplies digits II, III, IV, and V, with frequent variations regarding the division of tendons to the second and fifth digits.

In addition to these digital extensors, there is a variable number of others that represent the separation of a deep stratum from the primitive common extensor sheet (Howell and Straus 1933b). These are represented by the proper extensors and the long pollical extensor in *Papio*. In *Pan* and *Homo* these are the minimus extensor, long pollical extensor, and the extensor to the index finger. Also, in these forms the short pollical extensor has differentiated from the long one, while it is absent in *Papio*. In *Papio* these deeper extensors to digits II, III, IV, and V are shown in the insert. Note that there are but two muscle bellies, each of which divide into two tendons supplying the four ulnar digits.

The long abductor of the thumb, a large muscle representing the deepest layer of forearm extensors, is present in all three forms. Its tendon is often split, thus enjoying a double insertion into the trapezoid and base of the first metacarpal. A sesamoid bone is present in the tendon.

The supinator, not shown here, lies deep to the proper extensors as it sweeps around the proximal part of the radius. The deep branch of the radial nerve (Plate 70) either passes between its two lamina of fibers, as in *Homo* and *Pan,* or pierces the muscle, as in *Papio*.

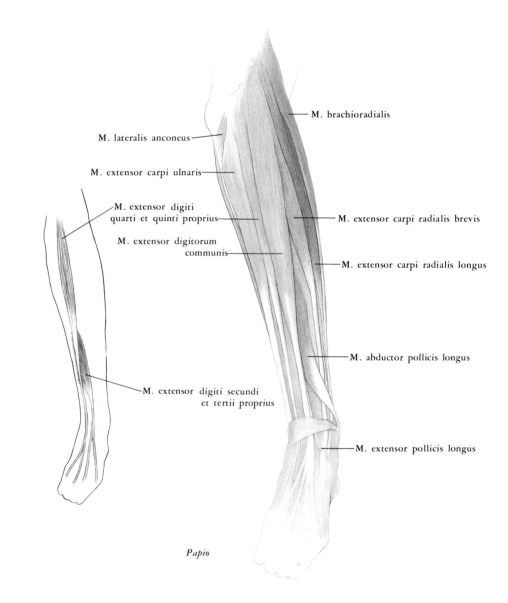

M. brachioradialis

M. lateralis anconeus

M. extensor carpi ulnaris

M. extensor digiti quarti et quinti proprius

M. extensor digitorum communis

M. extensor carpi radialis brevis

M. extensor carpi radialis longus

M. abductor pollicis longus

M. extensor digiti secundi et tertii proprius

M. extensor pollicis longus

Papio

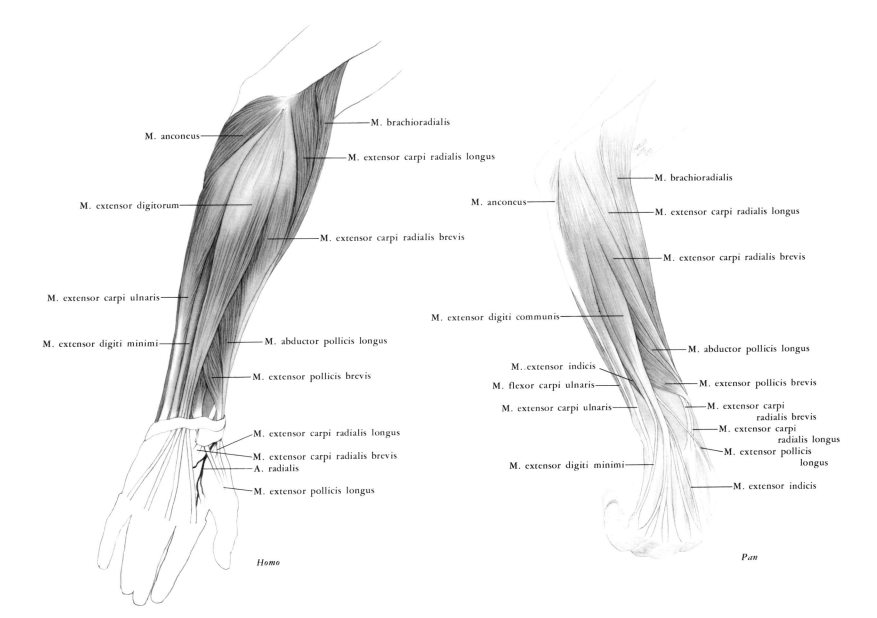

M. anconeus

M. brachioradialis

M. extensor carpi radialis longus

M. extensor digitorum

M. extensor carpi radialis brevis

M. extensor carpi ulnaris

M. extensor digiti minimi

M. abductor pollicis longus

M. extensor pollicis brevis

M. extensor carpi radialis longus

M. extensor carpi radialis brevis

A. radialis

M. extensor pollicis longus

Homo

M. brachioradialis

M. anconeus

M. extensor carpi radialis longus

M. extensor carpi radialis brevis

M. extensor digiti communis

M. abductor pollicis longus

M..extensor indicis

M. flexor carpi ulnaris

M. extensor pollicis brevis

M. extensor carpi ulnaris

M. extensor carpi radialis brevis

M. extensor carpi radialis longus

M. extensor pollicis longus

M. extensor digiti minimi

M. extensor indicis

Pan

PLATE 76

Topography of Hand

The primate hand has tenaciously retained the common plan of mammalian palmar pads: primitive pentadactylism and the basic phalangeal formula, $3 > 4 > 2 > 5 > 1$, with the third digit as the functional axis.

The pad distribution consists of a series of five primary terminal nail pads, three or four interdigital pads, and two more proximally situated pads, the thenar and hypothenar. Of these, the hypothenar is frequently divisible into two elements, proximal and distal, as shown in *Papio*. This separation is usually discernible to some degree among all primates, except for prosimians, who possess a single elevation when the lemurs are excluded (Midlo and Cummins 1942). According to these investigators, the great apes and man have flattened hypothenar pads, which tend to obscure their separate definition.

The palmar integument presents configurations of ridges and sulci, the dermatoglyphics, whose variegated patterns have been widely studied among the primates (Whipple 1904; Midlo and Cummins 1942; Biegert 1961). Similar functions are ascribed to epidermal ridges irrespective of whether they are on the hands or feet. The two most important are the increase in friction during locomotion and prehension and the enhancement of tactile sensibility. The skin over the dorsum of the hand may be manipulated and slipped in any direction, whereas on the palmar or flexor surface it is much less lax, being almost impossible to grasp or elevate.

Flexure lines are creases of the skin resulting from compression during movement. Several such lines are especially well developed on the palmar surface of primate hands. One in particular, the distal transverse flexure line, warrants attention. It lies proximal to digits III, IV, and V, and passes obliquely across the palmar surface to terminate in the second interdigital space. This is the usual condition in *Homo;* however, occasionally in this species and characteristically in *Papio* and *Pan* the line extends across the entire palm and is referred to as the "simian line."

One final word: apart from the aye-aye and marmoset, all living primates possess flattened nails on all their digits. This development is associated with the increasing functional importance of the terminal portions of the digits (Le Gros Clark 1960).

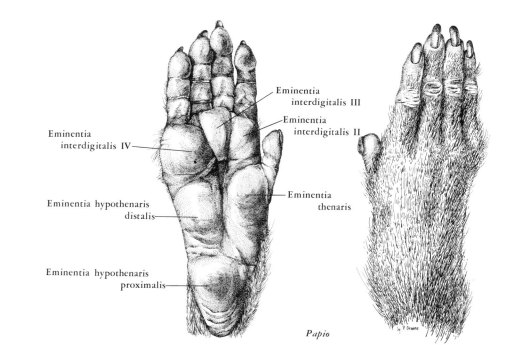

Eminentia interdigitalis III

Eminentia interdigitalis II

Eminentia interdigitalis IV

Eminentia thenaris

Eminentia hypothenaris distalis

Eminentia hypothenaris proximalis

Papio

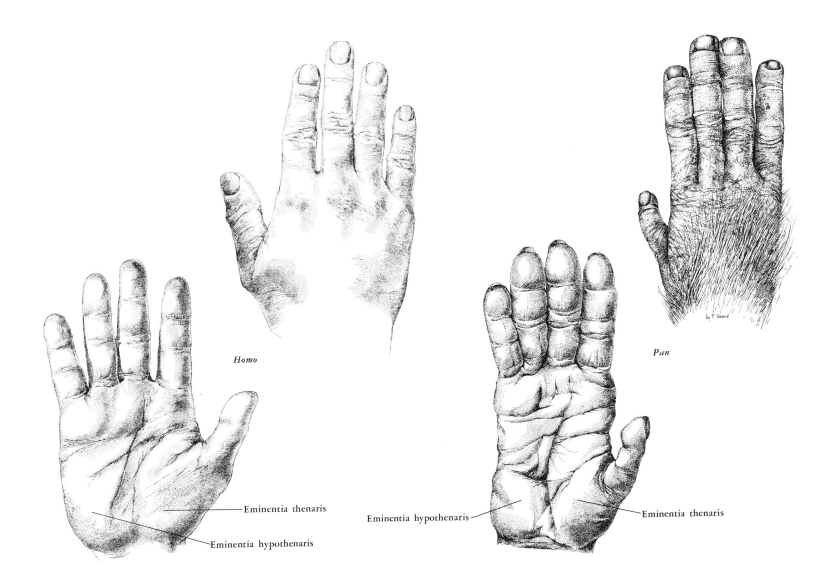

Homo

Pan

Eminentia thenaris

Eminentia hypothenaris

Eminentia hypothenaris

Eminentia thenaris

by P. Greene

PLATE 77

Palmar Hand I

For convenience, the intrinsic muscles of the hand may be subdivided into three groups: (1) muscles of the pollex, which produce the thenar eminence; (2) muscles of the fifth digit, which produce the hypothenar eminence; (3) those muscles occupying the central region of the palm. In this plate the palmar aponeurosis is removed from the three hands, while the thin, flat palmaris brevis muscle is shown only in *Pan*. For an excellent study of the intrinsic muscles of the hand of *Pan*, see Tuttle 1965.

The thenar muscles are associated functionally with the thumb and are more or less similarly disposed in the three primates. The short abductor of the thumb arises broadly from the carpal region to attach by a narrow tendon to the first phalanx of the thumb. The opponens pollicis is well formed in *Homo*, and normally present in all primates (Howell and Straus 1933b). The short flexor of the pollex is bicipital, and enjoys a dual innervation, median and ulnar, in these three primates.

The hypothenar muscles are differentiated into three well-developed muscles, of which two are shown here. The opponens lies deep to the abductor and flexor of the little finger.

The muscles of the central compartment are here represented by the four lumbricals shown arising from the tendons of the deep flexor digitorum in *Papio*. In all three, the radial two muscles are innervated by the median nerve, and the ulnar two by the deep branch of the ulnar nerve.

There is a single palmar arterial arch in *Papio*, rather than two as in *Pan* and *Homo*. This single arch results from the union of the superficial palmar branch of the radial with the superficial branch of the ulnar. It therefore corresponds to the superficial arch of *Pan* and *Papio*. The deep arch is absent in *Papio* and other cercopithecoids (Manners-Smith 1912). Interestingly, the gorilla is reported to lack the superficial palmar arch (Sonntag 1924).

Note the vulnerable muscular branch of the median nerve curving superficially on the surface of the thenar muscles. It is the sole innervation of these muscles.

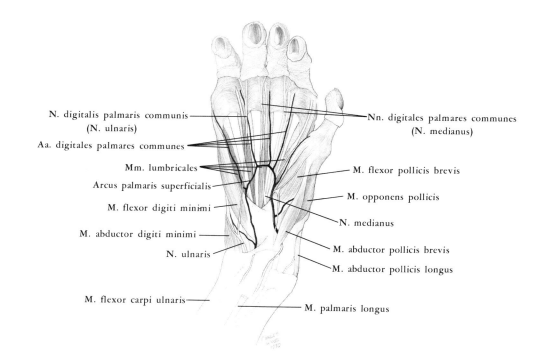

N. digitalis palmaris communis (N. ulnaris)
Aa. digitales palmares communes
Mm. lumbricales
Arcus palmaris superficialis
M. flexor digiti minimi
M. abductor digiti minimi
N. ulnaris
M. flexor carpi ulnaris

Nn. digitales palmares communes (N. medianus)
M. flexor pollicis brevis
M. opponens pollicis
N. medianus
M. abductor pollicis brevis
M. abductor pollicis longus
M. palmaris longus

Papio

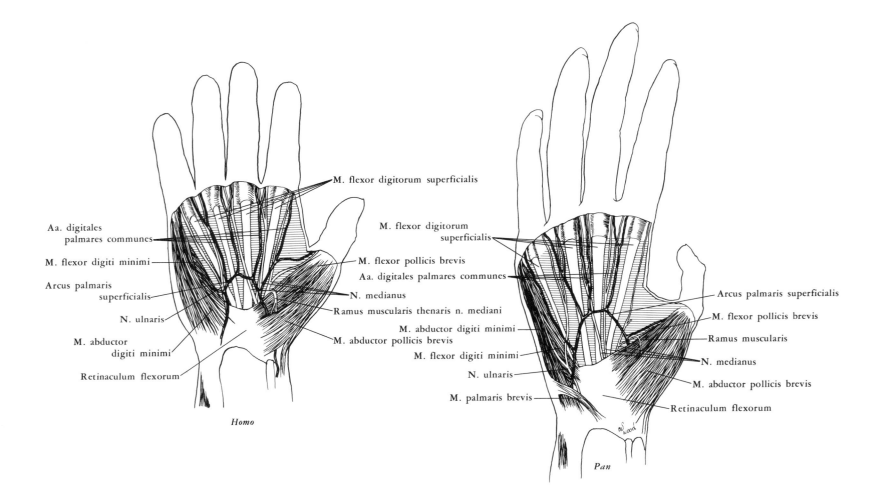

M. flexor digitorum superficialis

Aa. digitales
palmares communes

M. flexor digiti minimi

Arcus palmaris
superficialis

N. ulnaris

M. abductor
digiti minimi

Retinaculum flexorum

M. flexor pollicis brevis

N. medianus

Ramus muscularis thenaris n. mediani

M. abductor pollicis brevis

Homo

M. flexor digitorum
superficialis

Aa. digitales palmares communes

M. abductor digiti minimi

M. flexor digiti minimi

N. ulnaris

M. palmaris brevis

Arcus palmaris superficialis

M. flexor pollicis brevis

Ramus muscularis

N. medianus

M. abductor pollicis brevis

Retinaculum flexorum

Pan

PLATE 78

Palmar Hand II

The flexor tendons and lumbricals are reflected, exposing a deeper stratum of muscles. In *Papio* and *Pan* these are represented by the adductor of the pollex and the contrahentes, while in *Homo* the latter have disappeared.

In *Papio* three contrahentes are usually present. They attach to the second, fourth, and fifth digits, having originated from a common aponeurotic band in the center of the palm. The ones to the fourth and fifth digits are large; indeed, the muscle to the fifth digit frequently has two heads of origin. The contrahens of the second digit is small, largely aponeurotic, and practically covered by the adductor pollicis.

In *Pan* the contrahentes are represented by those to the fourth and fifth fingers, the one to the second being absent. They are usually rather small muscles and, as in *Papio,* they have a common tendon of origin. The adductor pollex is usually well developed among all primates; in all higher forms the muscle has differentiated into two heads, oblique and transverse. Both heads converge to attach to the base of the proximal phalanx of the thumb. The adductor is the sole remaining representative of the contrahentes complex in *Homo*.

The interossei muscles are shown here, but discussion of them is delayed until the next plate.

The deep and superficial heads of the short flexor of the thumb are clearly visible arising from the retinaculum in *Papio*. It is normally much stronger in *Homo* than in other primates.

Note the deep branch of the ulnar nerve disappearing deep to the contrahentes group. The nerve is better seen in the next plate.

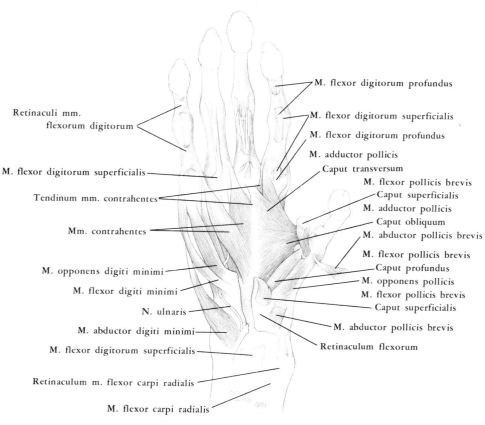

Retinaculi mm.
flexorum digitorum

M. flexor digitorum superficialis

Tendinum mm. contrahentes

Mm. contrahentes

M. opponens digiti minimi

M. flexor digiti minimi

N. ulnaris

M. abductor digiti minimi

M. flexor digitorum superficialis

Retinaculum m. flexor carpi radialis

M. flexor carpi radialis

M. flexor digitorum profundus

M. flexor digitorum superficialis

M. flexor digitorum profundus

M. adductor pollicis

Caput transversum

M. flexor pollicis brevis

Caput superficialis

M. adductor pollicis

Caput obliquum

M. abductor pollicis brevis

M. flexor pollicis brevis

Caput profundus

M. opponens pollicis

M. flexor pollicis brevis

Caput superficialis

M. abductor pollicis brevis

Retinaculum flexorum

Papio

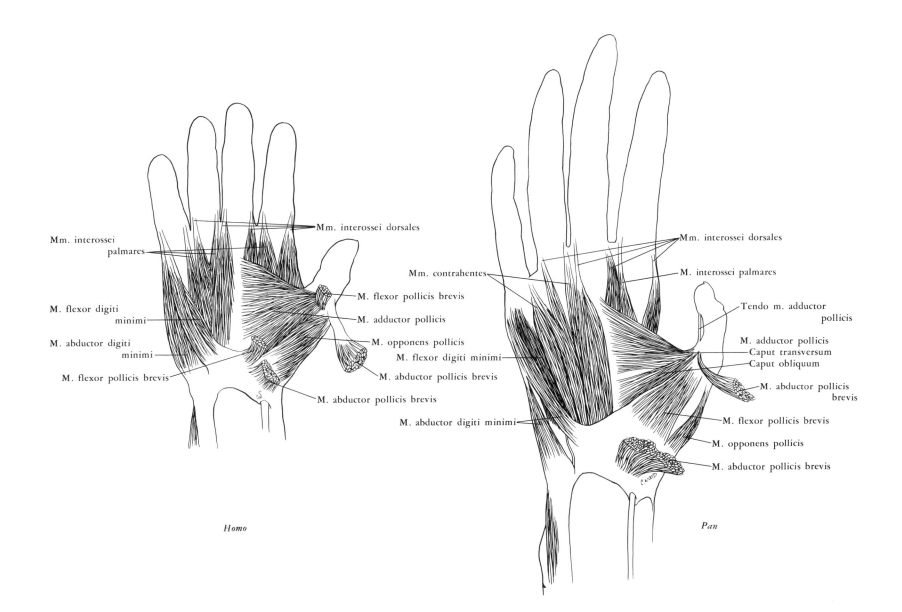

Mm. interossei
palmares

M. flexor digiti
minimi

M. abductor digiti
minimi

M. flexor pollicis brevis

Mm. interossei dorsales

M. flexor pollicis brevis
M. adductor pollicis
M. opponens pollicis
M. flexor digiti minimi
M. abductor pollicis brevis
M. abductor pollicis brevis

Homo

Mm. contrahentes

Mm. interossei dorsales

M. interossei palmares

Tendo m. adductor
pollicis

M. adductor pollicis
Caput transversum
Caput obliquum

M. abductor pollicis
brevis

M. abductor digiti minimi

M. flexor pollicis brevis

M. opponens pollicis

M. abductor pollicis brevis

Pan

PLATE 79

Palmar Hand III

The deepest stratum of palmar muscles is presented here. These muscles are the interossei. For an excellent discussion of these muscles see Lewis 1965.

According to Howell and Straus (1933b), there are four dorsal interossei in all primates, while the palmar number varies anywhere from three to seven. The former number is usually found in *Homo,* who has incorporated several palmar interossei into the dorsal series.

In *Papio* the arrangement is variable and must be worked out very carefully for each animal. There are four dorsal interossei, which can be seen from the dorsum of the hand between the metacarpals. Each muscle attaches to the proximal phalanx of its respective side. Thus, the ones to the second and fourth digits pass to one side, while the muscle to the third finger passes to each side, thereby producing the functional axis through the third digit, as in *Pan* and *Homo.* There are usually seven palmar interossei in *Papio,* which are associated with the second, third, fourth, and fifth digits. In all three animals, the dorsal interossei abduct, while the palmar ones adduct through the third finger.

Note the deep branch of the ulnar nerve passing across the surface of the interossei in *Papio* and *Homo.* In *Pan* the nerve passes deep to the interossei of the second and third digits. In all three forms, the nerve innervates the interossei.

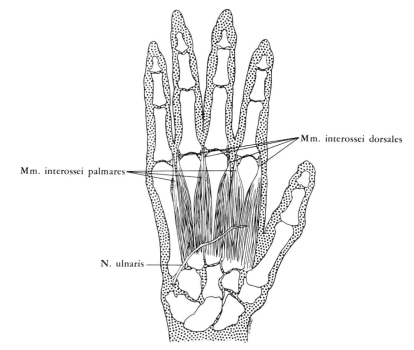

Mm. interossei dorsales

Mm. interossei palmares

N. ulnaris

Papio

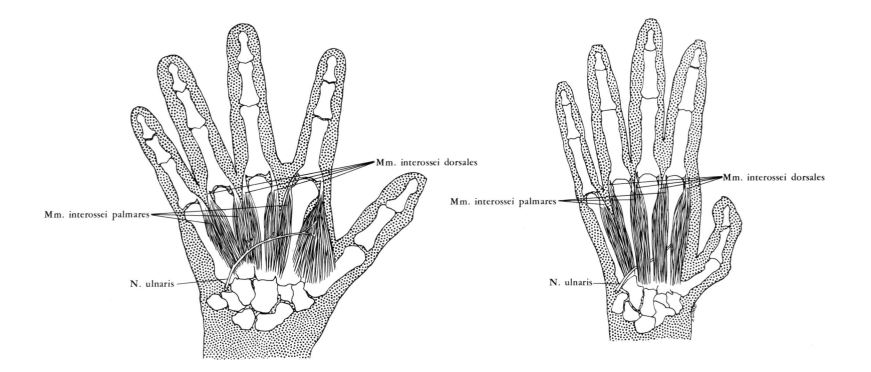

Mm. interossei dorsales

Mm. interossei palmares

N. ulnaris

Homo

Mm. interossei dorsales

Mm. interossei palmares

N. ulnaris

Pan

Part 4

BACK

PLATE 80

Back and Shoulder

The muscles of the back are divided into (1) the intrinsic dorsal musculature, the muscles innervated by the dorsal rami of the spinal nerves; and (2) the muscles belonging to the ventrolateral thoracic and upper extremity, innervated by the ventral rami of the spinal nerves. The intrinsic muscles are considered on the next plate. The ventrolateral and upper extremity muscles have secondarily migrated onto the neck and overlie the intrinsic group. In addition to these, *Papio* displays two other muscles, the platysma and panniculus carnosus. Deep to the skin, these are the most superficial muscles encountered, and are shown on the left side of *Papio*.

The panniculus carnosus (dermohumeralis) overlies and is more or less coextensive with the latissimus dorsi. Muscle fibers are variously developed throughout the sheet, being thickest ventrally. It is inserted to the proximal part of the humerus by a flat tendon. The platysma is a facial muscle that in *Papio* attaches to the ligamentum nuchae in the midline of the nape. From here it sweeps ventrally to the lateral side of the face and neck (Plate 31). Dorsally, it is composed of two thin, superficial muscle sheets. The panniculus carnosus is absent in *Homo*, and either lacking or much reduced in *Pan*. The platysma is present in *Homo* and *Pan*, but is limited to the face and ventral neck.

The latissimus dorsi is a broad, flat muscle arising from the spines of T5 or T6, distally to the lumbar region, where it attaches to the thoracolumbar fascia. The fibers are directed craniolaterally toward the axilla, where they attach by a flat tendon to the humerus. In *Papio* the cranial portion of the muscle is continued as a tendon that joins the flat tendon of the teres major (Ashton and Oxnard 1963; Hill 1970). This arrangement is also present in *Macaca mulatta* (Howell and Straus 1933b). The trapezius extends from the occipital bone to T9 or T10 in *Papio*, and to T12 in *Pan* and *Homo*. The muscle has two parts, an occipitocervical and a thoracic, with fibers passing toward the shoulder to attach to the scapula or clavicle.

Note the cutaneus nerves piercing the muscles to course in the superficial fascia. These represent the medial and lateral branches of the dorsal rami of the spinal nerves. In the cranial portion of the trunk the lateral branches are muscular, while the medial branches provide both muscular and cutaneus innervation. In the more caudal portion of the trunk, the reverse is true. Each nerve is usually accompanied by a small artery and vein.

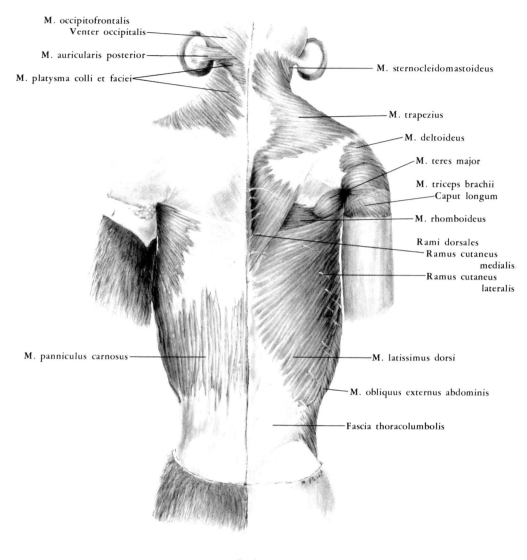

M. occipitofrontalis
Venter occipitalis
M. auricularis posterior
M. platysma colli et faciei

M. sternocleidomastoideus
M. trapezius
M. deltoideus
M. teres major
M. triceps brachii
Caput longum
M. rhomboideus
Rami dorsales
Ramus cutaneus medialis
Ramus cutaneus lateralis

M. panniculus carnosus
M. latissimus dorsi
M. obliquus externus abdominis
Fascia thoracolumbolis

Papio

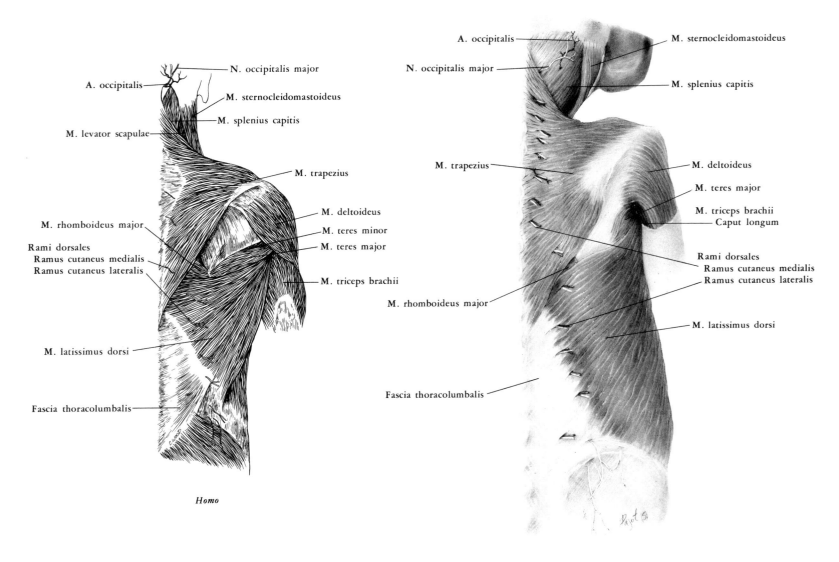

N. occipitalis major

A. occipitalis

M. sternocleidomastoideus

M. splenius capitis

M. levator scapulae

M. trapezius

M. deltoideus

M. rhomboideus major

M. teres minor

M. teres major

Rami dorsales

Ramus cutaneus medialis

Ramus cutaneus lateralis

M. triceps brachii

M. latissimus dorsi

Fascia thoracolumbalis

Homo

A. occipitalis

M. sternocleidomastoideus

N. occipitalis major

M. splenius capitis

M. trapezius

M. deltoideus

M. teres major

M. triceps brachii

Caput longum

Rami dorsales

Ramus cutaneus medialis

Ramus cutaneus lateralis

M. rhomboideus major

M. latissimus dorsi

Fascia thoracolumbalis

Pan

PLATE 81

Back Muscles

The intrinsic back muscles are shown on the right side of the animal. They lie deep to the serratus posterior superior and serratus posterior inferior. On the left side, the muscles are on a more superficial stratum and will be considered first.

In *Papio* the levator scapulae of *Homo* and *Pan* is represented by two muscles, the atlantoscapularis anterior and posterior. Both of these muscles originate from the atlas and pass caudodorsally to attach to the scapula. In *Homo* and *Pan* the levator scapulae attaches to the first four or five cervical vertebrae and passes to the vertebral border of the scapula. Note the suprascapular artery passing over the dorsal border of the scapula in *Papio*. The suprascapular nerve accompanies the artery.

The rhomboid muscle is usually less differentiated in *Papio* and *Pan* than it is in *Homo*. In the latter form there are normally two muscles, a minor and major rhomboid, arising from the lower cervical and upper thoracic vertebrae. In *Pan* the origin is similar, but there is a single, undivided muscle sheet. In *Papio* the more cranial fibers arise from the occipital bone (rhomboideus capitis) deep to the trapezius. The remainder of the muscle comes from the ligamentum nuchae and the anterior thoracic vertebrae. In all three, the muscle attaches along the vertebral border of the scapula.

The serratus posterior superior and inferior muscles lie deep to the rhomboid and latissimus dorsi muscles, respectively. They probably represent the differentiation of a single muscle anlage (Satoh 1969 and 1970). Both muscles have flat, aponeurotic origins, with muscle fibers appearing in their lateral portions. As mentioned above, the intrinsic back muscles lie deep to this stratum.

The intrinsic back muscles are usually separated into a superficial longitudinal group termed the erector spinae, and a deep group, the transversospinal system. The erector spinae is divisible into three long muscles: the spinalis, longissimus, and iliocostalis. The major mass of these muscles has a common origin in the lower lumbar and sacral regions. From here, the three systems proceed cranially for various distances, the longissimus being the only member to reach the skull. A cervical portion of the iliocostalis is present in *Homo*, but not in the other forms. The spinalis cervicis and capitis are inconstant muscles in the three primates.

The transversospinal system is extremely intricate and almost impossible to separate into its various elements (George 1968). The semispinalis capitis lies deep to the splenius capitis and is a thick, well-developed muscle (Plate 82). The multifidus and rotator muscles compose the deepest layers and are not shown.

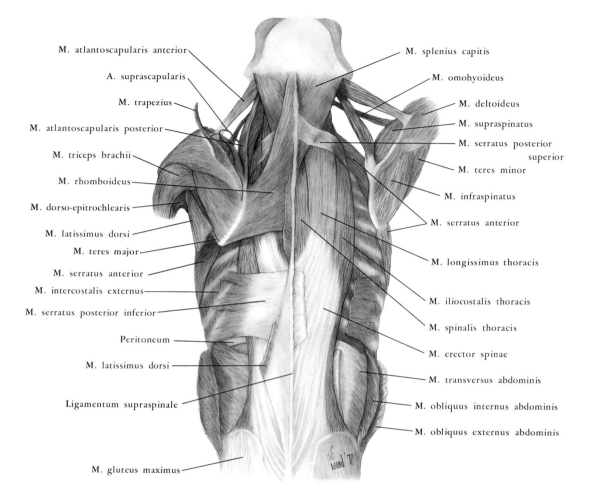

Papio

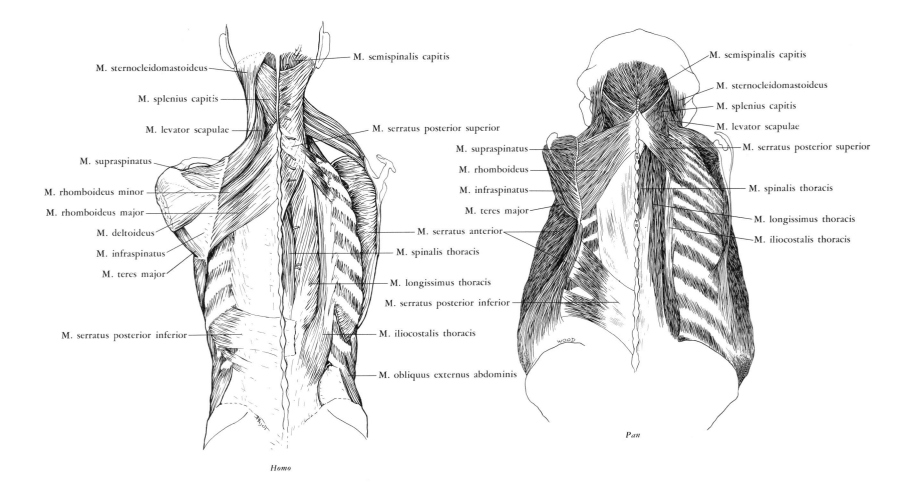

M. sternocleidomastoideus

M. semispinalis capitis

M. splenius capitis

M. levator scapulae

M. serratus posterior superior

M. supraspinatus

M. rhomboideus minor

M. rhomboideus major

M. deltoideus

M. infraspinatus

M. teres major

M. serratus anterior

M. spinalis thoracis

M. longissimus thoracis

M. serratus posterior inferior

M. iliocostalis thoracis

M. obliquus externus abdominis

Homo

M. semispinalis capitis

M. sternocleidomastoideus

M. splenius capitis

M. levator scapulae

M. serratus posterior superior

M. supraspinatus

M. rhomboideus

M. infraspinatus

M. teres major

M. spinalis thoracis

M. longissimus thoracis

M. iliocostalis thoracis

M. serratus posterior inferior

Pan

PLATE 82

Suboccipital I

In *Papio* the splenius capitis is a thick, flat muscle that
wraps around the nape of the neck deep to the trapezius.
It arises from the spines of the cranial four or five thoracic
vertebrae and the ligamentum nuchae. The muscle inserts
as a continuous attachment along the superior nuchal line
from near the midline to the mastoid process. There is no
cervical portion. In *Homo* this portion of the muscle is
present, while in *Pan,* if present, it is usually fused with the
levator scapulae.

The semispinalis capitis, as noted earlier, belongs to
the transversospinal muscles. It lies deep to the splenius
capitis and medial to the longissimus capitis. The muscle
is structurally complicated, especially in *Papio* and *Homo.*
In these forms it has two parts: a medial or biventer
cervicis portion, and a lateral or complexus division. The
amount of separation between the two parts exhibits a great
deal of individual variation. The muscle is usually not
separable into these two portions in *Pan* (Sonntag 1923).

Note the occipital artery (a branch of the external
carotid) emerging from beneath the longissimus capitis.
At this location, the artery pierces the fascial attachment of
the trapezius to continue in a tortuous course in the
superficial fascia of the scalp. Its terminal portion is
accompanied by the greater occipital nerve.

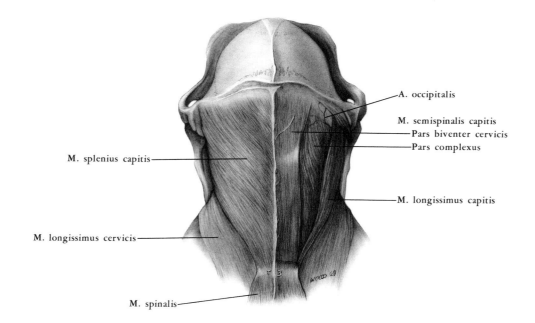

Papio

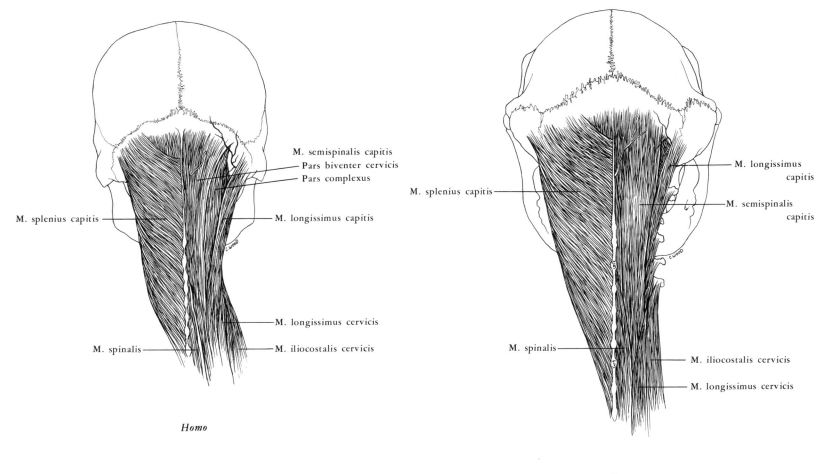

M. semispinalis capitis
Pars biventer cervicis
Pars complexus

M. splenius capitis

M. longissimus capitis

M. longissimus cervicis

M. spinalis
M. iliocostalis cervicis

Homo

M. splenius capitis

M. longissimus capitis

M. semispinalis capitis

M. spinalis

M. iliocostalis cervicis

M. longissimus cervicis

Pan

PLATE 83

Suboccipital II

The four suboccipital muscles lie deep to the semispinalis capitis and longissimus capitis. Of these four muscles, three delineate the suboccipital triangle. The base is formed by the inferior oblique, the lateral boundary by the superior oblique, and the medial border by the rectus capitis posterior major. The fourth muscle, the rectus capitis posterior minor, lies medial and deep to the rectus major. The triangular space contains a large amount of dense, fatty connective tissue, which must be removed to expose the suboccipital nerve (first cervical). This nerve innervates the suboccipital muscles. Observe the greater occipital nerve (second cervical) curving around the caudal border of the inferior oblique. It joins the occipital artery and travels with it in the superficial fascia of the scalp (Plate 80).

In *Pan* there is a muscle passing from the transverse process of the third cervical vertebra to the transverse process of the atlas. It lies dorsal to the intertransversarii muscles, which are located between the transverse processes of the vertebrae. Sonntag (1923) described this muscle and thought it probably represented an individual peculiarity. Since it is present in our specimens, it is likely more than an aberrant anomaly.

The semispinalis cervicis is shown lying deep to the semispinalis capitis. Note that it passes cranially only as far as the axis.

The vertebral artery is shown traversing the foramen transversarium of a cervical vertebra. The artery passes through the foramina of the first six cervical vertebrae to enter the cranium by way of the foramen magnum (Plate 4).

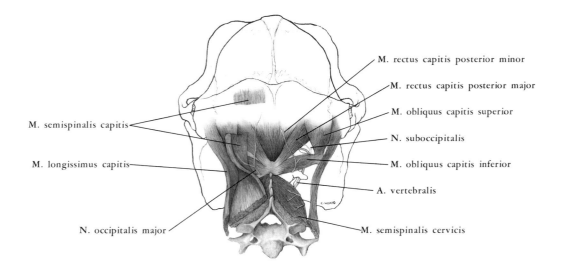

Papio

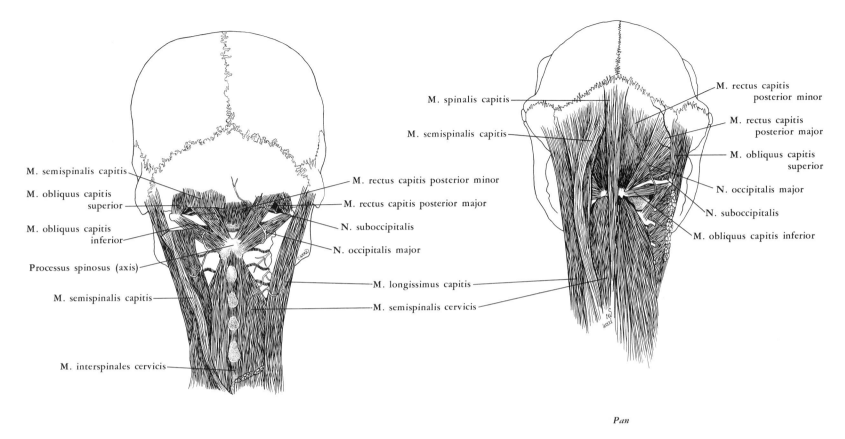

M. semispinalis capitis

M. obliquus capitis
superior

M. obliquus capitis
inferior

Processus spinosus (axis)

M. semispinalis capitis

M. interspinales cervicis

M. rectus capitis posterior minor

M. rectus capitis posterior major

N. suboccipitalis

N. occipitalis major

M. longissimus capitis

M. semispinalis cervicis

Homo

M. spinalis capitis

M. semispinalis capitis

M. rectus capitis
posterior minor

M. rectus capitis
posterior major

M. obliquus capitis
superior

N. occipitalis major

N. suboccipitalis

M. obliquus capitis inferior

Pan

Part 5

THORAX

PLATE 84

Thoracic Wall I

The most superficial muscles encountered on the ventral wall of the chest are not thoracic muscles but rather muscles belonging to the superior member. These muscles are the subclavius, pectoralis major, pectoralis minor, and pectoralis abdominis. The latter muscle is present in *Papio* but absent in *Pan* and *Homo*.

The pectoralis major is a powerful, trilaminated muscle in *Homo* whose overlapping layers are spread out like a fan covering the ventral wall of the chest. In *Pan* and *Papio* the muscle is less powerful, although occupying a prominent position on the chest wall. The muscle enjoys an extensive attachment to the clavicle in *Homo* and *Pan*, while the most cranial fibers in *Papio* reach only to the sternoclavicular joint. *Pan* does not have the separation between the clavicular and sternal parts that is found in *Homo*. In all three primates, the caudal border of the muscle is folded back, or cranially upon itself. In *Papio* and *Homo* the separation between the pectoralis major and deltoid is the deltopectoral triangle and contains the cephalic vein. The groove is often absent in *Pan;* in either case, the cephalic vein is absent (Bland-Sutton 1884; Sonntag 1924).

The deeper-lying pectoralis minor varies considerably among the three primates, especially regarding its insertion. In *Homo* the muscle inserts to the coracoid process, while in *Pan* and *Papio* this attachment may be to the capsule of the shoulder joint, coracoid process, or both (Lander 1918; Sonntag 1923; Hill 1970). Also, in *Pan* the cranial part of the muscle, as well as the tendon, is occasionally double, as shown here. Sonntag (1924) described this situation in *Pan* and *Gorilla*.

The deepest stratum is the pectoralis abdominis and it is present only in *Papio*. The muscle arises from the aponeurosis of the external oblique and the rectus sheath. It passes cranially to form an aponeurotic sheet, which attaches to the humerus, joint capsule, or coracoid process.

In *Papio* the well-developed subclavius is visible deep to the cranial border of the pectoralis minor. Also, observe the more cranial attachment of the rectus abdominis in *Papio* than in the other forms. This is shown in more detail on the next plate.

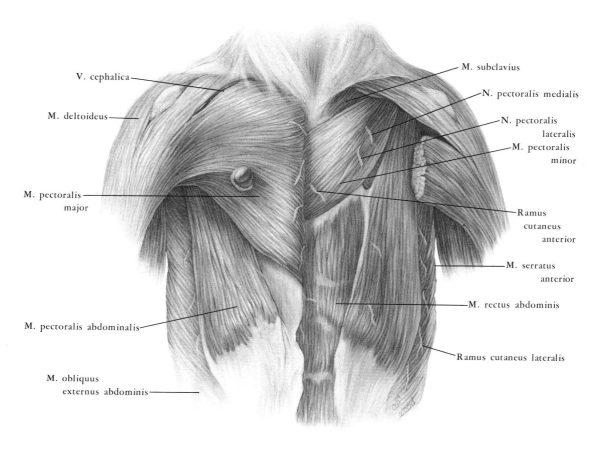

Papio

176

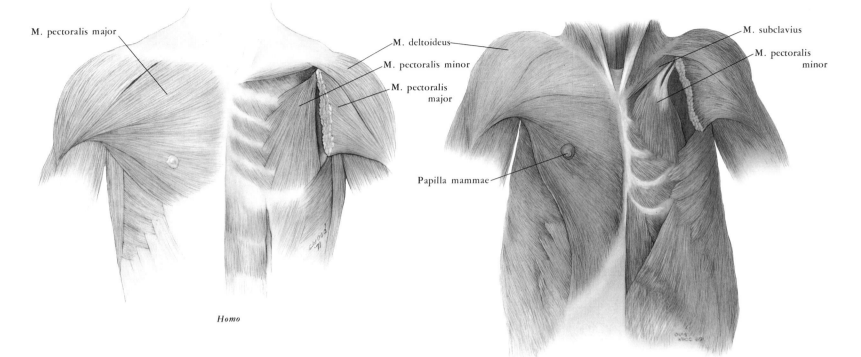

M. pectoralis major

M. deltoideus

M. pectoralis minor

M. pectoralis major

Homo

M. subclavius

M. pectoralis minor

Papilla mammae

Pan

PLATE 85

Thoracic Wall II

The intrinsic thoracic muscles are situated between the ribs and are disposed in two layers, the external and internal intercostals. Some students recognize two distinct layers of the internal layer, and the deepest layer is then called the innermost intercostal muscle. The intercostals are similarly arranged in the three primates. Note that the external intercostal muscle fibers are replaced near the sternum by the anterior intercostal membrane, while dorsally the internal intercostal fibers are replaced by the posterior intercostal membrane near the angle of the ribs. An intercostal nerve, artery, and vein course within each intercostal space.

The transverse thoracic muscle is visible in the window cut in the left side of the thoracic wall. The muscle represents the deepest stratum of intrinsic thoracic musculature and lies upon the dorsal side of the ventral thoracic wall. Observe the internal thoracic vessels running between the muscles and thoracic wall. Between the fifth and sixth interspaces the artery divides into two terminal branches, the superior epigastric and the musculophrenic arteries.

A well-developed sternocostal muscle is present in *Papio*. It passes from the cranial portion of the sternum laterally to attach to the first rib. The muscle is usually absent in *Pan* and *Homo* (Howell and Straus 1933b).

There are three scalene muscles present in these primates. According to Howell and Straus (1933a) these muscles are very complex in Old World monkeys and it is possible that the scalene posterior of *Homo* is not represented in the other primates. Observe the long scalene of *Papio* which may reach as far as the fifth rib. In *Homo* and *Pan* the caudal attachments of the scalene muscles are limited to the first two ribs. The muscles arise from the transverse processes of the cervical vertebrae.

In *Papio* the rectus abdominis has a much more cranial attachment than in the other primates, although the attachment varies considerably within the genus (Hill 1970). In the majority of the present sample, the muscle fibers attached to the second or third ribs, while the aponeurosis extended as far as the manubrium. Note that the more lateral muscle fibers always extend more cranially than the medial ones.

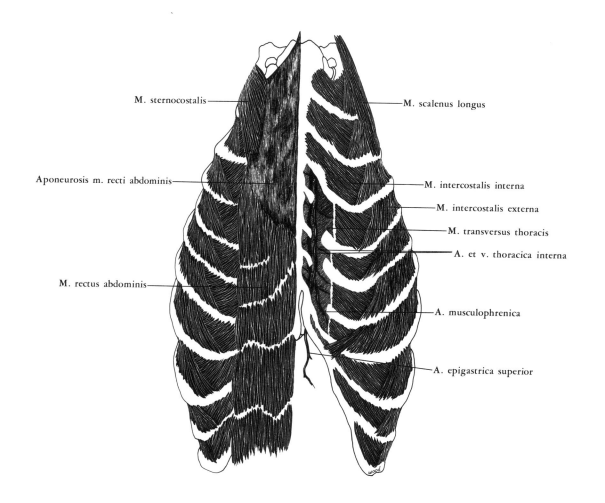

M. sternocostalis

M. scalenus longus

Aponeurosis m. recti abdominis

M. intercostalis interna

M. intercostalis externa

M. transversus thoracis

A. et v. thoracica interna

M. rectus abdominis

A. musculophrenica

A. epigastrica superior

Papio

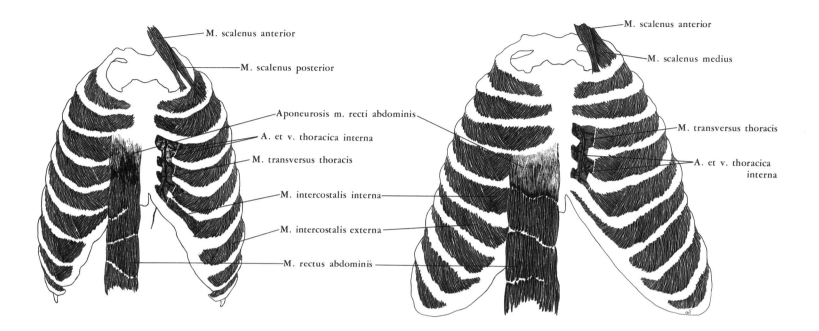

M. scalenus anterior

M. scalenus posterior

Aponeurosis m. recti abdominis

A. et v. thoracica interna

M. transversus thoracis

M. intercostalis interna

M. intercostalis externa

M. rectus abdominis

M. scalenus anterior

M. scalenus medius

M. transversus thoracis

A. et v. thoracica interna

Homo

Pan

PLATE 86

Thoracic Wall III

The major difference here is the extent of the transverse thoracic muscle. In *Papio* and *Pan* the muscle normally reaches the first or second intercostal space, whereas in *Homo* the muscle attaches from the third to sixth ribs. In all three primates, the fibers run obliquely from the sternum to the costal cartilages (Satoh 1971).

The internal thoracic artery arises from the caudal border of the subclavian near the thyrocervical trunk. The artery descends from this cervical origin into the thorax, where it lies on the cartilages of the ribs and the internal intercostal muscles. The transverse thoracic muscle covers it dorsally for much of its thoracic course, especially in *Papio* and *Pan*. The anterior intercostal arteries arise from the internal thoracic and are distributed to the cranial five or six intercostal spaces. These arteries anastomose with the corresponding posterior (aortic) intercostal arteries. The musculophrenic artery provides the anterior intercostal branches to the more caudal intercostal spaces. The posterior intercostals arise from the thoracic aorta except for those to the cranial two intercostal spaces, which arise from the supreme intercostal artery from the costocervical trunk. Within the intercostal space the artery runs along the costal groove between the intercostal vein cranially and the intercostal nerve caudally. The pattern is similar in the three primates.

The intercostal nerves are similarly disposed in the three primates. In *Papio* and *Homo* there are twelve thoracic nerves, while in *Pan* there are usually thirteen. The subcostal nerve is thus T13 rather than T12.

Note the attachment of the strap muscles, sternohyoid and sternothyroid, to the deep surface of the manubrium and first rib. In addition, the more superficial sternomastoid and subclavius muscles are depicted in *Papio*.

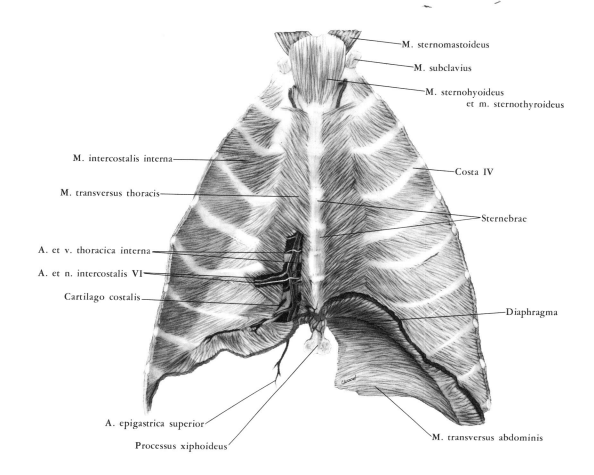

Papio

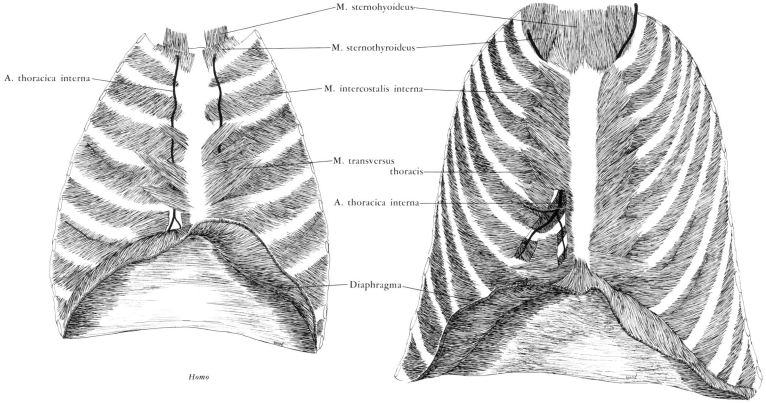

M. sternohyoideus

M. sternothyroideus

A. thoracica interna

M. intercostalis interna

M. transversus thoracis

A. thoracica interna

Diaphragma

Homo

Pan

PLATE 87

Thymus Gland

The thymus is a lobated gland of irregular shape occupying a cervicothoracic position. In all three primates it is largest during adolescence, and in *Homo* it quickly regresses after puberty. In *Papio* and *Pan* the organ atrophies with advancing age, although at a slower pace than in *Homo*. In all, the parenchyma is gradually replaced by fat.

When large, the thymus extends caudally over much of the fibrous pericardium, particularly in *Papio* and *Pan*. The cranial extension follows along the trachea and may reach the lower border of the thyroid. As shown in *Papio,* this more often involves the left lobe. The caudal portion lies deep to the sternum and broadens out in *Papio* and *Pan,* frequently achieving the fourth or fifth costal interspace. In *Pan* the caudal part of the gland is decidedly bifurcated, a fact that suggests double origin from the third pharyngeal cleft. Dorsally the thymus is intimately applied to the great vessels in the superior mediastinum. In adult *Homo* the gland is largely restricted to the superior and anterior mediastina.

The vascular supply is mainly by the internal thoracic and the inferior thyroid arteries. Numerous veins drain from the thymus to the brachiocephalic, internal thoracic, and inferior thyroid systems. Its innervation is by the vagus via numerous branches that can be seen entering the gland. An essential function of the gland is to produce lymphocytes; however, recent studies have also shown it to be an important manufacturer of thymocytes and a vital source in the cellular immune system (Chapman and Allen 1971).

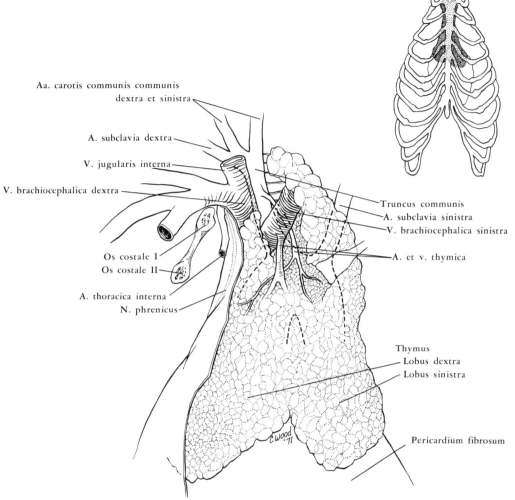

Aa. carotis communis communis dextra et sinistra

A. subclavia dextra

V. jugularis interna

V. brachiocephalica dextra

Os costale I
Os costale II

A. thoracica interna
N. phrenicus

Truncus communis
A. subclavia sinistra
V. brachiocephalica sinistra

A. et v. thymica

Thymus
Lobus dextra
Lobus sinistra

Pericardium fibrosum

Papio

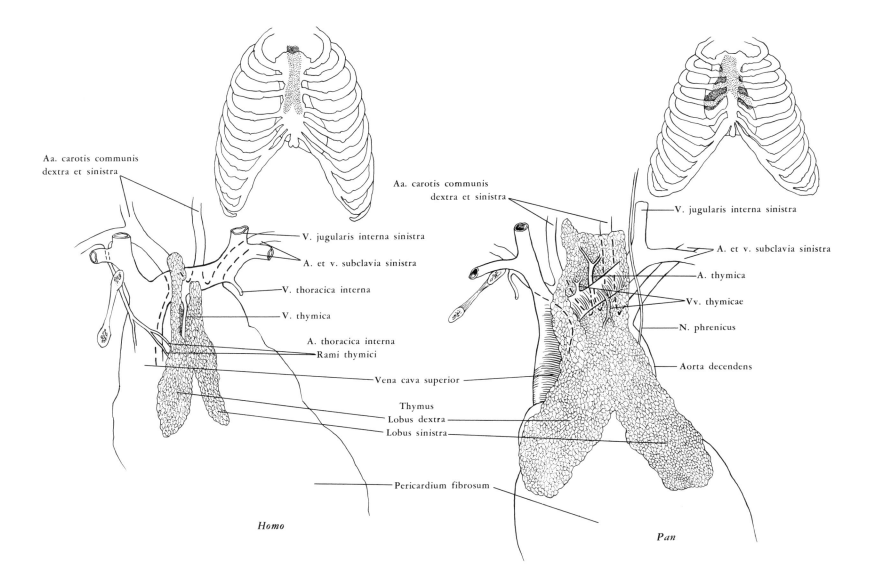

Aa. carotis communis
dextra et sinistra

Aa. carotis communis
dextra et sinistra

V. jugularis interna sinistra

V. jugularis interna sinistra

A. et v. subclavia sinistra

A. et v. subclavia sinistra

V. thoracica interna

A. thymica

V. thymica

Vv. thymicae

A. thoracica interna
Rami thymici

N. phrenicus

Aorta decendens

Vena cava superior

Thymus
Lobus dextra
Lobus sinistra

Pericardium fibrosum

Homo

Pan

PLATE 88

Relations of Pericardium and Lungs to the Thoracic Wall

The long, narrow thorax of *Papio* is particularly obvious in this plate. Note also the much wider intercostal spaces and the long, attenuated sternum of *Papio* when compared with *Pan* and *Homo*.

The pericardium outlines the heart and great vessels within the thorax. The positions of these structures were drawn from formalin preparations and, therefore, do not represent the exact location of the organs in the living animal. However, from the examination of radiographs of *Papio* it is clear that the position of a particular viscus is usually not off by more than a single intercostal space. Also, there is a certain amount of intraspecific variability in organ position within the thorax or, for that matter, within any anatomical region. In *Papio* the apex of the heart lies to the left of the sternum at the level of the sixth intercostal space or deep to the sixth rib. The base of the heart is located only slightly to the right of the sternum occupying the second and third interspaces. In *Pan* and *Homo* the geographic position of the heart is normally somewhat more cranial. Also, the long axis of the heart is oriented more in a craniocaudal direction in *Papio* than it is in the other two primates. This condition is found in most groups of Old World monkeys (Straus 1936). Note that the pericardium is separated from the diaphragm in *Papio,* but adheres strongly to the central part of the diaphragm in *Pan* and *Homo*. For an excellent study of the primate heart, see Frick 1960.

The lungs are shown on each side of the thoracic cavity. They are separated for the most part by the mediastinal partition. The pleurae invest the surfaces of the lungs but have been removed in order to demonstrate the lobation of the lungs. The left lung of *Papio* has three lobes and the right one, four lobes. The fourth lobe of the right lung is the mammalian azygos lobe, which is absent in *Pan* and *Homo* (Plate 89). In the latter two forms, the normal formula is L2, R3.

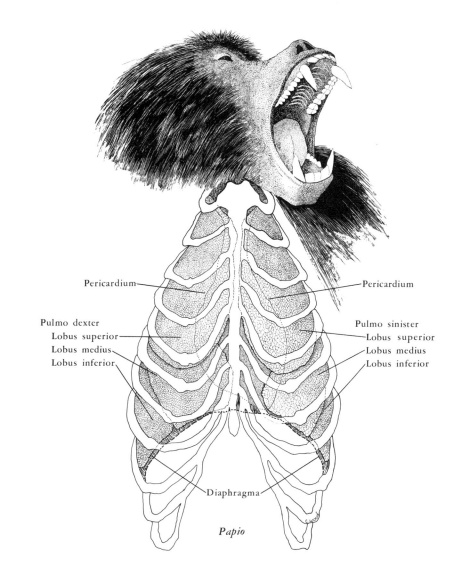

Pericardium

Pericardium

Pulmo dexter
Lobus superior
Lobus medius
Lobus inferior

Pulmo sinister
Lobus superior
Lobus medius
Lobus inferior

Diaphragma

Papio

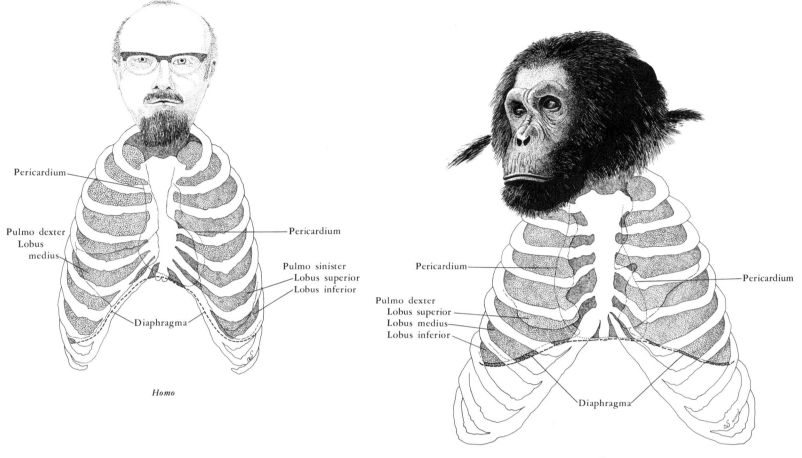

Pericardium

Pulmo dexter
Lobus
medius

Pericardium

Pulmo sinister
Lobus superior
Lobus inferior

Diaphragma

Homo

Pericardium

Pulmo dexter
Lobus superior
Lobus medius
Lobus inferior

Pericardium

Diaphragma

Pan

PLATE 89

Right Lung Mediastinal Surface

The lungs are conically shaped organs presenting a base, an apex, and three surfaces—costal, mediastinal, and diaphragmatic. The lungs of *Papio* are much more elongated than they are in *Pan* or *Homo;* in fact, the dorsal part of the inferior lobe is usually a long, attenuated process conforming with the elongated thorax of *Papio.* The lobar formula for *Papio* is R4, L3, and in *Pan* and *Homo* it is R3, L2.

The right lung of *Papio* is shown separated into its major lobes. As noted previously, the right lung of *Papio* has the infracardiac or azygos lobe, which is absent in *Pan* and *Homo* (Sonntag 1923; Straus 1936). The azygos lobe lies caudal to the root of the lung and is attached to the inferior lobe. This attachment may be in the form of a pedicle of pulmonary tissue surrounding blood vessels and bronchi, as in our specimens, or the connection may be solely by blood vessels and bronchi (Hill 1970). The lobe is usually well developed and *in situ* it occupies a pleural space directed toward the mediastinum dorsal to the vena cava and pericardium.

The trachea divides into the right and left primary bronchi in a similar fashion in the three primates. The eparterial bronchus arises immediately from the right bronchus cranial to the pulmonary artery. This bronchial tube is shown in *Pan* but lies hidden within the superior lobe in *Papio* and *Homo.* Additional bronchial rami pass to the middle and inferior lobes, and in *Papio* the azygos lobe is supplied by a ramus from the bronchus to the inferior lobe.

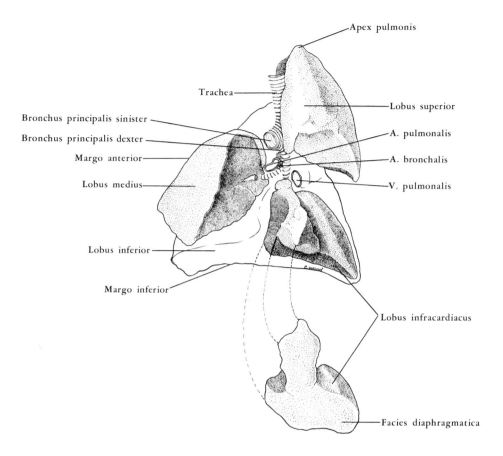

Apex pulmonis

Trachea

Bronchus principalis sinister

Bronchus principalis dexter

Margo anterior

Lobus medius

Lobus inferior

Margo inferior

Lobus superior

A. pulmonalis

A. bronchalis

V. pulmonalis

Lobus infracardiacus

Facies diaphragmatica

Papio

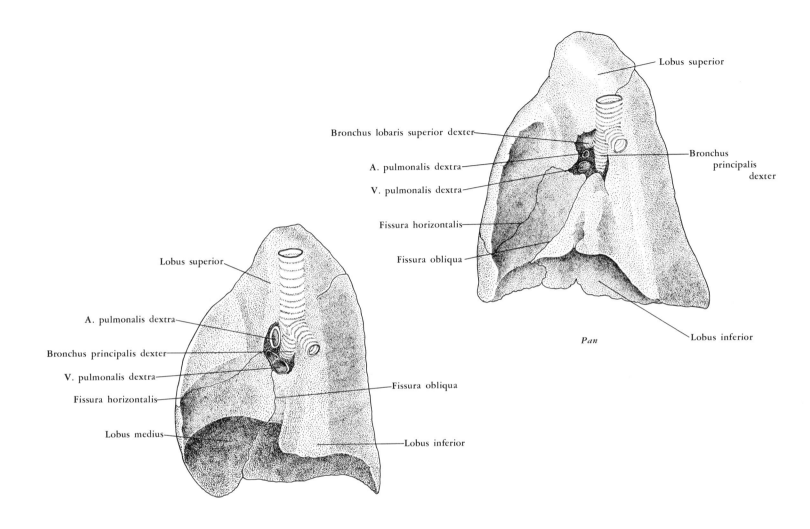

Lobus superior

Bronchus lobaris superior dexter

A. pulmonalis dextra

V. pulmonalis dextra

Bronchus principalis dexter

Fissura horizontalis

Fissura obliqua

Lobus inferior

Pan

Lobus superior

A. pulmonalis dextra

Bronchus principalis dexter

V. pulmonalis dextra

Fissura horizontalis

Fissura obliqua

Lobus medius

Lobus inferior

Homo

PLATE 90

Left Lung Mediastinal Surface

The pulmonary lobation of the left lung is normally three lobes in *Papio* and two in *Pan* and *Homo*. The lung of *Pan* depicted here, with three lobes rather than the usual two, is apparently extremely rare in *Pan*, although Mayer reported three lobes in a specimen he dissected in 1856 (reported in Sonntag 1923). The general trend toward numerical lobar reduction manifest in living primates reaches its ultimate expression in the orang, whose lungs are regularly devoid of any gross lobation (Straus 1936; Hayek 1960).

The presence of a middle lobe is the result of a deep fissure passing horizontally from the hilus of the lung to the anterior margin of the lung. In *Papio* this creates a rather small middle lobe tightly insinuated between the superior and inferior lobes. It should be mentioned that the interlobar clefts of the left lung of *Papio* display considerable intraindividual variability regarding their depth and length. Thus, the lobes of the left lung are frequently less distinct or isolated when compared with the lobes of the right lung.

In *Homo* the normal condition is two lobes as shown here. The oblique interlobar fissure of the left lung is more variable in its craniocaudal course than its counterpart in the right lung (Schaeffer and Ramsay 1966).

As shown here, the disposition of the bronchial tubes and pulmonary vessels at the hilus of the lung is similar in the three primates.

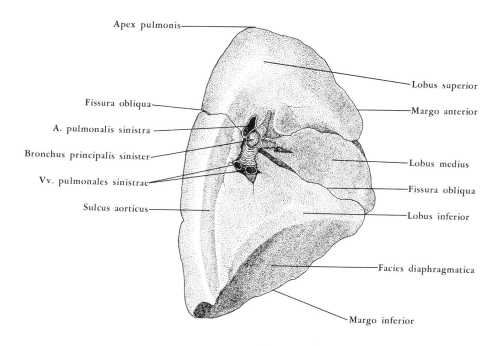

Apex pulmonis

Fissura obliqua

A. pulmonalis sinistra

Bronchus principalis sinister

Vv. pulmonales sinistrae

Sulcus aorticus

Lobus superior

Margo anterior

Lobus medius

Fissura obliqua

Lobus inferior

Facies diaphragmatica

Margo inferior

Papio

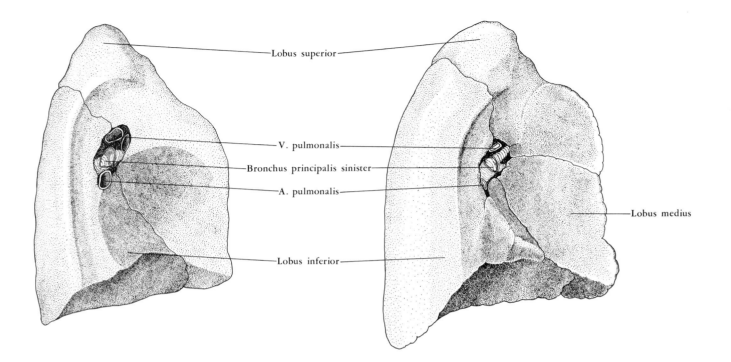

Lobus superior

V. pulmonalis

Bronchus principalis sinister

A. pulmonalis

Lobus medius

Lobus inferior

Homo

Pan

PLATE 91

Sternocostal Surface of Heart

The fibrous pericardium has been removed to facilitate viewing the structures depicted. It should be noted that the relations of the fibrous pericardium to the central tendon of the diaphragm are more variable in *Papio* than in *Pan* and *Homo*. In *Papio* the fibrous pericardium may be separated or in contact with the central tendon. In the latter arrangement, there is usually a small amount of areolar tissue interposed. In *Pan* and *Homo* its connection to the central tendon is intimate, especially in the region of the caval opening.

In all three animals the heart is less elongated craniocaudally than it is in the arboreal monkeys. The sternocostal surface of the heart is convex and in *Papio* it presents mostly the right and left ventricles, although the two small auricles are usually visible peeking over the base of the heart. In all three forms, the apex is made up entirely of the thick muscular wall of the left ventricle.

The left coronary artery is larger than the right. The stem of the artery is shorter in *Papio* than it is in *Pan* or *Homo*—that is, in *Papio* the artery divides almost immediately after arising from the left aortic sinus into its two principal branches, the anterior interventricular and circumflex arteries. The former lies in the interventricular sulcus and passes toward the apex; the latter passes around the left side toward the dorsal aspect of the heart. In its course it gives off small branches to the left atrium and ventricle.

The right coronary artery swings laterally around the base of the heart. In its course it gives rise to several ventricular branches before giving rise to a sizable right marginal artery. On the dorsal aspect of the heart the right coronary passes caudally to become the dorsal interventricular artery. Prior to this caudal bend in the artery, a communicating branch, which anastomoses with the left coronary, may be given off.

The cardiac venous system is very similar in all three forms. The superior vena cava is a large vessel lying to the right of the aortic arch. The vessel is somewhat longer in *Papio* than in *Pan* and *Homo*, and in all three it is formed by the confluence of the right and left brachiocephalic veins. The tributaries of those two major vessels are for the most part similar in the three primates.

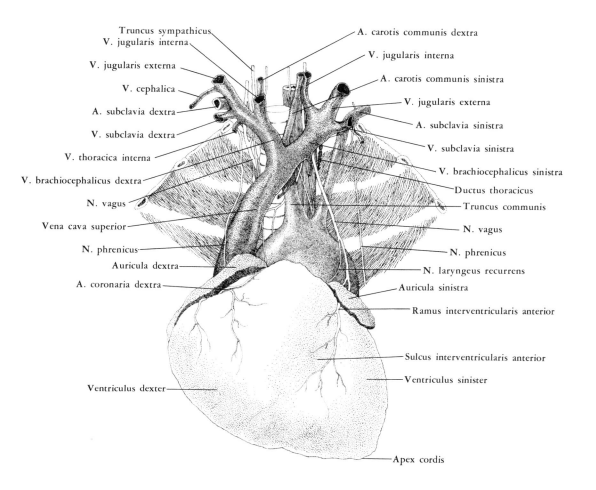

Papio

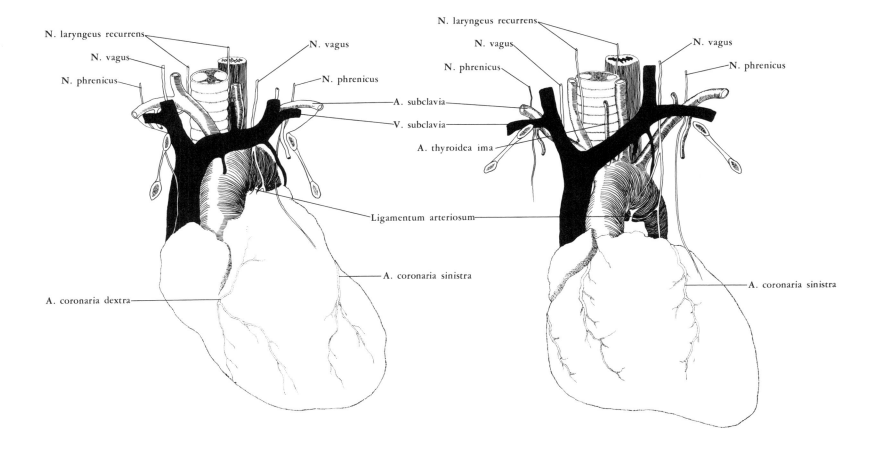

N. laryngeus recurrens

N. vagus

N. phrenicus

N. vagus

N. phrenicus

A. subclavia

V. subclavia

Ligamentum arteriosum

A. coronaria sinistra

A. coronaria dextra

Homo

N. laryngeus recurrens

N. vagus

N. phrenicus

N. vagus

N. phrenicus

A. thyroidea ima

A. coronaria sinistra

Pan

PLATE 92

Aortic Arch

In all three primates, the aortic arch lies in the superior mediastinum dorsal to the manubrium sternum. The arch proper lies somewhat more caudally within the thorax in *Papio*. Its position is deep to the third costal cartilage rather than the second, as in *Homo* and *Pan*. In all three, the arch passes to the left side of the trachea and esophagus.

In *Papio* the aortic arch normally has two major branches. The first, the truncus communis, is the larger of the two and runs a rather long course before dividing into the right subclavian and the left and right common carotids. The smaller second branch, the left subclavian, arises a short distance from the common trunk and passes cranially for some distance before passing from the thorax over the first rib. The two-branched aortic arch is common in many primates and occurs in man as a variant (Lineback 1933). For a detailed study of the aortic arch in the baboon and other primates, the reader is referred to the work of De Garis (1935).

The branching pattern of the aortic arch in *Pan* and *Homo* is usually different from the condition just described in *Papio*. Here the mean number of aortic branches is three, although a fourth branch, the thyroid ima, occurs with regular frequency in *Pan*. This pattern is considered rare in *Homo* (Glidden and De Garis 1936). The thyroid ima may, as shown here, spring from the aortic arch, or it may occasionally arise from the base of the left common carotid. For an excellent discussion of the different aortic branching patterns in the chimpanzee consult Glidden and De Garis 1936.

The most common pattern in *Homo*, which is depicted here, consists of a right brachiocephalic, a left common carotid, and a left subclavian. This pattern occurs in about 70 percent of specimens (Leichtz, Shields, and Anson 1957). A variant met with in *Homo* is the left vertebral artery arising from the arch between the left subclavian and left common carotid arteries.

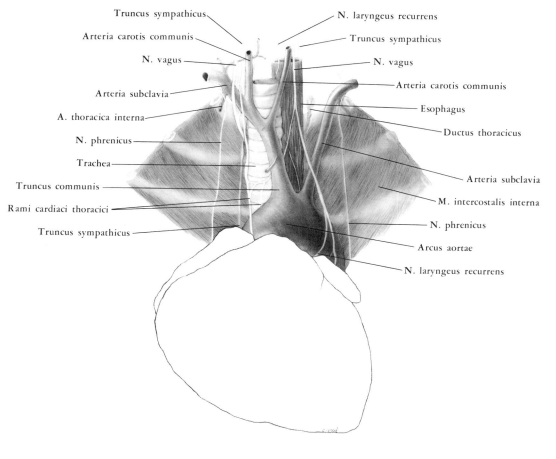

Papio

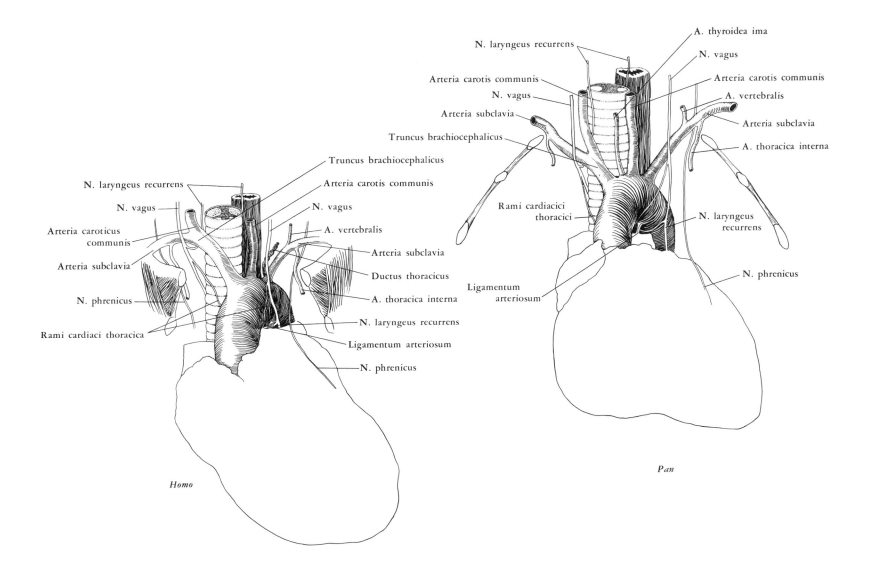

N. laryngeus recurrens

Arteria carotis communis

N. vagus

Arteria subclavia

Truncus brachiocephalicus

Rami cardiacici
thoracici

Ligamentum
arteriosum

A. thyroidea ima

N. vagus

Arteria carotis communis

A. vertebralis

Arteria subclavia

A. thoracica interna

N. laryngeus
recurrens

N. phrenicus

Pan

N. laryngeus recurrens

N. vagus

Arteria caroticus
communis

Arteria subclavia

N. phrenicus

Rami cardiaci thoracica

Truncus brachiocephalicus

Arteria carotis communis

N. vagus

A. vertebralis

Arteria subclavia

Ductus thoracicus

A. thoracica interna

N. laryngeus recurrens

Ligamentum arteriosum

N. phrenicus

Homo

PLATE 93

Interior of Heart

The heart is opened to expose the internal structures in the right and left ventricles. The arrangement of the internal structures is similar in the three animals, particularly between *Pan* and *Homo*.

The wall of the right ventricle is thicker than that of the atria, but not as thick as that of the left ventricle. The semilunar valves surrounding the pulmonary ostium are the right, left, and anterior. When approximated, they prevent regress of blood to the ventricle during diastole. The ventricular wall is relatively smooth caudal to the semilunar valves, and the conus pulmonalis is located in this wall. It is partially separated from the remainder of the ventricle by the supraventricular crest. One of the papillary muscles, the septal, originates from the caudal end of the crest. The anterior papillary muscle arises from the sternocostal wall, while the posterior papillary muscle is more variable. It is often composed of several separate muscles arising from the diaphragmatic wall of the ventricle. In this plate, three are present in *Papio*. The chordae tendinae stretch from the papillary muscles to the three cusps, guarding the right atrioventricular ostium. The ventricular wall is composed of numerous myocardial ridges, the trabeculae carneae. The septomarginal ridge is well developed in this heart of *Papio*. It extends from the septal wall to the anterior papillary muscles and consists of myocardium. This structure is apparently quite variable in *Papio,* since Hill (1970) did not find it in *Papio ursinus,* but Frick (1960) reported it in *Papio hamadryas.* It is present in our sample, thus suggesting some degree of interspecific variability. Note that this structure was formally called the moderator band and was thought to prevent overdistention of the ventricular wall.

The wall of the left ventricle is thicker than that of the right. There are two cusps and normally two papillary muscles forming the mitral valve. The muscles are the anterior and posterior and they connect with the anterior and posterior cusps via the shroudlike chordae tendinae.

The interiors of the atria are not shown here, but they differ little among the three species. The right one is larger than the left; however, both are less capacious than the ventricles. Projecting from each atrium is a large auricle which partially surrounds the pulmonary artery and aorta.

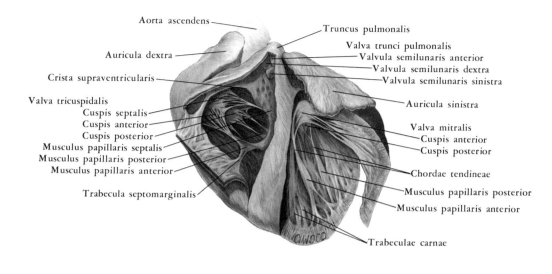

Papio

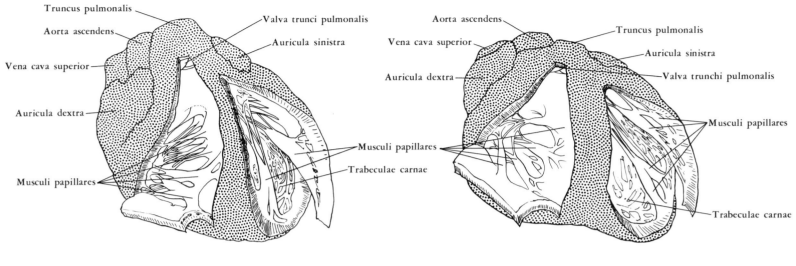

Truncus pulmonalis

Aorta ascendens

Vena cava superior

Auricula dextra

Musculi papillares

Valva trunci pulmonalis

Auricula sinistra

Musculi papillares

Trabeculae carnae

Homo

Aorta ascendens

Vena cava superior

Auricula dextra

Truncus pulmonalis

Auricula sinistra

Valva trunchi pulmonalis

Musculi papillares

Trabeculae carnae

Pan

PLATE 94

Dorsal View of Pericardial Cavity

The heart is removed in order to demonstrate the attachments of the major vessels and the pericardial reflections. The reflection of the epicardial covering of the heart and its continuity with the pericardium at the venous and arterial vessels is similar in the three primates. The major differences involve sizes and proportions.

In *Papio* the oblique sinus assumes a shallow, oblong pocket extending cranially upon the dorsal surface of the atria between the right and left pulmonary veins. This cul-de-sac is more extensive in *Pan* and *Homo*, being deepest in the latter form. An explanation for these proportional differences is suggested in the plate, notably, the more caudally positioned attachments of the right and left pulmonary veins within the pericardial cavity in *Papio*. This positional shift creates what Hill (1970) has called an "incipient oblique sinus" in *Papio*.

Commensurate with the anatomic condition just described is the very broad transverse sinus of *Papio*. The sinus extends laterally between the reflections of the epicardium at the arterial and venous attachments of the heart. The sinus connects the right and left sides of the pericardial cavity. With the heart *in situ* the sinus lies dorsal to the pulmonary artery and the aorta, and ventral to the superior vena cava and left atrium. As shown here, the sinus is much narrower in *Pan* and *Homo,* although it permits the intrusion of the index finger during examination.

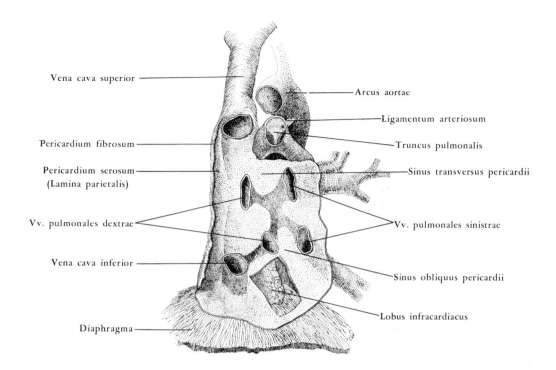

Vena cava superior

Arcus aortae

Ligamentum arteriosum

Pericardium fibrosum

Truncus pulmonalis

Pericardium serosum
(Lamina parietalis)

Sinus transversus pericardii

Vv. pulmonales dextrae

Vv. pulmonales sinistrae

Vena cava inferior

Sinus obliquus pericardii

Lobus infracardiacus

Diaphragma

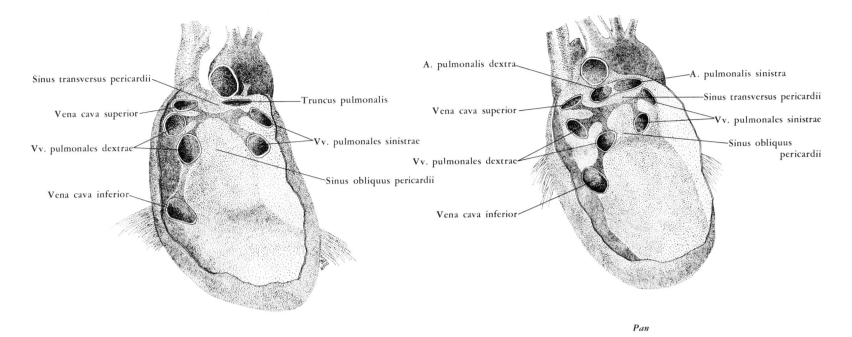

Sinus transversus pericardii

Vena cava superior

Vv. pulmonales dextrae

Vena cava inferior

Truncus pulmonalis

Vv. pulmonales sinistrae

Sinus obliquus pericardii

Homo

A. pulmonalis dextra

Vena cava superior

Vv. pulmonales dextrae

Vena cava inferior

A. pulmonalis sinistra

Sinus transversus pericardii

Vv. pulmonales sinistrae

Sinus obliquus pericardii

Pan

PLATE 95

Superior Mediastinum

The heart is removed so that the roots of the great vessels, as well as the bifurcation of the trachea, are exposed. The general disposition of these structures is similar in the three animals. Thus, the arrangement of the major vessels around the division of the trachea is practically identical.

The ligamentum arteriosum is seen passing from the concavity of the aortic arch to the left pulmonary artery. Note the position of the left recurrent laryngeal nerve passing to the left of the ligamentum arteriosum and then dorsally to the aortic arch coming to lie in the groove between the trachea and the esophagus. The right recurrent laryngeal nerve is shown looping around the right subclavian artery in Plate 52. Both of these topographic relations are constant in these primates.

The caudal continuation of the two vagi is shown here in *Papio,* as the ventral and dorsal vagi occupying those respective surfaces of the esophagus. This relation is maintained throughout the thorax.

The trachea is the most prominent structure in the neck. It commences at the cricoid cartilage and terminates at its bifurcation in the superior mediastinum. Throughout its course the trachea is composed of cartilaginous plates that encircle a muscular tube and fail to join dorsally. Because of this lack of fusion the trachea of *Papio* as well as of cercopithecoids generally is considered to resemble the trachea of all higher primates or hominoids. The eparterial bronchus, although not visible in this plate, usually departs from the right bronchus almost immediately after its separation from the trachea. The left bronchus normally travels a longer course before giving rise to additional bronchi.

Note the right phrenic nerve traveling its solitary course through the mediastinum to the diaphragm. The course is similar in the three primates. The left phrenic nerve is shown in Plate 51.

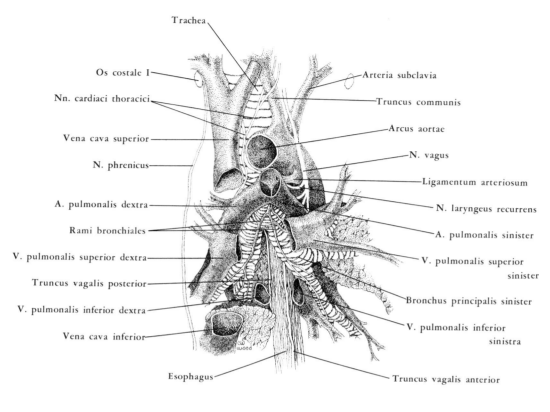

Papio

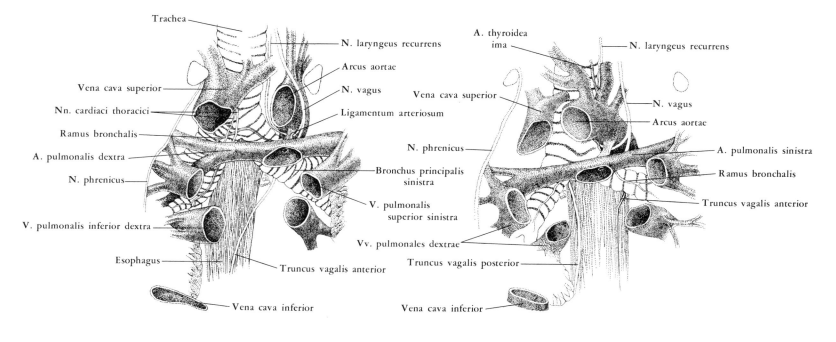

Trachea

N. laryngeus recurrens

Arcus aortae

Vena cava superior

N. vagus

Nn. cardiaci thoracici

Ligamentum arteriosum

Ramus bronchalis

A. pulmonalis dextra

N. phrenicus

Bronchus principalis
sinistra

V. pulmonalis inferior dextra

V. pulmonalis
superior sinistra

Esophagus

Truncus vagalis anterior

Vena cava inferior

Homo

A. thyroidea
ima

N. laryngeus recurrens

Vena cava superior

N. vagus

Arcus aortae

N. phrenicus

A. pulmonalis sinistra

Ramus bronchalis

Truncus vagalis anterior

Vv. pulmonales dextrae

Truncus vagalis posterior

Vena cava inferior

Pan

PLATE 96

Azygos System

This drainage system is composed of longitudinal channels lying in the posterior mediastinum of the thorax that collect the blood from the intercostal veins and the vertebral venous plexus. There are usually three major channels: the hemiazygos and accessory hemiazygos on the left side of the vertebral column, and the azygos and right superior intercostal veins disposed to the right side of the column.

The azygos vein originates at the level of the twelfth thoracic vertebra, which represents the cranial continuation of the ascending lumbar vein. It is closely applied to the vertebral bodies as it passes cranially through the thorax. Near its cranial end the azygos vein curves over the root of the right lung to empty into the superior vena cava. The right superior intercostal vein drains the second, third, and fourth intercostal spaces before passing into the arch of the azygos vein. The vein may receive the first intercostal vein; if not, the right highest intercostal vein is responsible for draining the first intercostal space. The highest right intercostal usually empties into the right brachiocephalic vein. This is the situation found in all three primates, but one must constantly be on guard for minor intraspecific variations.

The hemiazygos, when present, is composed of the left ascending lumbar vein and the more caudal left thoracic segmental veins. The number of segmental veins received by the hemiazygos is extremely variable. In *Papio* a true hemiazygos was not encountered in the dissections; rather, the right and left ascending lumbars drained into either the eleventh or twelfth thoracic intercostals, which in turn coalesced to form the azygos vein proper. In *Pan* and *Homo* the hemiazygos is present and enters the azygos system at the level of the eighth or ninth thoracic vertebra. In a study of human cadavers, Seib (1934) found the hemiazygos to be continuous with the accessory hemiazygos in approximately 40 percent of cases.

The accessory hemiazygos, like the hemiazygos, is variable in origin. In *Papio* it is absent, whereas in *Pan* and *Homo* it lies to the left of the vertebral column between the ninth and fifth thoracic vertebrae. It empties into the azygos vein via a trunk passing dorsal to the aorta. Both the hemiazygos and accessory hemiazygos veins are present in *Macaca mulatta* (Lineback 1933). Hill (1970) does not mention the azygos system in his discussion of the anatomy of *Papio*.

The left superior intercostal vein drains the second, third, and fourth intercostal spaces before terminating in the left brachiocephalic vein. In all three species it frequently communicates with the azygos system. The left highest intercostal vein drains the first intercostal space (and on occasion the second also) prior to passing into the left brachiocephalic vein in *Pan* and *Homo,* and into the left subclavian vein in *Papio*.

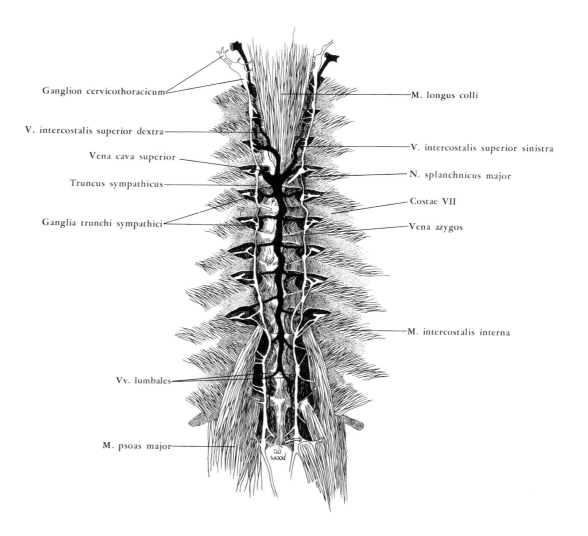

Ganglion cervicothoracicum
M. longus colli
V. intercostalis superior dextra
V. intercostalis superior sinistra
Vena cava superior
N. splanchnicus major
Truncus sympathicus
Costae VII
Ganglia trunchi sympathici
Vena azygos
M. intercostalis interna
Vv. lumbales
M. psoas major

Papio

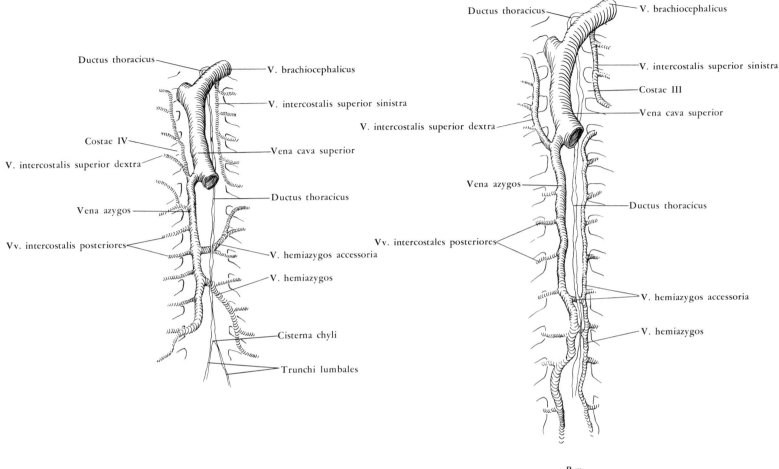

Ductus thoracicus

V. brachiocephalicus

V. intercostalis superior sinistra

Costae IV

V. intercostalis superior dextra

Vena cava superior

Ductus thoracicus

Vena azygos

Vv. intercostalis posteriores

V. hemiazygos accessoria

V. hemiazygos

Cisterna chyli

Trunchi lumbales

Homo

Ductus thoracicus

V. brachiocephalicus

V. intercostalis superior sinistra

Costae III

Vena cava superior

V. intercostalis superior dextra

Vena azygos

Ductus thoracicus

Vv. intercostales posteriores

V. hemiazygos accessoria

V. hemiazygos

Pan

Part 6

ABDOMEN

PLATE 97

Ventral Abdominal Wall

The abdominal musculature consists of the external and internal oblique muscles, the transverse abdominis, the rectus, pyramidalis, and cremaster muscles.

In *Papio* the rectus abdominis is a broad, straplike muscle extending from the manubrium cranially to the pubic symphysis caudally. In *Pan* and *Homo* the muscle attaches cranially only as far as the xiphoid process. The muscle presents an inconstant number of transverse tendinous inscriptions. The rectus is ensheathed by the aponeuroses of the three flat abdominal muscles as follows. In *Papio* the aponeuroses of the external and internal oblique muscles pass ventral to the rectus throughout its extent. The aponeurosis of the transverse muscle forms the dorsal wall of the rectus sheath. At a variable distance between the umbilicus and pubis this dorsal lamina passes ventrally, joining the aponeuroses of the external and internal oblique muscles. This results in the formation of the arcuate line. From this line caudally the dorsal wall is formed by the fascia transversalis.

In *Pan* and *Homo* the major difference is that the aponeurosis of the internal oblique divides into a ventral and dorsal lamina, which pass to the respective surfaces of the rectus muscle. Otherwise, the mode of formation of the rectus sheath is similar. Observe the details on the left side of each specimen.

The well-formed cremaster muscle of *Papio* is shown draping over the spermatic cord as it issues through the abdominal inguinal ring. The muscle is continuous with the internal oblique and transverse abdominal muscles. For an excellent study of the inguinal canal of primates, see Miller 1947.

The development of the pyramidalis muscle, shown here in *Papio* and *Homo,* is variable in primates (Ashley-Montagu 1939). Observe the inferior and superior epigastric arteries in *Papio*. These are branches of the external iliac and internal thoracic arteries, respectively. The epigastrics pass within the rectus sheath along the dorsal surface of the rectus muscle, where they ramify and inosculate.

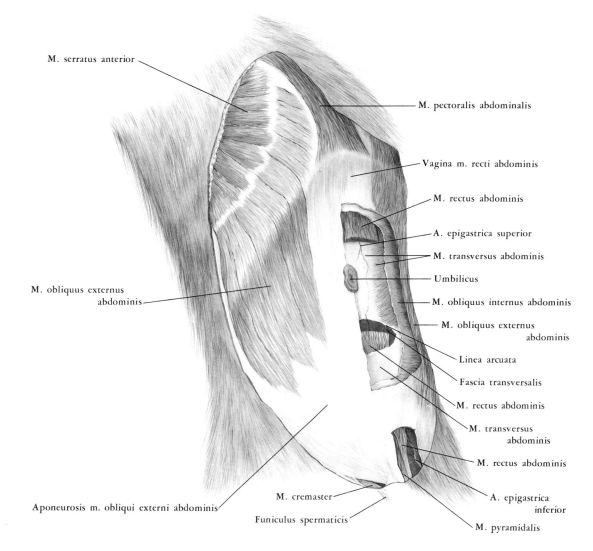

M. serratus anterior

M. pectoralis abdominalis

Vagina m. recti abdominis

M. rectus abdominis

A. epigastrica superior

M. transversus abdominis

Umbilicus

M. obliquus externus abdominis

M. obliquus internus abdominis

M. obliquus externus abdominis

Linea arcuata

Fascia transversalis

M. rectus abdominis

M. transversus abdominis

M. rectus abdominis

Aponeurosis m. obliqui externi abdominis

M. cremaster

A. epigastrica inferior

Funiculus spermaticis

M. pyramidalis

Papio

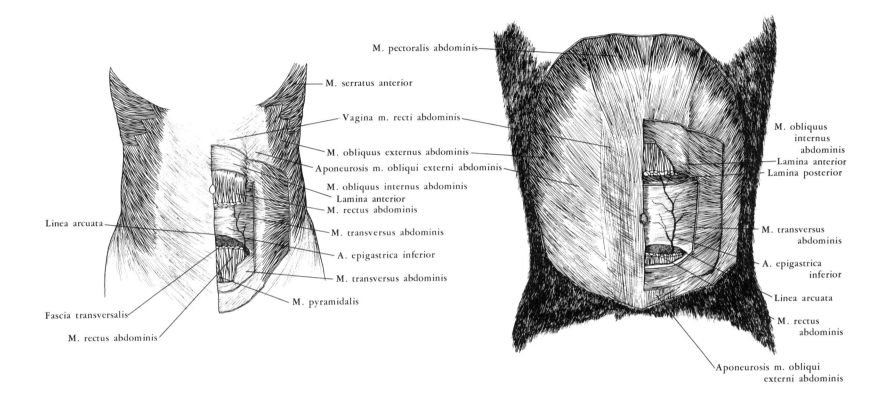

M. pectoralis abdominis

M. serratus anterior

Vagina m. recti abdominis

M. obliquus externus abdominis

Aponeurosis m. obliqui externi abdominis

M. obliquus internus abdominis

Lamina anterior

M. rectus abdominis

M. transversus abdominis

A. epigastrica inferior

M. transversus abdominis

M. pyramidalis

Linea arcuata

Fascia transversalis

M. rectus abdominis

M. obliquus internus abdominis

Lamina anterior

Lamina posterior

M. transversus abdominis

A. epigastrica inferior

Linea arcuata

M. rectus abdominis

Aponeurosis m. obliqui externi abdominis

Homo

Pan

PLATE 98

Abdominal Viscera I

The abdominal wall is reflected laterally, exposing the abdominal viscera *in situ*. The most conspicuous structure is the large liver occupying the cranial portion of the abdominal cavity. In *Pan* and *Homo* it is located mainly in the right side of the abdominal cavity, while in *Papio* the gland extends much farther to the left because of the well-developed left lobe. The liver is in contact with the diaphragm cranially, and several abdominal viscera caudally. The falciform ligament is a fold of peritoneum assisting in the support of the liver. The round ligament of the liver is located in the free caudal margin of the falciform ligament and represents the obliterated fetal left umbilical vein.

The stomach is visible running along the caudal margin of the liver. The lesser omentum is well developed and passes from the lesser curvature of the stomach to the liver. Its attachment to the stomach is from the esophageal junction to just distal to the pyloroduodenal junction, where it forms the ventral boundary of the epiploic foramen. The greater omentum is suspended in an apronlike fashion from the greater curvature of the stomach. This membrane is extremely large in *Papio*, extending into all regions of the abdomen and pelvis. In older animals it often forms adhesions with the peritoneum lining the walls of the abdominal and pelvic cavities.

Parts of the small and large intestines are visible lying dorsal to the greater omentum. Observe the spleen lying to the left side of the stomach. It is particularly large and elongated in *Papio*.

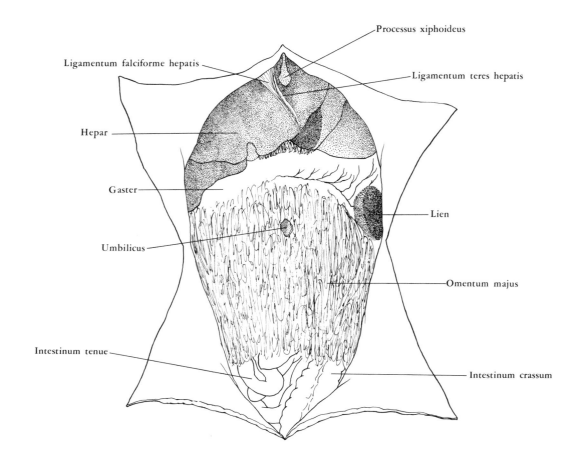

Papio

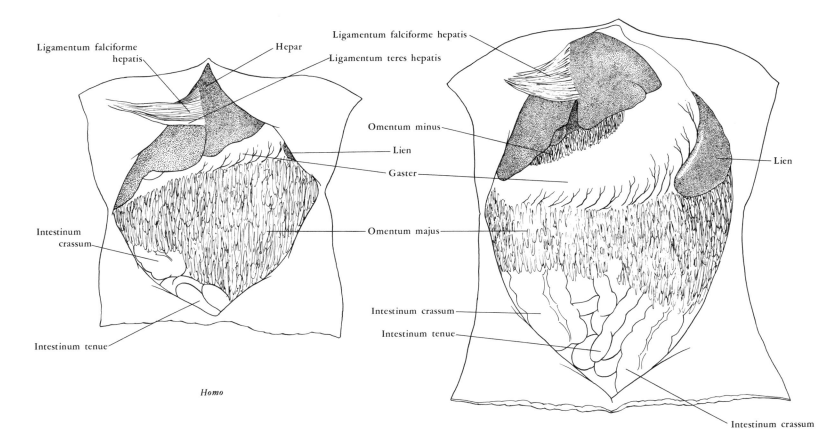

Ligamentum falciforme
hepatis

Hepar

Ligamentum falciforme hepatis

Ligamentum teres hepatis

Omentum minus

Lien

Gaster

Intestinum
crassum

Omentum majus

Intestinum tenue

Intestinum crassum

Intestinum tenue

Lien

Intestinum crassum

Homo

Pan

PLATE 99

Abdominal Viscera II

The intestine extends from the stomach to the anus.
It is separated into small and large intestines, which in turn
are divided into different segments.

   The duodenum is considered in Plate 102. The jejunum
commences at the duodenojejunal flexure and usually
occupies much of the left side of the abdominal cavity.
The ileum continues as the caudal portion of the small
intestine and terminates at the ileocecal junction. Many of
its coils lie in the right portion of the abdominal cavity.
The transition from jejunum to ileum is gradual with no
definite line of demarcation. The jejunum and ileum share
a common free mesentery with the ascending colon in
Papio (see insert). In *Pan* and *Homo* a secondary support
for the jejunum and ileum is present in the form of the
mesentery, a structure peculiar to the apes and man
(Straus 1936). It extends from the duodenojejunal flexure
to the ileocecal junction (see inserts). The mesentery
contains the vessels and structures passing to and from
the intestine.

   The large intestine begins with the cecum and ends
at the anal canal. It is very different in appearance from
the small intestine since it possesses sacculations, termed
haustra. These are produced by three muscular bands,
teniae coli, which run longitudinally from the cecum to the
rectum. The colon of *Papio* is especially well marked by
sacculations, which are usually larger along the ascending
colon. In *Papio* the entire colon is intraperitoneal, but the
ascending colon may display some degree of fixation
(ibid.). In *Pan* and *Homo* the ascending and descending
parts of the colon tend to lose their peritoneal supports and
become fixed to the dorsal body wall. The transverse
mesocolon, however, is long and well developed (see
inserts). In *Papio* there is no sigmoid colon, since the
descending colon presents a series of loops that move
to the midline as they approach the pelvis and become
fixed to the sacrum. Here the colon becomes the rectum.
In *Pan* and *Homo* the sigmoid portion possesses its own
mesocolon.

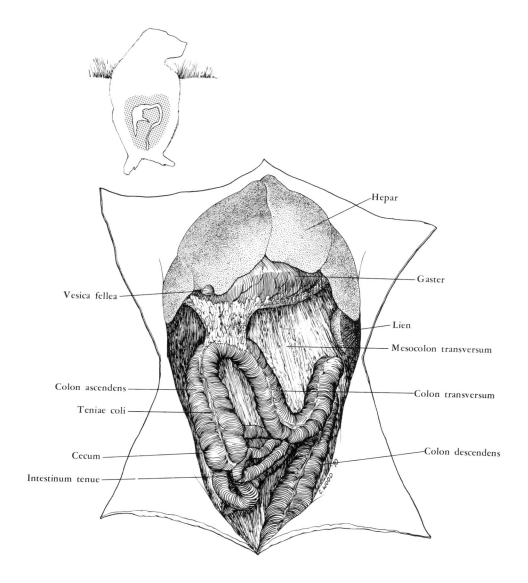

Papio

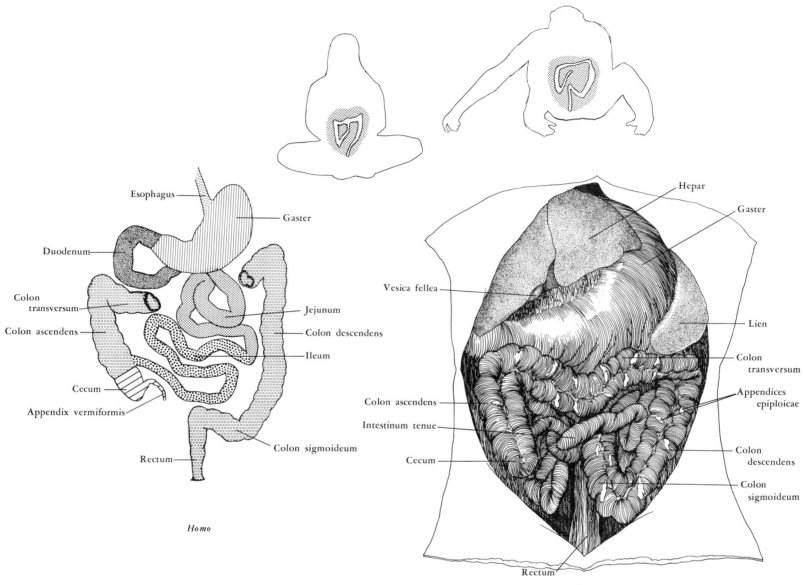

Esophagus

Gaster

Duodenum

Colon
transversum

Colon ascendens

Jejunum

Colon descendens

Ileum

Cecum

Appendix vermiformis

Colon sigmoideum

Rectum

Homo

Hepar

Gaster

Vesica fellea

Lien

Colon
transversum

Colon ascendens

Appendices
epiploicae

Intestinum tenue

Colon
descendens

Cecum

Colon
sigmoideum

Rectum

Pan

PLATE 100

Abdominal Viscera III

The gastric morphology of these three primates is very similar, being divisible into fundus, body, and pyloric segments (Straus 1936; Hill 1957). The fundus lies against the left surface of the diaphragm and the left lobe of the liver. The body of the stomach lies between the fundus and pyloris making up a large portion of the greater curvature of the stomach. The pyloric section is thick-walled and more tubular than the other portions. The pyloric sphincter is usually marked by an external annular sulcus.

The lesser omentum represents the primitive ventral mesogastrium extending from the stomach and duodenum to the liver. It consists of two parts. The cranial portion is the hepatogastric ligament connecting the lesser curvature of the stomach with the liver. The caudal part forms the hepatoduodenal ligament running between the pyloris and cranial part of the duodenum and the liver. Its free margin forms the ventral border of the epiploic foramen. Between the layers of the ligament pass the common bile duct, hepatic artery, and portal vein.

The liver of *Papio* consists of all four primitive lobes: central, left lateral, right lateral, and Spigelian. The central lobe is the largest of the four, being demarcated between the right and left lateral lobes by deep fissures. The left lobe is the smallest, and it is almost completely separated from the central lobe. Its visceral surface forms part of the gastric impression. The right lobe is larger than the left and somewhat overlaps the central lobe. Its visceral surface is in contact with the right kidney. Observe the gall bladder lying in a deep fossa on the quadrate area of the central lobe. Its fundus usually does not reach the caudal margin of the liver. In this view the Spigelian complex lies behind the lesser omentum and is not shown. It consists of the caudate lobe and papillary process, which form an oblong area between the inferior vena cava on the right and a deep fissure separating it from the left lobe. It is better observed from the visceral aspect of the liver.

The livers of *Pan* and *Homo* are characterized by a reduction in lobation and are topographically very similar (Sonntag 1923; Straus 1936). The central lobe has disappeared as a distinct structure, having fused with adjacent parts of the lateral lobes forming the right and left lobes of *Pan* and *Homo* (Straus 1936). The result is four lobes: right, left, caudate, and quadrate.

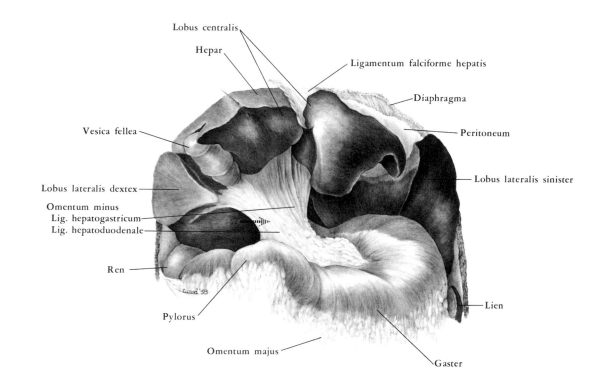

Lobus centralis

Hepar

Ligamentum falciforme hepatis

Diaphragma

Vesica fellea

Peritoneum

Lobus lateralis dextex

Lobus lateralis sinister

Omentum minus
Lig. hepatogastricum
Lig. hepatoduodenale

Ren

Lien

Pylorus

Omentum majus

Gaster

☆ Foramen epiploicum

Papio

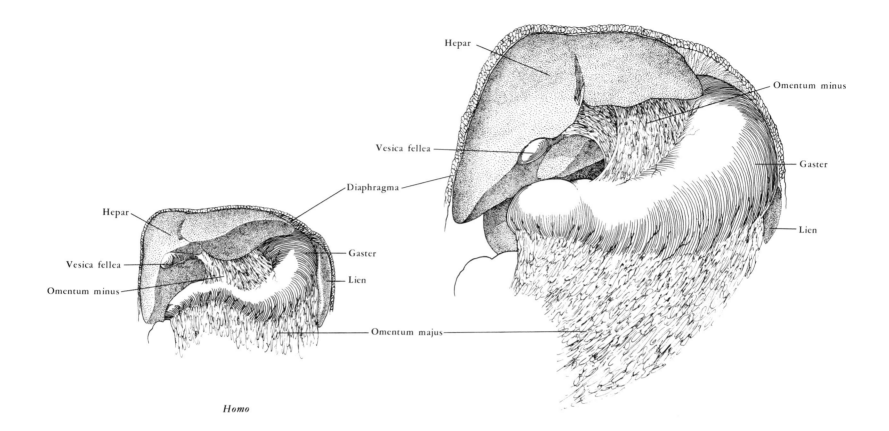

Hepar

Vesica fellea

Diaphragma

Gaster

Lien

Omentum minus

Gaster

Lien

Hepar

Vesica fellea

Omentum minus

Omentum majus

Homo

Pan

ABDOMEN 211

PLATE 101

Celiac Artery

The celiac artery is the first visceral branch of the abdominal aorta. It arises from the ventral surface of the aorta as the vessel passes between the crura of the diaphragm. The celiac trunk supplies the liver, gall bladder, stomach, pancreas, duodenum, and spleen. Variational patterns of the celiac trunk are legion in *Homo,* as Michels (1955) has so aptly demonstrated. A high degree of variation is also to be expected in catarrhine monkeys (Rojecki 1889; Grzybowski 1926).

In *Papio* the celiac usually bifurcates into the left gastric and hepatosplenic arteries. The latter divides almost immediately into the hepatic and splenic arteries. In *Pan* and *Homo* the celiac trifurcates in the majority of cases into the left gastric, splenic, and hepatic arteries. Other arterial variations occurred, but these were the two most frequently encountered in the present sample.

In *Papio* the left gastric is a large artery that gives off a long branch passing toward the proximal end of the stomach. Several esophageal branches arise from it along the cardiac portion of the stomach. Shortly thereafter, the left gastric divides into a large dorsal and a small ventral branch. These supply numerous rami to the respective surfaces of the stomach. The hepatic courses toward the liver through the free border of the lesser omentum. The gastroduodenal is usually the first branch of the hepatic, and it may give rise to the right gastric, as shown in *Papio,* or the right gastric may originate from the proper hepatic, as depicted in *Pan* and *Homo.* The cystic artery arises from the right hepatic to pass directly to the gall bladder. The splenic is uncoiled in *Papio* and runs along the cranial border of the pancreas toward the spleen. In *Pan* and *Homo* the artery is often markedly tortuous, especially in older individuals. The left gastroepiploic arises from the splenic to anastomose with the right gastroepiploic along the greater curvature of the stomach. Several short gastric arteries pass directly from the splenic to the fundus of the stomach.

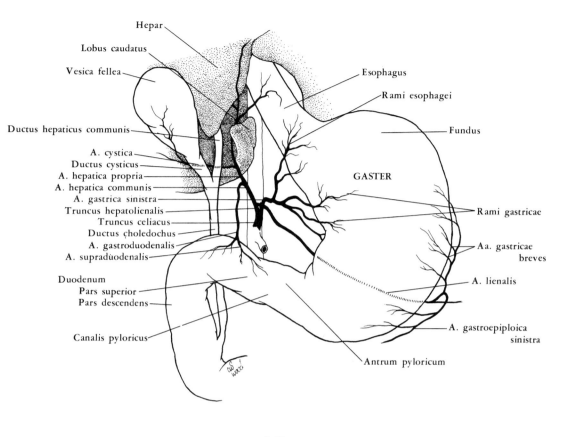

Papio

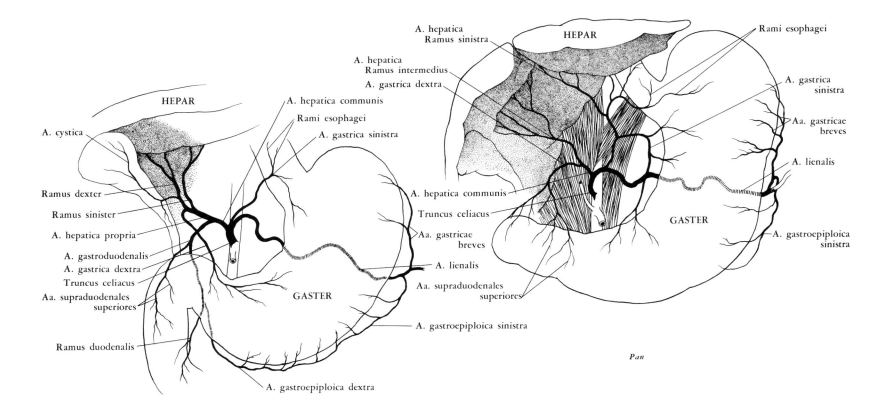

A. cystica

HEPAR

A. hepatica communis

Rami esophagei

A. gastrica sinistra

A. hepatica
Ramus sinistra

A. hepatica
Ramus intermedius

A. gastrica dextra

Rami esophagei

HEPAR

A. gastrica
sinistra

Aa. gastricae
breves

A. lienalis

Ramus dexter

Ramus sinister

A. hepatica propria

A. gastroduodenalis

A. gastrica dextra

Truncus celiacus

Aa. supraduodenales
superiores

Ramus duodenalis

GASTER

A. hepatica communis

Aa. gastricae
breves

A. lienalis

Aa. supraduodenales
superiores

A. gastroepiploica sinistra

A. gastroepiploica dextra

Truncus celiacus

GASTER

A. gastroepiploica
sinistra

Homo

Pan

PLATE 102

Pancreas, Duodenum, and Superior Mesenteric Artery

The pancreas is an elongated gland extending transversely along the dorsal wall of the abdomen from the spleen to the duodenum. For the most part it is completely retroperitoneal. There are three parts to the pancreas: the head, the body, and the tail. The head lies within the duodenal loop and lacks the uncinate process in *Papio*. The body is directed to the left and is usually on a somewhat more cranial level than the head. The tail is variable in form but is usually blunted and passes ventrally. It is invariably in contact with the medial surface of the spleen. Note that the splenic vessels may cross ventral or dorsal to the tail of the pancreas on their way to the spleen.

There are two pancreatic ducts, the principal and the accessory. Boyden (1955, 1966) has worked out the details of these ducts regarding their formation, course, and entrance into the duodenum for *Papio* and *Pan*. The usual termination of the biliary and pancreatic ducts are as follows. The major pancreatic duct joins the common bile duct to penetrate the duodenal wall. Inside the duodenum they terminate on the major duodenal papilla either by a common aperture or separately. Note that in *Pan* the pancreatic duct widens into what Boyden (1955) calls "a sinus pancreaticus," while the bile duct narrows at its confluence with the sinus. If present, the accessory pancreatic duct passes separately into the duodenum to open on the minor papilla.

The arterial supply of the pancreas is from the splenic artery by way of its pancreatic branches, and from the superior mesenteric and hepatic by the superior and inferior pancreaticoduodenal arteries.

The duodenum extends from the pylorus to the duodenojejunal flexure. In *Pan* and *Homo* it is typically C-shaped, while in *Papio* it invariably lacks the fourth part, thus displaying a J-shaped contour (Hill 1970). In all three primates, the duodenum is almost entirely retroperitoneal.

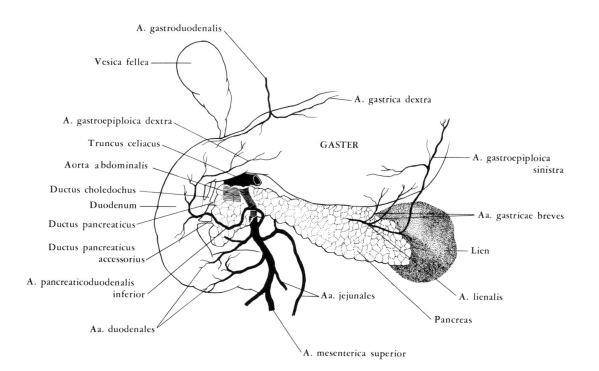

Papio

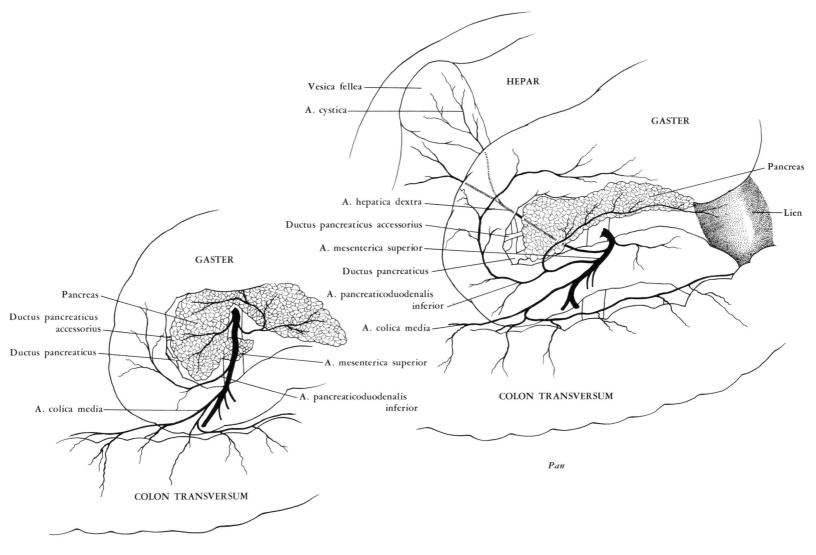

Vesica fellea

A. cystica

HEPAR

GASTER

Pancreas

Lien

A. hepatica dextra

Ductus pancreaticus accessorius

A. mesenterica superior

Ductus pancreaticus

A. pancreaticoduodenalis inferior

A. colica media

GASTER

Pancreas

Ductus pancreaticus accessorius

Ductus pancreaticus

A. mesenterica superior

A. pancreaticoduodenalis inferior

A. colica media

COLON TRANSVERSUM

Pan

COLON TRANSVERSUM

Homo

PLATE 103

Superior and Inferior Mesenteric Arteries

The superior and inferior mesenteric arteries carry blood to the gut from the duodenum to the rectum. In addition, the superior mesenteric is responsible for a part of the pancreas, where it anastomoses with branches of the celiac artery.

In *Papio* the superior mesenteric arises as it does in the other primates just caudal to the celiac and passes dorsal to the pancreas and ventral to the duodenum. It gives off one or two pancreaticoduodenal branches before entering the mesentery. The intestinal arteries arise from the superior mesenteric within the mesentery. Their number varies from twelve to twenty-five as they radiate into the mesentery, forming primary loops or arcades. From the final arcades arise straight terminal branches, vasa recti, which pass directly to the walls of the small intestine. In *Papio* there is a large right colic branch which passes toward the middle of the ascending colon. There is no middle colic in *Papio,* although it is usually present in *Pan* and *Homo.* In the absence of the middle colic, the right colic courses along the margin of the colon to anastomose with the ascending branch of the left colic artery. The superior mesenteric ends as the iliocolic artery, which passes toward the iliocolic junction and cecum.

The inferior mesenteric artery is the third unpaired branch of the abdominal aorta. It arises caudal to the gonadal arteries and runs obliquely caudal and to the left. It supplies the large intestine from the left colic flexure to the rectum, where it terminates as the superior rectal artery. In *Papio* the inferior mesenteric courses in the descending mesocolon, while in *Pan* and *Homo* its path is essentially retroperitoneal. In *Pan* and *Homo* the inferior mesenteric has three branches: the left colic, sigmoid, and superior rectal. In *Papio* there is no true sigmoid colon; therefore, sigmoid arteries are not present.

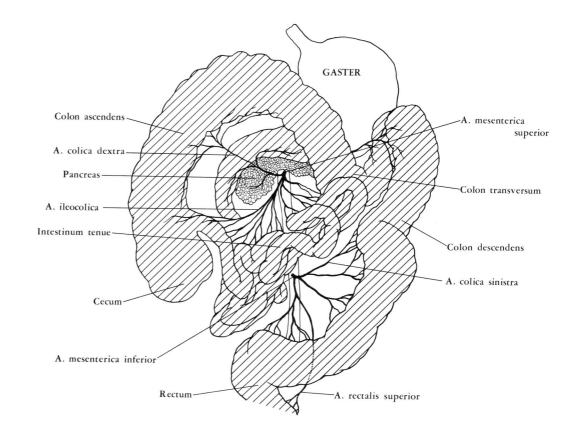

Papio

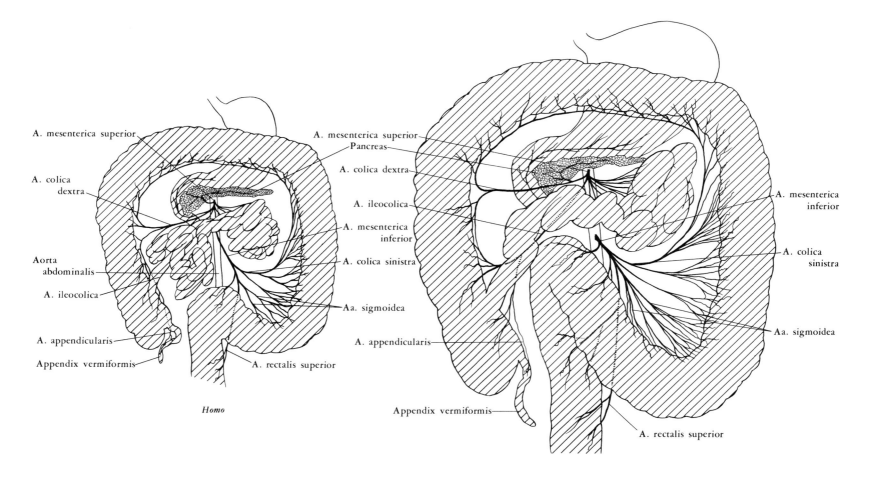

A. mesenterica superior

A. colica
dextra

Aorta
abdominalis

A. ileocolica

A. appendicularis

Appendix vermiformis

A. mesenterica superior
Pancreas

A. colica dextra

A. ileocolica

A. mesenterica
inferior

A. colica sinistra

Aa. sigmoidea

A. rectalis superior

Homo

A. mesenterica
inferior

A. colica
sinistra

Aa. sigmoidea

A. appendicularis

Appendix vermiformis

A. rectalis superior

Pan

PLATE 104

Portal System

The portal system is an anatomically unique drainage pattern since blood from the intestinal arteries traverses two distinct sets of capillaries before returning to the heart. Blood is conveyed from the caudal esophagus, abdominal and pelvic intestines, pancreas, spleen, and gall bladder to the liver. The veins transporting the blood from these diverse locations constitute the portal system. They are the superior mesenteric, inferior mesenteric, splenic, and portal veins. The latter is normally formed by the union of the superior mesenteric and splenic veins. Note that the inferior mesenteric vein usually drains into the splenic, although on occasion it may join the superior mesenteric vein.

The description of the portal system as just presented obtains in all primates. Minor variations are to be expected, especially when dealing with the venous side of the cardiovascular system. A functionally important and vital part of the portal pattern is concerned with collateral circulation, which involves the anastomoses between tributaries of the portal and caval systems. These are of paramount importance in diseases of the liver, which obstruct normal blood flow to the heart. Several sites are described in the literature, and three important ones are: (1) tributaries of portal vein with paraumbilical veins; (2) superior rectal veins and internal iliac tributaries; and (3) esophageal tributaries of the azygos and left gastric veins. What evidence there is suggests that these anatomic locations are similar in the three animals and, certainly, portal-systemic shunts have been validated in cercopithecoids (Waldhausen, Abel, and Pearce 1967).

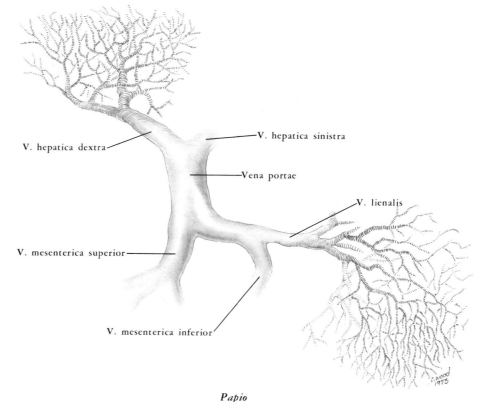

V. hepatica dextra

V. hepatica sinistra

Vena portae

V. lienalis

V. mesenterica superior

V. mesenterica inferior

Papio

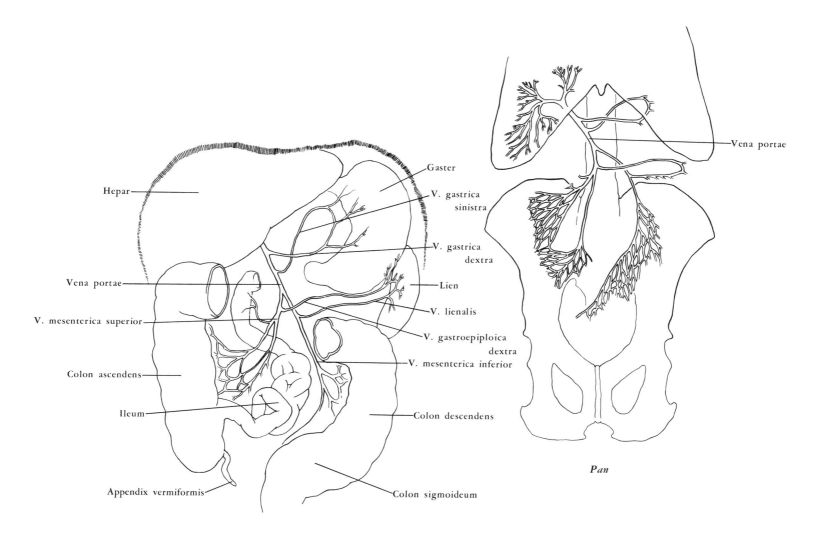

Hepar

Gaster

V. gastrica sinistra

V. gastrica dextra

Vena portae

Lien

V. mesenterica superior

V. lienalis

V. gastroepiploica dextra

Colon ascendens

V. mesenterica inferior

Ileum

Colon descendens

Appendix vermiformis

Colon sigmoideum

Homo

Vena portae

Pan

PLATE 105

Ileocecal Junction

The cecum and related structures have been extensively studied by Straus (1936), Hill and Rewell (1948), and Hill (1957). The shape and general configuration of the cecum varies a great deal depending upon the physiological condition at the time of death.

In *Papio* the cecum is rather long, forming a rounded distal portion and a proximal segment with three or four well-formed haustra. The three teniae pass on to the distal portion of the cecum, where they often expand to form a continuous muscular coat. There is usually some degree of asymmetry in the cecum of *Papio.* The magnitude of this bowing increases as the animal advances in age (Hill 1957). The appendix is absent in *Papio;* indeed, among the primates the organ is present only in the lemur *(Nycticebus),* the four anthropoid apes, and man (Lineback 1933). The appendix of *Pan* is much longer than it is in *Homo,* and often presents several coils. In both, the appendix may be retrocecal.

The ileocolic artery passes from the superior mesentery to supply the cecum, ileum, and appendix (when present). The appendicular artery is usually a branch of the posterior cecal, although it may arise from the ileal, anterior cecal, or directly from the ileocolic. In *Papio* the posterior cecal is large and usually supplies the majority of the cecum.

The cecum is completely covered by peritoneum, and in *Papio* there is a well-formed triangular flap of peritoneum connecting the medial surface of the cecum with the ileum. This has been referred to as the mesotyphlon (Hill 1957, 1970).

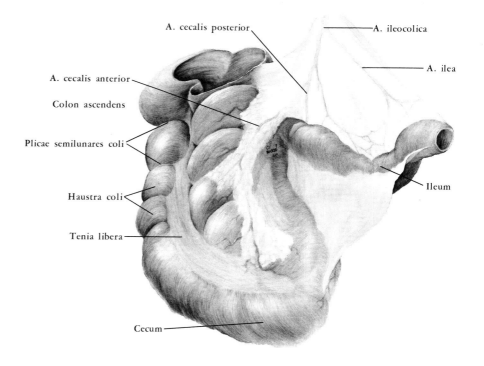

Papio

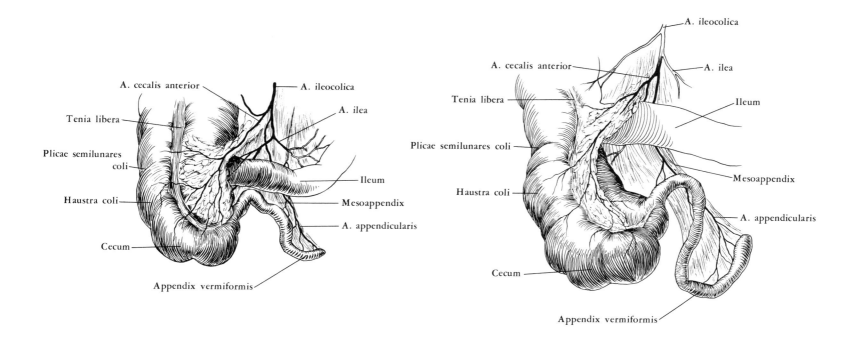

A. cecalis anterior

Tenia libera

Plicae semilunares
coli

Haustra coli

Cecum

Appendix vermiformis

A. ileocolica

A. ilea

Ileum

Mesoappendix

A. appendicularis

Homo

A. ileocolica

A. cecalis anterior

A. ilea

Tenia libera

Ileum

Plicae semilunares coli

Mesoappendix

Haustra coli

A. appendicularis

Cecum

Appendix vermiformis

Pan

PLATE 106

Posterior Abdominal Wall

The abdominal aorta begins at the aortic hiatus of the diaphragm and ends by dividing into the right and left common iliac arteries. It is retroperitoneal and dorsal to the viscera throughout the abdomen. Its branches may be divided into parietal, visceral, and terminal groups. The three unpaired visceral branches are considered in detail in Plates 101, 102, and 103. The paired visceral branches are the gonadal, renal, and middle suprarenal arteries. The latter may not be present in *Papio*. The parietal arteries are the inferior phrenics, lumbars, and middle sacral (caudal). In *Papio* the inferior phrenics usually arise from the aorta, although Hill (1970) reports them originating from the left renal and left gastric arteries. In *Pan* and *Homo* there are usually four or five pairs of lumbar segmental arteries, while in *Papio* the common number is three.

The inferior vena cava is formed by the confluence of the right and left common iliac veins. In *Papio* this confluence occurs opposite the body of the third lumbar vertebra, while in *Pan* and *Homo* it is at the level of the fifth lumbar. From here the vein passes to the right of the aorta as far as the caval opening in the diaphragm. Tributaries to the inferior vena cava correspond with the branches of the abdominal aorta.

The kidneys are located in the posterior part of the abdomen, immediately dorsal to the peritoneum. In *Papio* the left kidney is more caudal than the right, whereas in *Pan* and *Homo* it is just the opposite. The medial border of the kidney is concave and presents an aperture, the hilus. The renal pelvis, vessels, and nerves enter and leave through the hilus. The ureters continue from the pelvis, passing caudally over the psoas muscle and ventral to the common iliac vessels to terminate in the dorsolateral surface of the urinary bladder.

The suprarenal glands normally cap the cranial pole of each kidney, although in *Papio* they are shown somewhat removed from this position. They are larger in younger animals, becoming smaller as the animal gets older, and resemble somewhat the shape of an olive (Hill 1970). They are richly supplied with arteries, while usually a single vein drains the gland. These glands receive more blood per gram of weight than any other organ in the body (Gardner 1966).

In *Papio* the spleen is extremely elongated and occupies much of the space between the left margin of the liver and the left kidney. The spleen is connected to the kidney by the lienorenal ligament, which is particularly well developed in *Papio* (Hill 1970).

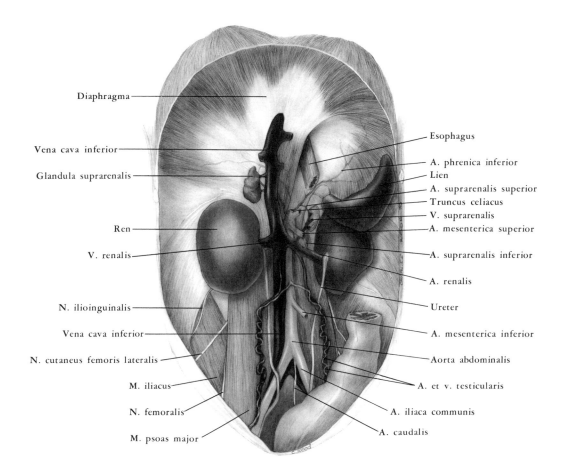

Papio

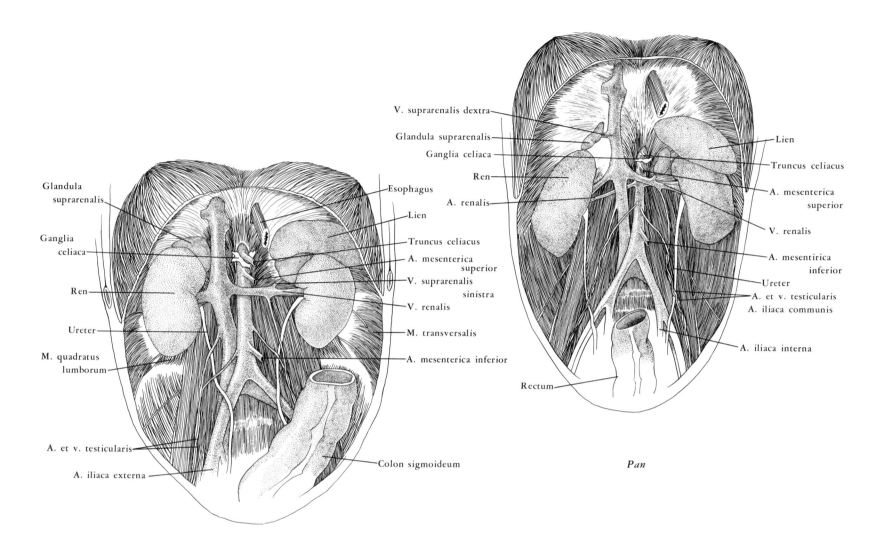

Glandula
suprarenalis

Ganglia
celiaca

Ren

Ureter

M. quadratus
lumborum

A. et v. testicularis

A. iliaca externa

Esophagus

Lien

Truncus celiacus

A. mesenterica
superior

V. suprarenalis
sinistra

V. renalis

M. transversalis

A. mesenterica inferior

Colon sigmoideum

Homo

V. suprarenalis dextra

Glandula suprarenalis

Ganglia celiaca

Ren

A. renalis

Lien

Truncus celiacus

A. mesenterica
superior

V. renalis

A. mesentirica
inferior

Ureter

A. et v. testicularis
A. iliaca communis

A. iliaca interna

Rectum

Pan

PLATE 107

Lumbosacral Plexus

Among primates there is a marked variability in the number of ventral primary rami of lumbar and sacral spinal nerves forming the lumbosacral plexus. Also, there is much variability concerning the participation of the spinal nerves to the various nerves emerging from the plexus. In *Papio* and *Homo* there are twelve pairs of ribs, whereas *Pan* has thirteen pairs. There are usually four lumbar vertebrae in *Pan,* five in *Homo,* and seven in *Papio.* These anatomical differences lead to numerous difficulties when enumerating the similarities and differences in the mode of formation of the plexus among these three primates (Zuckerman 1938; Gourmain 1966; Urbanowicz and Zaluska 1969).

The subcostal nerve joins with L1 to form the iliohypogastric nerve in the majority of cases in *Pan* and about 50 percent of the time in *Homo;* it remains independent of the lumbar plexus most of the time in *Papio* (Sonntag 1923; Francis 1966; Hill 1970). In *Papio* the iliohypogastric and ilioinguinal nerves are formed from L1 and L2, while L3 unites with L4 to form the large genitofemoral nerve. In *Homo* and *Pan* the three nerves are usually formed by T12 (T13) and L1, with the genitofemoral receiving a contribution from L2 in *Homo.* The femoral and obturator nerves are large in all three primates. In *Papio* they arise from L4-L6, although they have been reported as high as L2-L4 (Soutoul et al. 1966). In *Pan* they normally result from the union of L1-L3, while in *Homo* the usual mode of formation is L2-L4. The former condition is referred to as a prefixed plexus in anthropotomy.

The large lumbosacral trunk is mainly formed by L5-L7 and S1 in *Papio,* while in *Pan* it is made up of contributions from L3-L4 and S1-S2. In *Homo* this portion of the plexus is formed by L4-L5 and S1-S3. The important pudendal nerve is formed by S1-S2 in *Papio,* S2-S4 in *Homo,* and S2-S3 in *Pan.* In *Pan* the nerve may represent the single ventral primary ramus of S2 (Sonntag 1923). The extremely large sciatic nerve is composed of L5-L7 and S1 in *Papio.* In *Pan* it results from the union of L3-L4 and S1-S3. The major difference between *Pan* and *Homo* is that the cranial portion of *Homo*'s sciatic nerve is formed by L4 and L5.

Note the presence of two nerves in *Papio* that are not present in *Homo,* the flexores femoris and puboischiofemoris. The former nerve may be found in *Pan.* In both *Papio* and *Pan* the flexores femoris is simply a separate nerve from the ventral aspect of the sciatic which innervates the hamstring muscles (Howell and Straus 1933a) (Plate 121). In *Homo* and *Pan* the puboischiofemoris is represented by separate musclar rami to the short ischiopubofemoral musculature of the hip.

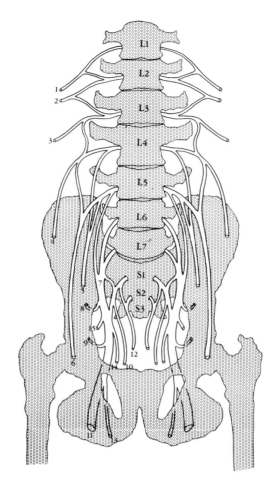

Papio

1   N. iliohypogastricus
2   N. ilioinguinalis
3   N. genitofemoralis
4   N. cutaneus femoris lateralis
5   N. obturatorius
6   N. femoralis
7   Truncus lumbosacralis
8   N. gluteus superior
9   N. gluteus inferior
10   N. cutaneus femoris posterior
11   N. ischiadicus
12   N. pudendus
13   N. flexores femoris
14   N. pubo-ischiofemoralis
15   Rami musculares (to M. piriformis)
16   Rami musculares (to Mm. obturatorius internus et gemellus superior)
17   Rami musculares (to Mm. quadratus femoris et gemellus inferior)

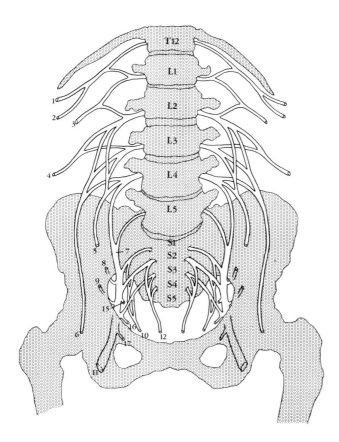

Homo

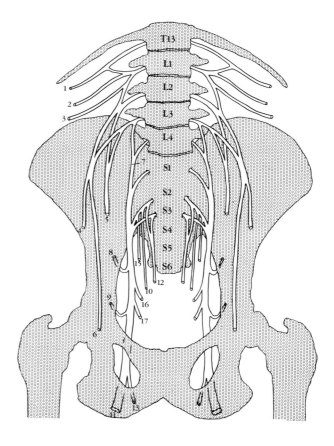

Pan

Part 7

PELVIS

PLATE 108

Male Pelvis

The urogenital organs of the pelvis lie in more or less similar positions in the three primates and will be discussed from ventral to dorsal.

The urinary bladder varies in size depending upon its state of distention. In *Pan* it is shown inflated, with much of the body occupying a suprapubic position. The muscular wall is thick and it is especially well developed in the region of the trigone.

The seminal vesicles lie on the dorsal surface of the urinary bladder. In *Papio* they are large, lobulated glands; in the adult animal they are relatively larger than in *Homo*. Each gland is made up of numerous coiled tubes held together by connective tissue forming a more complex structure than in *Homo* or *Pan*. They communicate with the vas deferens near the apex of the urinary bladder.

The prostate gland is well developed in the three primates; however, the large ventral lobe of *Homo* is absent in *Papio*. Consequently, the urethra is not completely surrounded by prostatic tissue. In *Pan* the gland unites anteriorly, although the ventral lobe is small. A similar arrangement is reported in the gorilla (Raven 1950). The prostate is divisible into four lobes in *Papio*, a conspicuous cranial and caudal lobe and two poorly differentiated lateral lobes. This configuration was first reported by Mijsberg (1923) and later by Hill (1970).

There are two large bulbo-urethral glands lying outside of the urogenital diaphragm in *Papio*. These glands are much smaller, and are situated within the urogenital diaphragm in *Pan* and *Homo*. They are particularly minute in *Pan,* and they are apparently absent in the gorilla (Raven 1950). Their small, thin ducts open into the bulbar portion of the urethra.

The penis of *Papio* is unusually long for catarrhines. The shaft is composed of erectile tissue, which is capped externally by a well-defined glans. The base or bulb of the penis contains a large amount of erectile tissue which is covered by the bulbocavernosus muscle. Note the levator penis muscle passing along the dorsum of the penis. It is absent in *Pan* and *Homo*.

The os penis or baculum is present in *Papio* and *Pan,* although it is not shown in the latter primate. It is embedded in the right side of the glans penis in *Papio*, whereas in *Macaca mulatta* it deviates to the left (Wislocki 1933).

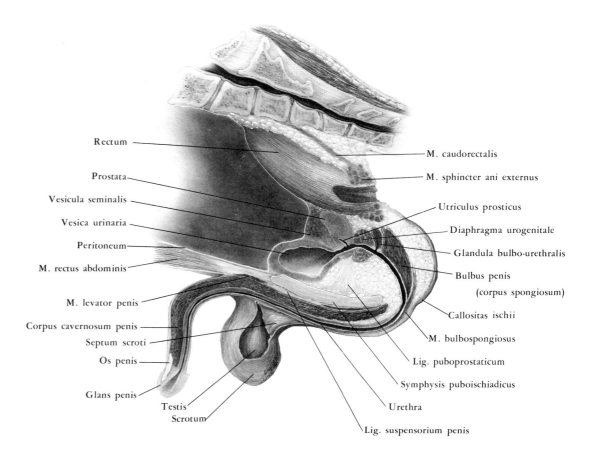

Papio

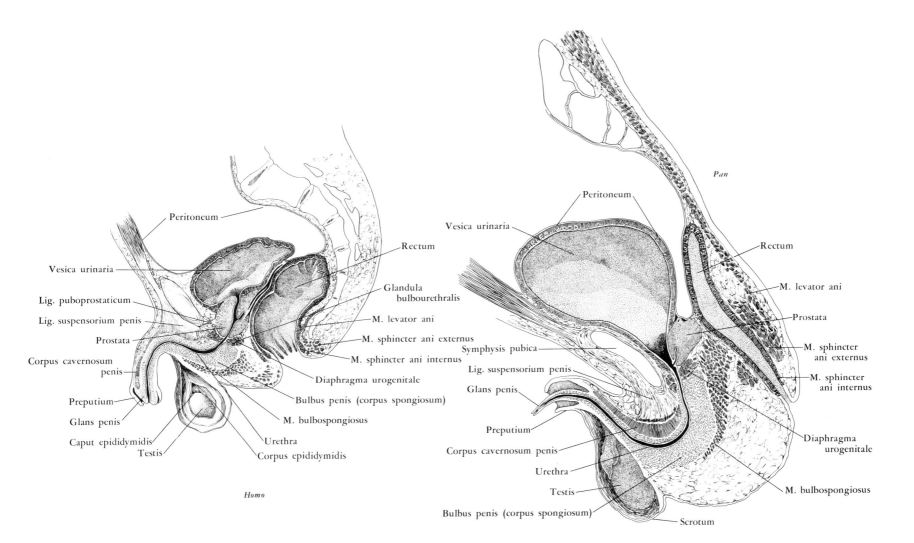

Peritoneum

Vesica urinaria

Lig. puboprostaticum

Lig. suspensorium penis

Prostata

Corpus cavernosum
penis

Preputium

Glans penis

Caput epididymidis

Testis

Rectum

Glandula
bulbourethralis

M. levator ani

M. sphincter ani externus

M. sphincter ani internus

Diaphragma urogenitale

Bulbus penis (corpus spongiosum)

M. bulbospongiosus

Urethra

Corpus epididymidis

Homo

Pan

Peritoneum

Vesica urinaria

Symphysis pubica

Lig. suspensorium penis

Glans penis

Preputium

Corpus cavernosum penis

Urethra

Testis

Bulbus penis (corpus spongiosum)

Rectum

M. levator ani

Prostata

M. sphincter
ani externus

M. sphincter
ani internus

Diaphragma
urogenitale

M. bulbospongiosus

Scrotum

PLATE 109

Female Pelvis

The urinary bladder of the female is a thick-walled organ lying dorsal to the pubic bone. In *Pan* the body of the bladder is more suprapubic in position than in *Papio* or *Homo,* and the urachus is absent. Sonntag (1923) also reported the absence of the urachus in a female *Pan.* The urethra is a short, muscular tube extending along the ventral wall of the vagina. It opens into the ventral portion of the genital passage, just dorsal to the clitoris. In adult female *Papio* the urethra is approximately an inch long, whereas it courses for five to eight inches in the male (Plate 108).

The uterus is piriform in outline and is extremely muscular. It is divided into two main portions, the body and the cervix. In *Papio,* and especially in *Pan,* the long axis of the uterus is inclined ventrally only slightly from the direction taken by the vagina. A similar orientation is reported in female gorillas (Atkinson and Elftman 1950). In *Homo* the uterus presents a marked ventral inclination at the junction between body and cervix.

The body of the uterus is covered with peritoneum that extends from the lateral sides of the uterus to the pelvic walls as the broad ligament. An additional uterine support, the round ligament, is shown only in *Papio.* This is a fibrous cord extending from the uterus ventrolaterally toward the abdominal inguinal ring. It passes through the inguinal canal to terminate in the labia majora.

The ovaries are small, globular bodies located lateral to the sides of the uterus. They are attached to the broad ligament by the short mesovarium. In addition to this attachment, the ovaries are connected to the sides of the uterus by the ovarian ligament. The uterine tubes extend laterally from the sides of the uterus to the lateral wall of the pelvis, where they expand to form the infundibulae. The tubes are located in the free edge of the mesosalpinx, which is a fold of the peritoneum.

The vaginal portion of the cervix projects into the lumen of the vagina for some distance. In *Papio* the dorsal labium is much thicker and longer than the anterior lip; consequently, the dorsal fornix is deeper than the ventral one. In *Homo* the ventral labium is thicker than the dorsal labium. The uterine ostium is bounded by the two labia.

The vagina is a highly dilatable muscular canal extending from the uterus to the exterior. The interior of the vagina, lined with mucous membrane, is highly rugose, the folds being mainly directed longitudinally.

The external genitalia comprise the labia majora, labia minora, clitoris, and vestibule. The clitoris is especially well developed in *Papio* and *Pan,* reaching an inch or more in length in adult *Papio ursinus* (Hill 1970). Both labia majora and labia minora are present in the three primates, although the labia majora are not pronounced in *Papio.* The presence of a hymen is questionable in *Papio* and *Pan:* Sonntag (1923) did not find it in his young chimpanzee, nor were we able to detect it in our young specimens.

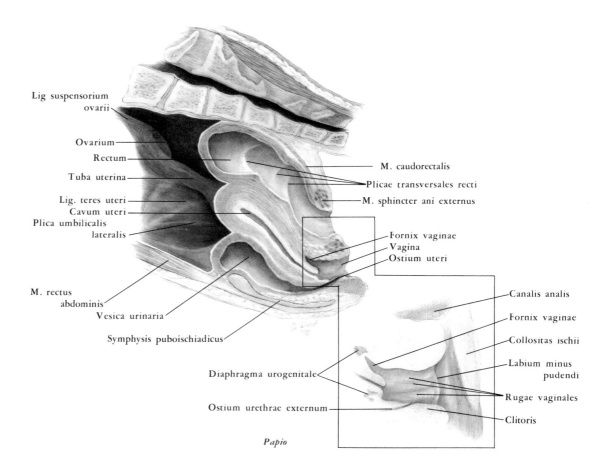

Papio

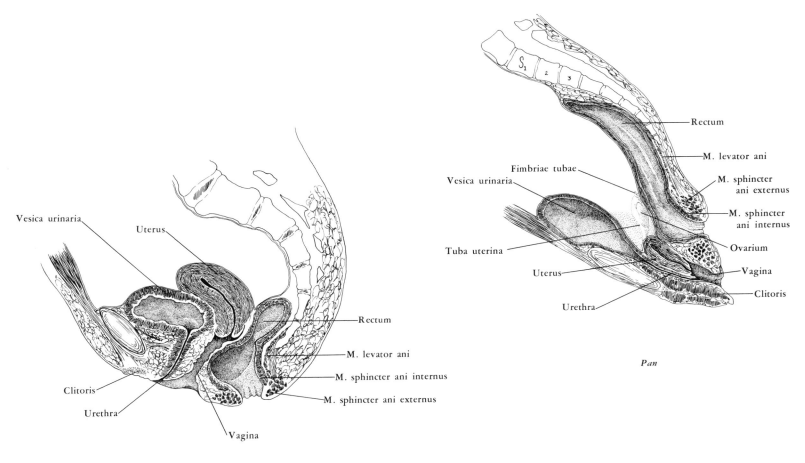

Vesica urinaria

Uterus

Rectum

M. levator ani

M. sphincter ani internus

M. sphincter ani externus

Clitoris

Urethra

Vagina

Homo

Fimbriae tubae

Vesica urinaria

Tuba uterina

Uterus

Urethra

Rectum

M. levator ani

M. sphincter ani externus

M. sphincter ani internus

Ovarium

Vagina

Clitoris

Pan

PLATE 110

Pelvis I

The arteries of the pelvis display considerable variability regarding their origins in all three primates. Also, the pattern is often different between the right and left sides of the same animal. Indeed, these differences of arterial patterns led Glidden and De Garis (1936) to state that this variability "may well be taken to signify the great lability of these regions in respect to vascular distribution" (p. 518).

In the caudal lumbar region the abdominal aorta bifurcates into the right and left common iliac arteries. These, in turn, pass a short distance before dividing into the external and internal iliacs. The external iliac runs along the medial side of the psoas muscle toward the thigh, where it becomes the femoral artery. In *Papio* and *Homo* there are normally two branches from the external iliac, the inferior epigastric and deep circumflex iliac. In *Pan* two additional arteries frequently arise from the external iliac, the medial femoral circumflex and the obturator. The former artery is extremely variable and has been observed arising from the external iliac, internal iliac, and obturator (ibid.).

The internal iliac divides into dorsal and ventral parts. In *Papio* the dorsal ramus constitutes the superior gluteal artery, whereas in *Pan* and *Homo* the lateral sacral and iliolumbar arteries also arise from this division. In *Papio* these arteries are usually branches of the middle sacral (caudal), which arises from the dorsal side of the aorta before its bifurcation.

The ventral division gives rise to all other branches of the internal iliac. The inferior gluteal and internal pudendal are the largest of these branches. The vesical arteries pass to the bladder, where they ramify upon the cranial and caudal surfaces of the organ. A small deferential artery accompanies the ductus deferens in the male. This artery is considered the homologue of the uterine artery of the female. A vaginal artery is also present in the female. The middle rectal arteries arise from the internal pudendal just before it passes out of the pelvis beneath the caudal border of the piriformis muscle. They anastomose with the superior and inferior rectals on the wall of the rectum. The obturator artery passes through the pelvis in company with the obturator nerve. Both exit the pelvis through the obturator foramen. Note that in *Papio* the medial femoral circumflex artery arises from the obturator. The umbilical artery is usually the first branch of the ventral ramus of the internal iliac, especially in *Homo*. In the adult animal, it is fibrous and lacks a lumen for most of its course to the umbilicus.

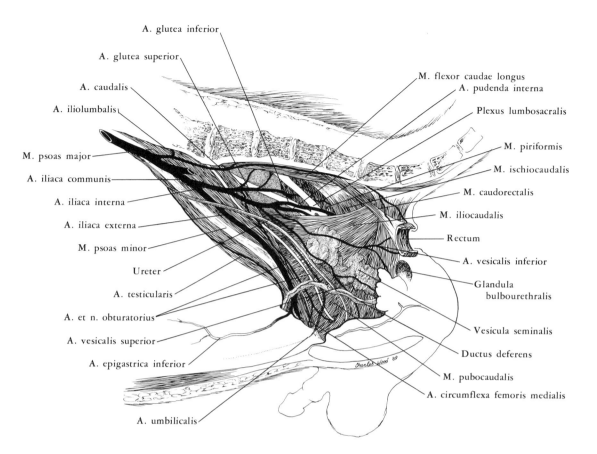

Papio

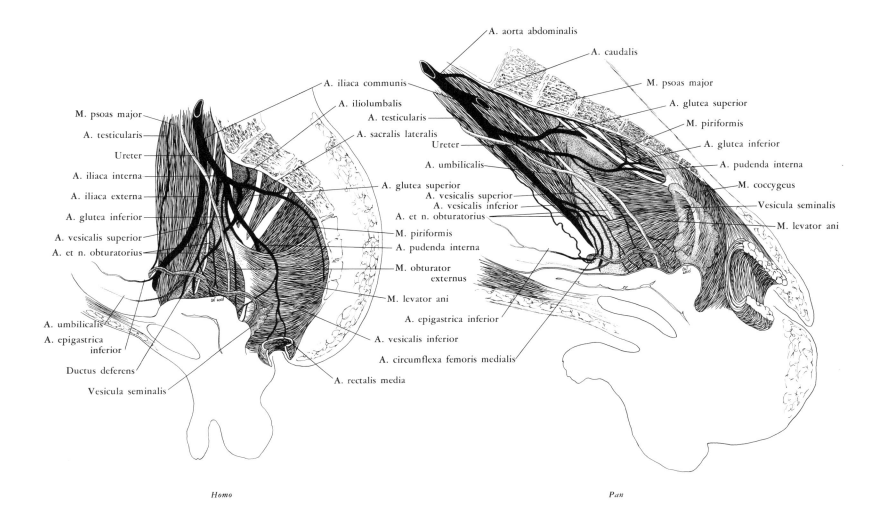

A. psoas major
A. testicularis
Ureter
A. iliaca interna
A. iliaca externa
A. glutea inferior
A. vesicalis superior
A. et n. obturatorius

A. umbilicalis
A. epigastrica
inferior
Ductus deferens
Vesicula seminalis

A. iliaca communis
A. iliolumbalis
A. testicularis
A. sacralis lateralis
A. glutea superior
M. piriformis
A. pudenda interna
M. obturator
externus
M. levator ani
A. epigastrica inferior
A. vesicalis inferior
A. circumflexa femoris medialis
A. rectalis media

Homo

A. aorta abdominalis
A. caudalis
M. psoas major
A. glutea superior
M. piriformis
A. glutea inferior
A. pudenda interna
M. coccygeus
Vesicula seminalis
M. levator ani

A. testicularis
Ureter
A. umbilicalis
A. vesicalis superior
A. vesicalis inferior
A. et n. obturatorius

Pan

PLATE 111

Pelvis II

The musculature of the pelvic outlet is substantially different in *Papio* than it is in *Pan* and *Homo*. *Papio* is a quadrupedal primate possessing a tail, and the functional relations of these muscles are primarily associated with the tail. In *Pan* and *Homo* these muscles are modified into a sling, or diaphragm, more intimately related to the pelvic viscera.

In *Papio* the iliocaudalis is a broad muscle running from the pelvic brim to the lateral side of the third caudal vertebra. The pubocaudalis has an aponeurotic origin from the medial surface of the puboischiadic symphysis. From this broad origin the fibers converge to attach to the second and third caudal vertebrae. Occasionally, fibers of this muscle attach to the rectum as shown here, thereby aiding in the support of this structure. The ischiocaudalis is a well-developed muscle lying dorsal to the iliocaudalis. It arises from the body of the ischium and the diminutive ischial spine, and passes toward the tail to attach to the last sacral and first two or three caudal vertebrae. These three muscles are abductors and flexors of the tail.

In the absence of a tail, the pubocaudalis and iliocaudalis attach to the rectum, forming the levator ani muscle in *Pan* and *Homo*. The muscle is divisible into three portions: an iliococcygeal, a pubococcygeal, and a puborectal. The two levator ani muscles arise from the pubis and the arcus tendineus and pass toward the midline, where the iliococcygeal fibers terminate in the anococcygeal ligament. The puborectal and pubococcygeal portions attach mainly to the rectum as well as forming a space through which pass the vagina and urethra in the female, and the lower part of the prostate and membranous urethra in the male. The ischiocaudalis of *Papio* is the coccygeus of *Pan* and *Homo*. Thus, the levator ani and coccygeus muscles of the two sides form a muscular support for the pelvic viscera.

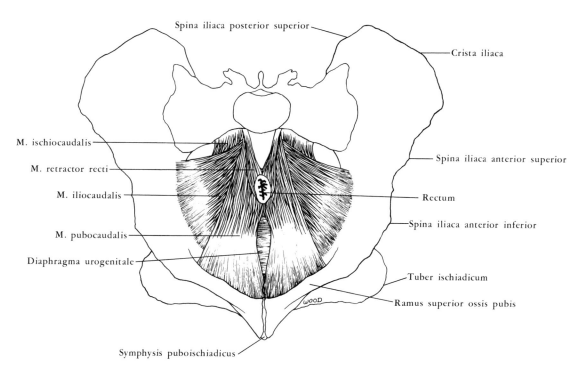

Papio

234

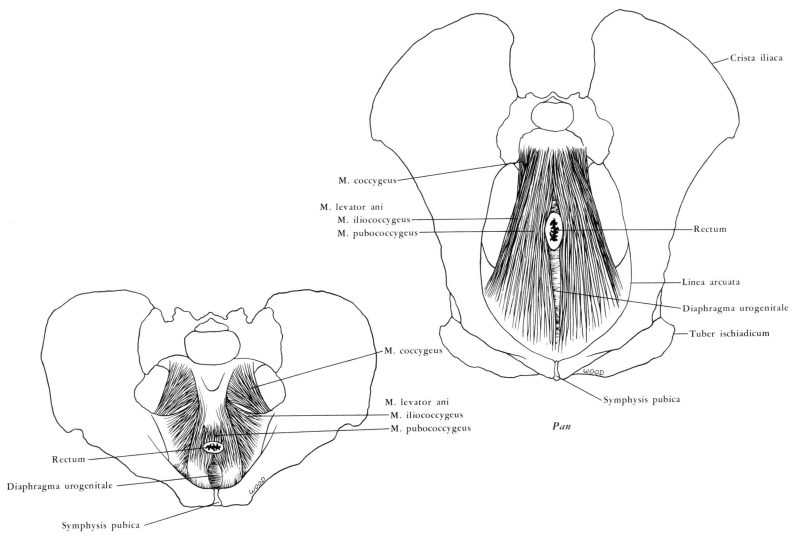

M. coccygeus

M. levator ani
M. iliococcygeus
M. pubococcygeus

Rectum

Crista iliaca

Rectum

Linea arcuata

Diaphragma urogenitale

Tuber ischiadicum

Symphysis pubica

Pan

M. coccygeus

M. levator ani
M. iliococcygeus
M. pubococcygeus

Rectum

Diaphragma urogenitale

Symphysis pubica

Homo

PLATE 112

Pelvis III

In *Papio,* the puboiliocaudal complex has been partially removed to expose the underlying obturator internus muscle. The counterpart of these muscles, the levator ani, has likewise been removed in *Pan* and *Homo.*

The obturator internus is a broad, flat, triangular muscle arising from the medial surface of the inferior ischiopubic rami and from the obturator membrane. In *Papio* the muscle is more or less divisible into two parts. The cranial or major portion converges to form a tendon that passes out of the pelvis caudal to the small ischial spine through the lesser sciatic notch. The caudal portion arises from the medial side of the ischial tuberosity to attach to the major tendon, which then passes to the medial side of the greater trochanter of the femur. The muscle is not divisible in *Pan* or *Homo.*

The piriformis is usually a distinct structure in all three primates, although in catarrhines it may not be completely differentiated from the gluteus medius (Howell and Straus 1933b). In *Papio* the muscle passes from the last two sacral vertebrae to the medial aspect of the greater trochanter.

In addition to these muscles, *Papio* possesses a retractor recti and caudorectalis. These muscles pass from the lateral sides of the first three or four caudal vertebrae to the rectum. In the female, some of the fibers of the retractor recti pass to the vagina. In *Macaca mulatta* these two muscles are composed entirely of smooth muscle fibers (ibid.).

A portion of the sacral plexus is shown lying on the medioventral surface of the piriformis muscle. The large sciatic nerve is hidden by the coccygeus muscle as it leaves the pelvis caudal to the piriformis. The pudendal nerve lies close to the sciatic as it exits the pelvic cavity on its way to the perineum.

Observe the obturator nerve passing along the lateral wall of the pelvis. In *Papio* the nerve courses between the iliocaudalis and pubocaudalis muscles before piercing the obturator internus to pass through the obturator foramen.

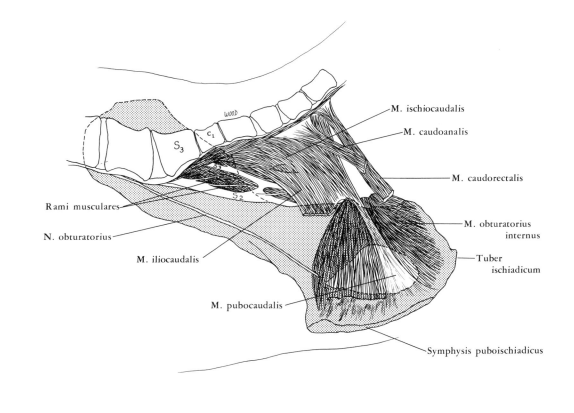

Papio

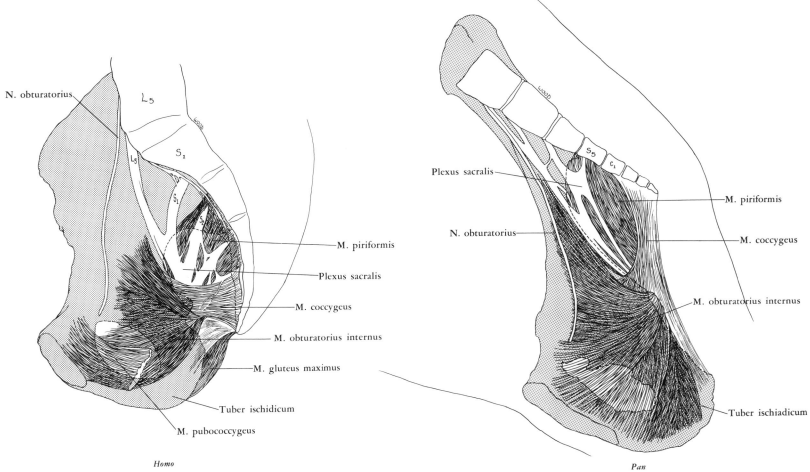

N. obturatorius

L₅

S₁

L₅

S₁

N. obturatorius

Plexus sacralis

Homo

M. piriformis

Plexus sacralis

M. coccygeus

M. obturatorius internus

M. gluteus maximus

Tuber ischidicum

M. pubococcygeus

S₅

C₁

M. piriformis

M. coccygeus

M. obturatorius internus

Tuber ischiadicum

Pan

Part 8

INFERIOR MEMBER

PLATE 113

Superficial Veins

The veins of the inferior member are divided into superficial and deep systems. The deep veins accompany their corresponding arteries and have similar names. Venae comitantes (companion veins) accompany these arteries. The superficial veins lie in the superficial fascia and begin in the plexuses of the foot. Two veins, the great and small saphenous, are much larger than the others and warrant special attention.

In *Homo* the great saphenous vein commences on the dorsomedial side of the foot and courses through the leg and thigh, receiving numerous cutaneous tributaries before joining the femoral vein. The small saphenous vein begins on the dorsolateral side of the foot and ascends along the posterior side of the leg to the popliteal fossa, where it normally drains into the popliteal vein.

The drainage pattern in *Papio* is different in that the great saphenous vein is normally absent. Lineback (1933) states, however, that it is "more constantly present" in *Macaca mulatta.* There are numerous superficial veins in the leg and thigh, but none of these ever forms a single vessel, as in man. Rather, on the medial side of the leg, venae comitantes accompany the saphenous artery. These normally drain into the femoral vein some distance proximal to the knee. A pronounced small saphenous vein is always present on the lateral side of the foot and leg. Indeed, this vessel drains the majority of the dorsal foot. As in man, it enters the popliteal vein.

Pan is more similar to *Homo* in drainage pattern, possessing both saphenous veins. In addition, there are venae comitantes accompanying the saphenous artery on the medial side of the foot and leg. They are similar in position to those in *Papio.*

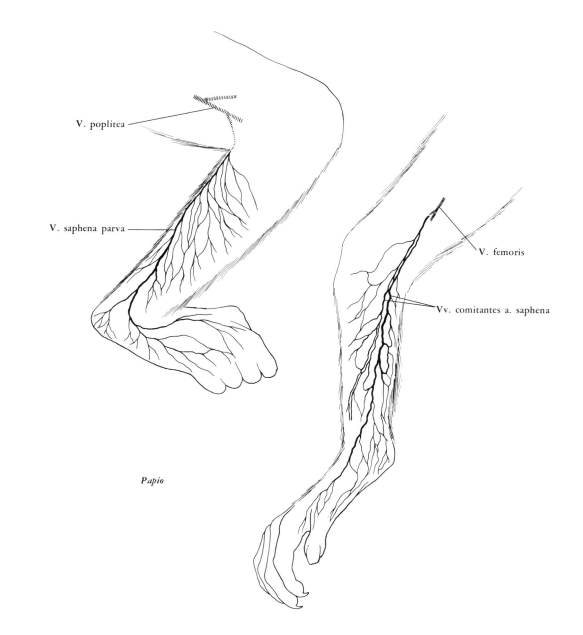

V. poplitea

V. saphena parva

V. femoris

Vv. comitantes a. saphena

Papio

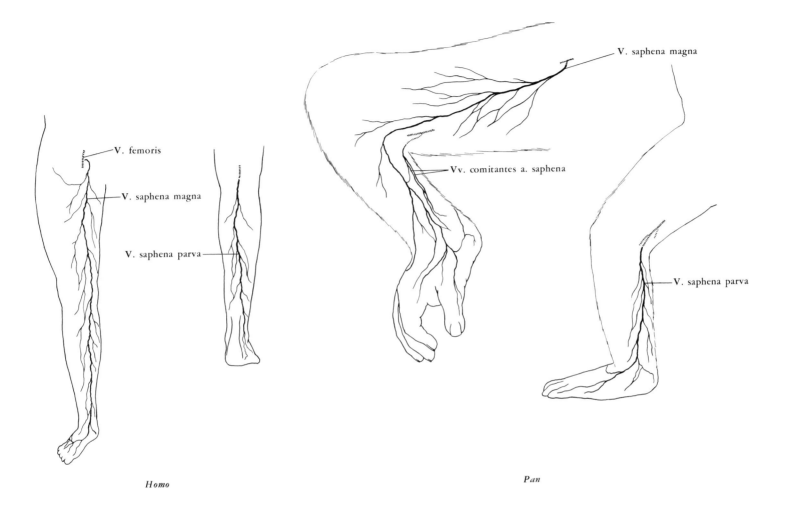

V. femoris

V. saphena magna

V. saphena parva

V. saphena magna

Vv. comitantes a. saphena

V. saphena parva

Homo

Pan

PLATE 114

Cutaneous Nerves

The cutaneous nerves are sensory branches of deeper-lying motor nerves. These branches appear subcutaneously at different locations throughout the inferior limb and thenceforth course in the superficial fascia to supply the skin. The formation, position, and distribution are variable, and the patterns depicted represent the most common arrangement observed. There is a general similarity in pattern among the three primates, although certain minor differences may be noted.

The cutaneous nerves on the ventral aspect of the inferior limb are similar in the three animals. Of the femoral branches supplying the skin of the ventral thigh, only the saphenous nerve passes distal to the knee. This nerve usually extends halfway along the medial border of the foot in the three primates. Occasionally, the cutaneous ramus of the obturator nerve extends to the calf in *Homo*. This was not observed in *Papio* or *Pan*. The remaining ventral cutaneous nerves are very similar in distribution.

On the posterior side of the inferior limb the posterior femoral cutaneous nerve in *Papio* becomes subcutaneous between the gluteus maximus muscle and the lateral margin of the ischial tuberosity and, therefore, occupies a more lateral position than in *Pan* or *Homo*. It supplies the ischial callosity as well as the skin of the lateral thigh.

The manner of formation of the sural nerve warrants attention. According to Huelke (1957), the sural nerve in *Homo* may be formed by: (1) the union of the medial sural cutaneous with the peroneal communicating branch of the common peroneal; (2) the continuation of the medial sural cutaneous nerve; (3) the continuation of the peroneal communicating branch. He found the first type of formation in some 80 percent of human cadavers. In *Papio* and *Pan* the medial sural and peroneal communicating branches remain separate, and the medial sural nerve is large. This arrangement was also noted by Howell and Straus (1933a) in *Macaca mulatta* and by Hill (1970) in *Papio*. The other nerves are very similar in their positions in the three primates.

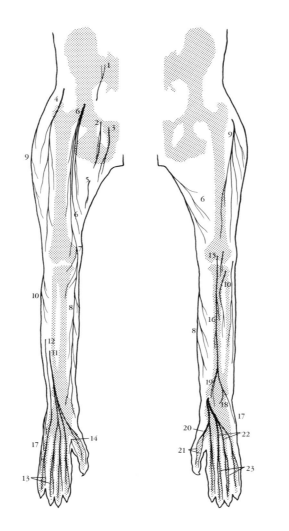

Papio

1 N. iliohypogastricus
2 N. ilioinguinalis
  N. genitofemoralis
3   Ramus femoralis
4 N. cutaneus femoris lateralis
  N. obturatorius
5   Ramus cutaneus
  N. femoralis
6   Rami cutanei anteriores
7   N. saphenus
8   Rami cutanei cruris medialis
9 N. cutaneus femoris posterior
  N. ischiadicus
  N. peroneus communis
10   N. cutaneus surae lateralis
  N. peroneus superficialis
11   N. cutaneus dorsales medialis
12   N. cutaneus dorsales intermedius
13   Nn. digitales dorsales pedis
  N. peroneus profundus
14   Nn. digitales dorsales pedis
  N. tibialis
15   N. cutaneus surae medialis
16   N. suralis
17   N. cutaneus dorsalis lateralis
18   Rami calcanei laterales
19   Rami calcanei mediales
  N. plantaris medialis
20   Nn. digitalis plantares communes
21   Nn. digitalis plantares proprii
  N. plantares lateralis
22   Nn. digitalis plantares communes
23   Nn. digitalis plantares proprii

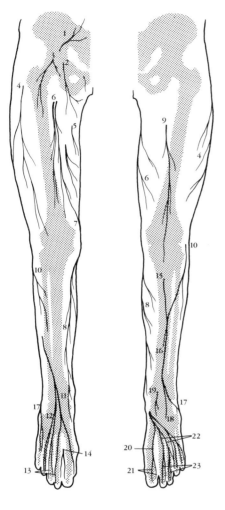

Homo

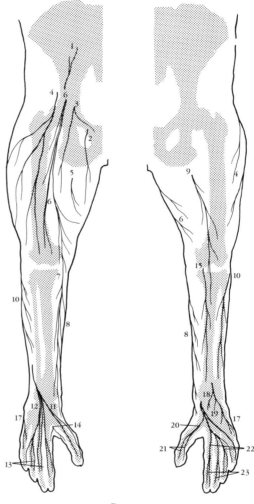

Pan

PLATE 115

Arterial Pattern

There is a great deal of intra- and interspecific variability regarding the mode of formation of these arteries. Only the major differences are considered here.

In the pelvis, the common iliac bifurcates into the internal and external iliacs. The external iliac continues onto the thigh as the femoral artery. The largest branch of the femoral artery is the deep femoral. In *Homo* it gives rise to the medial and lateral femoral circumflex arteries before passing distally through the thigh where it sends off several (usually four) perforating branches. In *Papio,* the medial femoral circumflex artery is a branch of the obturator artery from the internal iliac, although it may arise directly from the internal iliac in many cercopithecoids (Manners-Smith 1912). In *Pan* the medial femoral circumflex artery arises directly from the external iliac and takes over much of the obturator area of distribution (Glidden and De Garis 1936).

In *Homo* the descending genicular artery arises as the last branch of the femoral before it passes into the popliteal fossa to become the popliteal artery. The genicular artery gives a small, rather insignificant branch to the medial side of the knee and leg, the saphenous artery. The popliteal continues into the leg as the anterior and posterior tibial arteries. The posterior tibial gives rise to the large peroneal, which ends along the lateral surface of the calcaneus. At the ankle the anterior tibial becomes the dorsal pedal and the posterior tibial terminates as the medial and lateral plantar arteries. The lateral plantar anastomoses with the deep plantar branch of the dorsal pedal to form the plantar arch.

In *Papio* the saphenous artery arises directly from the femoral and is larger than the popliteal. It divides into anterior and posterior branches, which are the major sources of blood to the distal leg and foot. According to Manners-Smith (1912) and Hill (1970), the popliteal ends by dividing into the anterior tibial and peroneal arteries. Thus, there is no posterior tibial from the popliteal. In the present sample, a large branch from the popliteal was always observed passing distally through the posterior compartment of the leg. It terminates just proximal to the ankle. We believe this artery is the posterior tibial from its position and function, rather than designating the posterior tibial as the deep branch of the saphenous (Manners-Smith 1912; Hill 1970). Therefore, the medial and lateral plantar arteries are terminal branches of the posterior saphenous artery. The anterior tibial and peroneal arteries end just proximal to the ankle; the anterior saphenous gives rise to the superficial and deep dorsal pedal arteries. The plantar arch is present if there is an anastomosis between the lateral plantar artery and the perforating branch from the dorsal pedal.

Pan displays similarities with both of these patterns. Thus, there is a large saphenous as well as a large posterior tibial artery from the popliteal. The latter, however, forms the medial and lateral plantars. The anterior tibial terminates proximal to the ankle and the dorsal pedal arises from the saphenous as in *Papio*. The peroneal artery has a distribution similar to that in man.

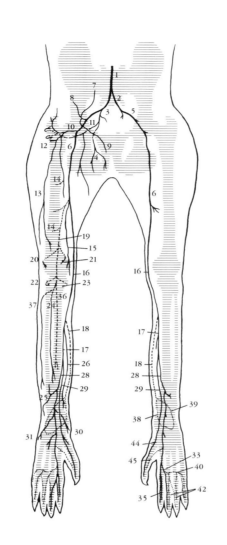

Papio

1 Aorta abdominalis
2 A. iliaca communis
3 A. iliaca interna
4 A. obturatoria
5 A. iliaca externa
6 A. femoralis
7 A. epigastrica superficialis
8 A. circumflexa ilium superficialis
9 A. pudenda externa
10 A. profunda femoris
11 A. circumflexa femoris medialis
12 A. circumflexa femoris lateralis
13 R. descendens
14 Aa. perforantes
15 A. genu suprema
16 A. saphena
17 R. anterior
18 R. posterior
19 A. poplitea
20 A. genus superior lateralis
21 A. genus superior medialis
22 A. genus inferior lateralis
23 A. genus inferior medialis
24 A. tibialis anterior
25 A. malleolaris lateralis
26 A. malleolaris medialis
27 A. dorsalis pedis
28 A. dorsalis pedis profundus
29 A. dorsalis pedis superficialis
30 A. tarsea medialis
31 A. tarsea lateralis
32 A. arcuata
33 R. plantaris profundus
34 Aa. metatarseae dorsales
35 Aa. digitales dorsales
36 A. tibialis posterior
37 A. peronea
38 A. plantaris medialis
39 A. plantaris lateralis
40 Arcus plantaris
41 Aa. metatarseae plantares
42 Aa. digitales plantares
43 Aa. perforantes
44 A. dorsalis hallucis
45 A. ventralis hallucis

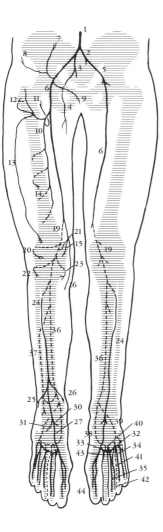

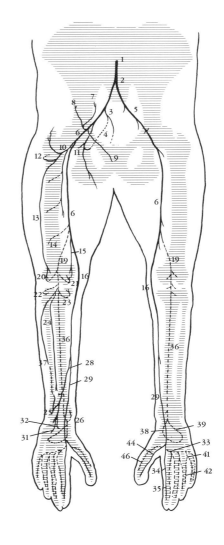

Homo

Pan

PLATE 116

Anterior Thigh I

The muscles of the anterior thigh (extensor group) are composed of the quadriceps femoris and the sartorius. The former is composed of the rectus femoris, vastus lateralis, vastus medialis, and vastus intermedius. With the exception of the sartorius and rectus femoris, these muscles are covered by a firm sheet of fascia in *Papio,* the iliotibial tract. In *Pan* and *Homo* the iliotibial tract is limited more to the lateral aspect of the thigh.

In *Homo* the sartorius arises from the anterior superior spine of the ilium, whereas its origin is caudal to the iliac crest along the acetabular border of the ilium in both *Papio* and *Pan* (Plate 144). The rectus femoris has two heads of origin in *Homo,* the "straight" head from the anterior inferior spine of the ilium and the "reflected" tendon from the cranial surface of the acetabulum. Normally, there is a single head of origin in *Papio* caudal to the anterior inferior spine. *Pan* also has a single head which has been noted by Champneys (1871) and Sonntag (1923). For a detailed discussion of muscle-bone homologies, see Benton and Gavan 1960. In the three animals, the quadriceps femoris terminates as the patella tendon, which is inserted to the tuberosity of the tibia.

Several muscles of the medial thigh (adductors) are visible in this plate. These muscles are considered in detail in Plate 118.

On the lateral side of the thigh, note the tensor fascia latae, and in *Papio,* the gluteus maximus. Both of these muscles belong to the posterior group and are discussed later. However, their anterior position should be noted in *Papio,* especially that of the gluteus maximus. These two muscles are fused in their upper portions, a condition only infrequently encountered in *Homo* and the anthropoids.

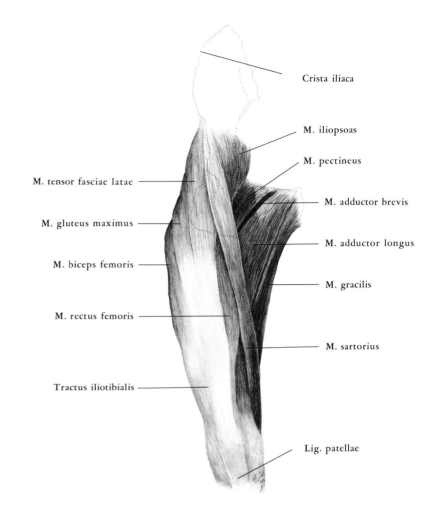

Crista iliaca

M. iliopsoas

M. pectineus

M. tensor fasciae latae

M. adductor brevis

M. adductor longus

M. gluteus maximus

M. gracilis

M. biceps femoris

M. rectus femoris

M. sartorius

Tractus iliotibialis

Lig. patellae

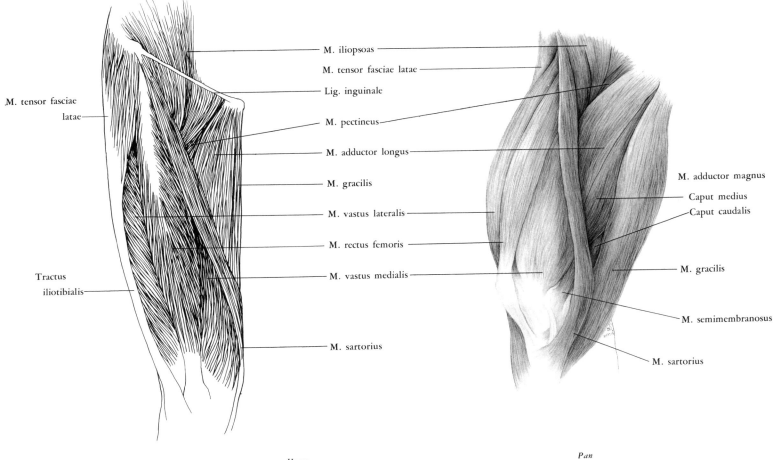

M. iliopsoas

M. tensor fasciae latae

Lig. inguinale

M. pectineus

M. adductor longus

M. gracilis

M. vastus lateralis

M. rectus femoris

M. vastus medialis

M. sartorius

M. tensor fasciae latae

Tractus iliotibialis

M. adductor magnus

Caput medius

Caput caudalis

M. gracilis

M. semimembranosus

M. sartorius

Homo

Pan

PLATE 117

Anterior Thigh II

According to Howell and Straus (1933b) the inguinal ligament is present only in man and gorilla. Miller (1947), on the other hand, says that it is absent in gorilla. In *Papio* and *Pan* a true inguinal ligament—the caudal free margin of the external oblique aponeurosis, extending from the anterior superior iliac spine to the pubic tubercle—is replaced by a series of aponeurotic crural arches (Straus 1929; Benton and Gavan 1960).

In *Pan* and *Papio* the lateral femoral cutaneous nerve appears in the thigh lateral to the origin of the sartorius muscle, near the lateral point of fixation of the crural arch. In *Homo* the nerve emerges from beneath the inguinal ligament medial to the sartorius.

In *Papio* the sartorius has been cut to show the subjacent structures lying within the femoral triangle. Note the lateral position of the femoral nerve compared to its position in *Pan* and *Homo*. The femoral vein has been removed from the medial side of the femoral artery. These vessels are very close together as they course through the femoral triangle. The medial femoral circumflex artery is shown descending from its pelvic origin in *Papio* (Plate 115). For most of its course through the thigh, the femoral artery lies deep to the sartorius; therefore, a femoral pulse is easier felt just distal to the emergence of the artery into the thigh. The deep femoral artery is observed giving rise to the lateral femoral circumflex artery before passing deep to the adductor longus muscle to supply the musculature in the posterior region. In addition, in *Homo* the medial femoral circumflex artery is usually a branch of the deep femoral or femoral.

The anterior division of the obturator nerve is visible between the adductor longus and gracilis muscles in *Papio*. This branch of the obturator lies dorsal to the pectineus and adductor longus, and ventral to the adductor brevis and adductor magnus muscles. The obturator supplies the adductor muscles.

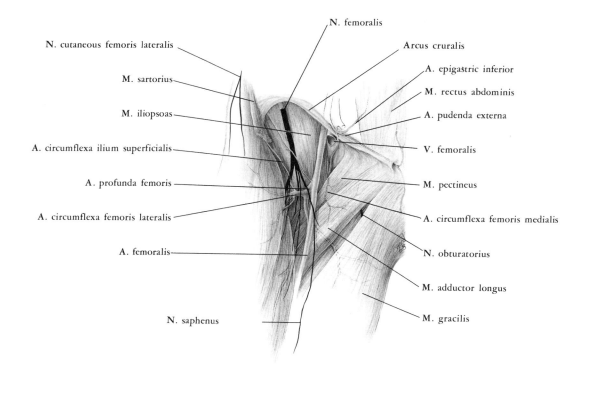

N. cutaneous femoris lateralis

M. sartorius

M. iliopsoas

A. circumflexa ilium superficialis

A. profunda femoris

A. circumflexa femoris lateralis

A. femoralis

N. saphenus

N. femoralis

Arcus cruralis

A. epigastric inferior

M. rectus abdominis

A. pudenda externa

V. femoralis

M. pectineus

A. circumflexa femoris medialis

N. obturatorius

M. adductor longus

M. gracilis

Papio

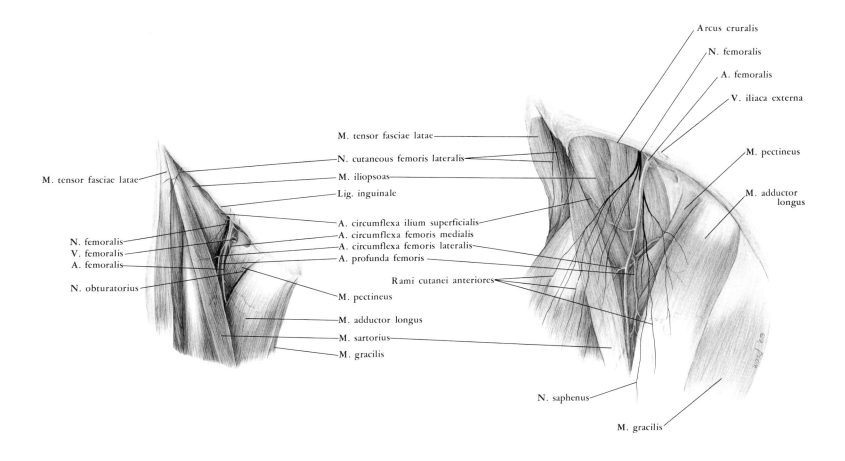

M. tensor fasciae latae

N. cutaneous femoris lateralis

M. iliopsoas

Lig. inguinale

A. circumflexa ilium superficialis

A. circumflexa femoris medialis

A. circumflexa femoris lateralis

A. profunda femoris

Rami cutanei anteriores

M. pectineus

M. adductor longus

M. sartorius

M. gracilis

M. tensor fasciae latae

N. femoralis

V. femoralis

A. femoralis

N. obturatorius

Homo

Arcus cruralis

N. femoralis

A. femoralis

V. iliaca externa

M. pectineus

M. adductor longus

N. saphenus

M. gracilis

Pan

PLATE 118

Medial Thigh I

Functionally, the major muscles of the medial thigh—the gracilis, pectineus, adductor longus, adductor brevis, and adductor magnus—are the adductors. In *Papio* the pectineus is supplied by the femoral nerve, the others by the obturator nerve. In *Pan* and *Homo* the pectineus receives motor fibers from both the femoral and obturator nerves. Also, the adductor magnus is dually innervated by the obturator and sciatic nerves since it represents the fusion of the semimembranosus accessorius with the adductor magnus element (Howell and Straus 1933b). The adductor magnus of the chimpanzee displays three heads of origin, of which the cranial and middle portions are united and attach to the femoral shaft, while the caudal head usually runs separately to the adductor tubercle. In *Papio* the adductor magnus is separated from the semi-membranosus accessorius and is usually divisible into two main portions. It should be noted that the semi-membranosus accessorius is named ischiocondyloideus by some students (Hill 1970; Uhlmann 1968). In *Papio* this muscle is clearly separate from the adductor magnus, and we follow Howell and Straus (1933b) in placing it with the hamstring muscles (ischiadic innervation) rather than with the adductor magnus (obturator innervation). As mentioned earlier, the muscle fuses with the adductor magnus in *Homo,* forming its distal portion.

The gracilis is a thin, wide muscle in *Papio* and *Pan,* especially in its cranial half. At its distal end the gracilis lies deep to the sartorius along the anteromedial border of the tibia.

The muscles of the anterior thigh are quite obvious in this view, particularly in *Papio* and *Homo*. They are less apparent in *Pan,* since the thigh is more laterally rotated when the animal is moving forward in its typical bent-knee gait. In this functional position, the broad gracilis, the cranial portion of the adductor magnus, and the semitendinosus stand out.

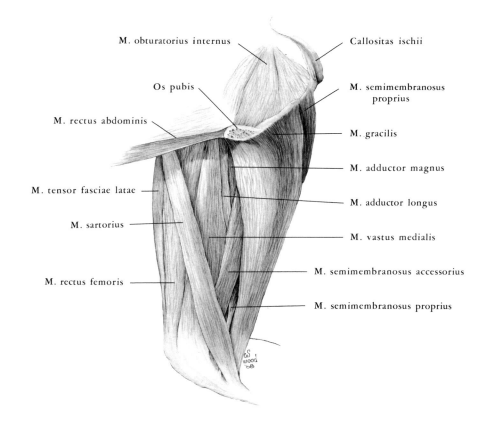

Papio

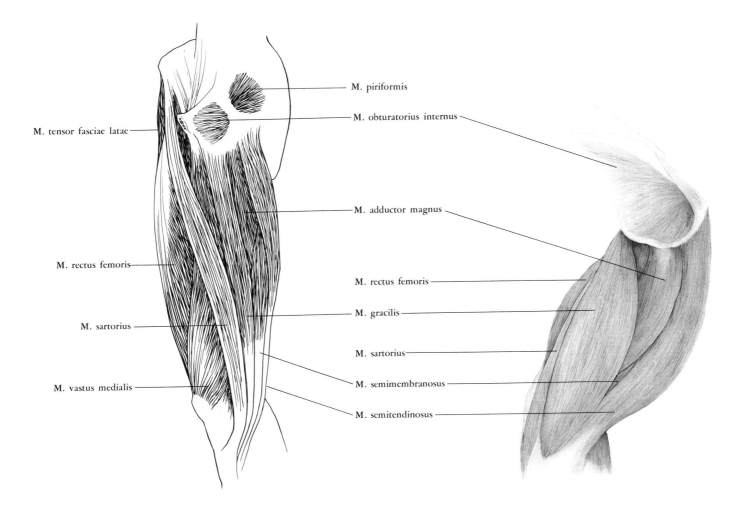

M. piriformis

M. obturatorius internus

M. tensor fasciae latae

M. adductor magnus

M. rectus femoris

M. rectus femoris

M. gracilis

M. sartorius

M. sartorius

M. semimembranosus

M. vastus medialis

M. semitendinosus

Homo

Pan

PLATE 119

Medial Thigh II

The more superficial muscles have been partly reflected or cut to expose the deeper-lying vessels and nerves. Observe the femoral artery disappearing cranial to the semimembranosus accessorius in *Papio* to become the popliteal artery on the posterior surface of the knee. In *Pan* the femoral vessels pass between the middle and caudal portions of the adductor magnus muscle to the popliteal space. These vessels pass through the adductor hiatus in *Homo*.

The saphenous nerve accompanies the femoral artery in its course deep to the sartorius (adductor canal) becoming superficial between the sartorius and gracilis to descend along the medial border of the tibia. In *Homo* a very small saphenous artery is closely associated with the nerve. The saphenous artery in *Papio* is large and departs directly from the femoral just as this vessel passes deep to the semimembranosus accessorius. In *Pan* the saphenous artery branches from the femoral as it courses between the middle and caudal heads of the adductor magnus. This artery is an important source of blood to the distal leg and foot in *Papio*, but less so in *Pan*.

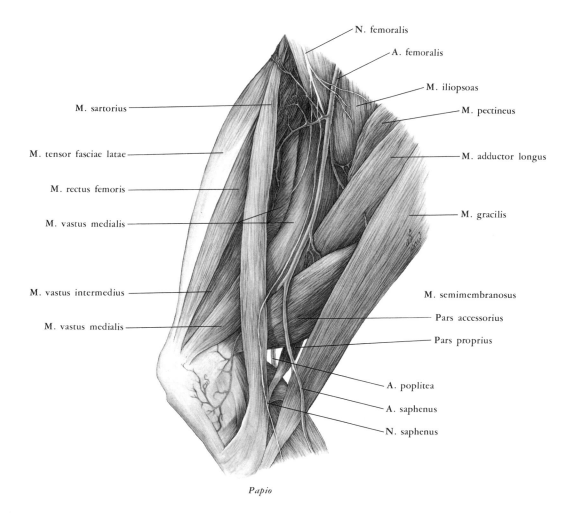

N. femoralis

A. femoralis

M. iliopsoas

M. pectineus

M. sartorius

M. adductor longus

M. tensor fasciae latae

M. rectus femoris

M. gracilis

M. vastus medialis

M. vastus intermedius

M. semimembranosus

Pars accessorius

M. vastus medialis

Pars proprius

A. poplitea

A. saphenus

N. saphenus

Papio

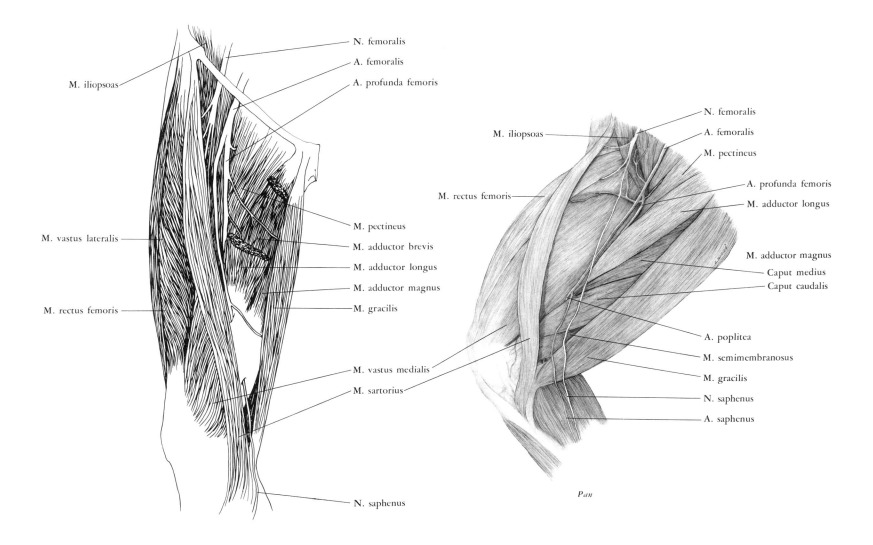

M. iliopsoas

N. femoralis

A. femoralis

A. profunda femoris

M. vastus lateralis

M. pectineus

M. adductor brevis

M. adductor longus

M. adductor magnus

M. gracilis

M. rectus femoris

M. vastus medialis

M. sartorius

N. saphenus

Homo

M. iliopsoas

M. rectus femoris

N. femoralis

A. femoralis

M. pectineus

A. profunda femoris

M. adductor longus

M. adductor magnus

Caput medius

Caput caudalis

A. poplitea

M. semimembranosus

M. gracilis

N. saphenus

A. saphenus

Pan

PLATE 120

Posterior Thigh

The muscles of the posterior thigh (hamstring group) are the semitendinosus, semimembranosus, and biceps femoris. They are primarily flexors of the leg, although when the knee is fixed, they also extend or retract the thigh.

The biceps femoris occupies much of the posterolateral aspect of the thigh, especially in *Papio*. In this species, as well as in all Old World monkeys, the biceps is not bicipital (Howell and Straus 1933b). Only the ischial or long head is present in these primates. The femoral or short head is present in *Pan* and *Homo,* making the muscle truly bicipital. It should be noted, however, that the biceps of *Papio* is partially separable throughout much of its extent; but if followed cranially, the muscle will be observed to converge to a single tendon of attachment to the ischial tuberosity. The muscle has a broad, extensive attachment to the fascia lata of the thigh and can be traced distally into the crural fascia nearly one-third of the way to the ankle. The cranial portion from the ischial tuberosity to the femur is often considered a separate muscle, the ischiofemoralis (see insert; also Uhlmann 1968; Hill 1970). Its distal extent is much less in *Pan* and *Homo*.

The semimembranosus and semitendinosus run along the posteromedial thigh. In *Papio* the former muscle is composed of two parts, a proper and accessory. Both arise from the ischial tuberosity, but the proper part attaches to the medial border of the tibia and the accessory portion to the medial shaft of the femur as far as the medial condyle. In *Homo* and *Pan* the accessory part is united with the adductor magnus, resulting in a compound muscle. The semitendinosus is intimately associated with the biceps femoris near their origins, but diverge quickly as they pass distally into the posterior thigh.

The gluteus maximus muscle is a powerful extensor of the thigh in *Homo,* whereas in nonhuman primates it is an abductor of the thigh. According to Sigmon and Robinson (1967) however, there is "no major difference in function of m. gluteus maximus in apes and in man" (p. 246). Note the different topographical position of the muscles in this posterior view.

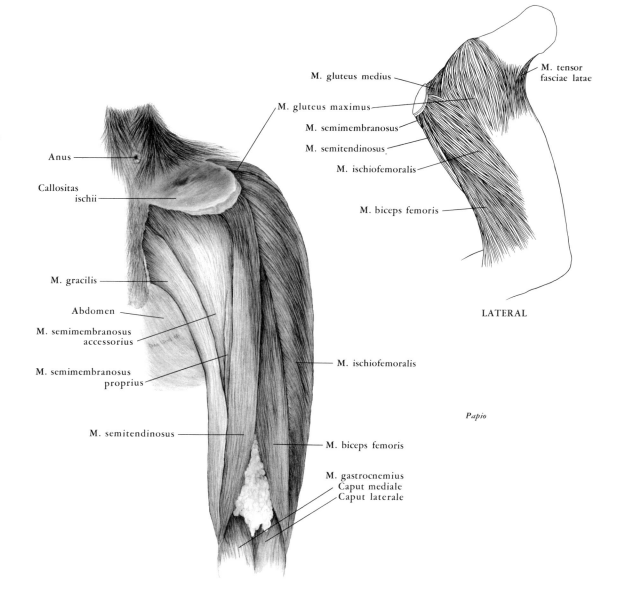

M. gluteus medius

M. tensor fasciae latae

M. gluteus maximus

M. semimembranosus

M. semitendinosus

M. ischiofemoralis

M. biceps femoris

Anus

Callositas ischii

M. gracilis

Abdomen

M. semimembranosus accessorius

M. semimembranosus proprius

M. ischiofemoralis

M. semitendinosus

M. biceps femoris

M. gastrocnemius
Caput mediale
Caput laterale

LATERAL

Papio

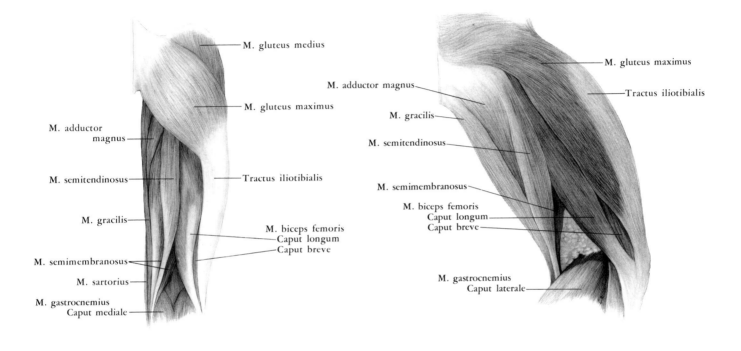

M. gluteus medius

M. gluteus maximus

M. adductor
magnus

M. semitendinosus

Tractus iliotibialis

M. gracilis

M. biceps femoris
Caput longum
Caput breve

M. semimembranosus

M. sartorius

M. gastrocnemius
Caput mediale

M. gluteus maximus

Tractus iliotibialis

M. adductor magnus

M. gracilis

M. semitendinosus

M. semimembranosus

M. biceps femoris
Caput longum
Caput breve

M. gastrocnemius
Caput laterale

Homo

Pan

PLATE 121

Gluteal Region

The gluteus maximus and medius muscles are cut, exposing the vessels and nerves as they exit the pelvic cavity via the greater sciatic foramen. The piriformis is cut in *Pan* and *Papio* but left intact in *Homo*.

The scansorius muscle is present along the ventrolateral border of the gluteus minimus in *Papio*. It is absent in *Pan* and *Homo*. There is a great deal of confusion in the literature about the presence or absence of this muscle in pongids. In an excellent study, Sigmon (1969) found it only as a separate muscle in the orang-utan among the anthropoids. She correctly points out that the "scansorius appears to be no more than the ventro-lateral part of gluteus minimus which in some primates is occasionally divided from the posterolateral portion of gluteus minimus" (p. 256).

The short puboischiofemoral muscles are rather constant in primates. The most variable of these are the gemelli, which may be absent or not completely differentiated into separate muscles. Both muscles are distinguished in *Papio*, although separation is somewhat tenuous. In *Pan* and *Homo* they are usually independent. The tendon of the obturator internus is insinuated between the gemelli and may be completely covered by them.

The vessels and nerves are similarly disposed in the three primates. The superior gluteal vessels and nerves appear cranial to the piriformis while the inferior gluteal vessels and nerves enter the gluteal region caudal to this muscle. The largest nerve in the body, the ischiadic, passes under the caudal border of the piriformis and gives off numerous branches while in the gluteal region. One of these, the flexores femoris, is always present in *Papio*. It is the motor nerve to the hamstring muscles, thus representing a separate portion of the tibial division of the ischiadic. In *Pan* and *Homo* the hamstrings are supplied by the ischiadic (tibial portion) as it passes through the thigh. Occasionally, the flexores femoris nerve is present in *Pan*.

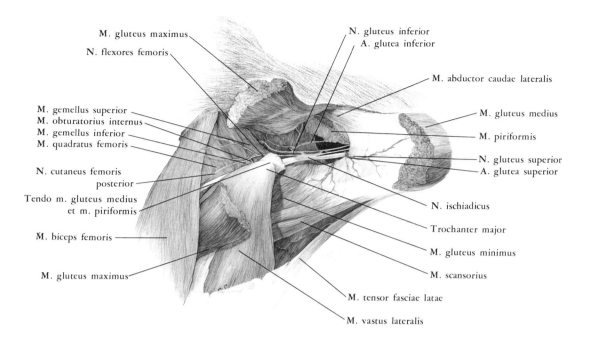

Papio

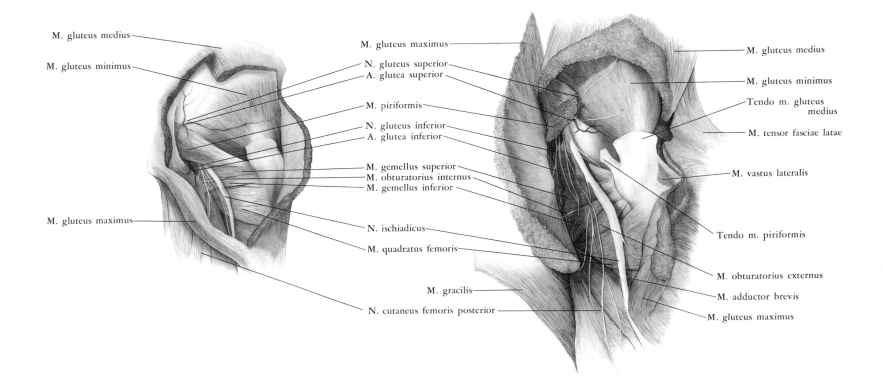

M. gluteus medius

M. gluteus minimus

M. gluteus maximus

M. gluteus maximus

N. gluteus superior

A. glutea superior

M. piriformis

N. gluteus inferior

A. glutea inferior

M. gemellus superior

M. obturatorius internus

M. gemellus inferior

N. ischiadicus

M. quadratus femoris

M. gracilis

N. cutaneus femoris posterior

M. gluteus medius

M. gluteus minimus

Tendo m. gluteus medius

M. tensor fasciae latae

M. vastus lateralis

Tendo m. piriformis

M. obturatorius externus

M. adductor brevis

M. gluteus maximus

Homo

Pan

PLATE 122

Popliteal Fossa I

The diamond-shaped popliteal fossa is behind the knee. It is demarcated on four sides by muscle: the biceps femoris proximolaterally; the semitendinosus and semi-membranosus proximomedially; the medial and lateral heads of the gastrocnemius distally. The major structures in the fossa are the popliteal vessels and the tibial and common peroneal nerves. These are embedded in a mass of fatty tissue, which has been removed.

In these three primates the ischiadic nerve normally bifurcates into the tibial and common peroneal at the proximal end of the popliteal space. On occasion, it may separate much more proximally or, in rare situations, the two portions may be independent from the sacral plexus. In such cases, the peroneal part usually pierces the piriformis muscle.

The tibial nerve passes out of the popliteal fossa between the two heads of the gastrocnemius and assumes a position deep to the soleus. It then continues distally through the leg between this muscle and the deep flexors to the medial malleolus, where it terminates as the medial and lateral plantar nerves. The medial sural cutaneous nerve arises from the tibial in the popliteal space. It continues distally on the surface of the gastrocnemius to about the middle of the calf, where in *Homo* it may unite with the peroneal anastomotic branch of the peroneal to form the sural nerve (Plate 114). In *Papio* and *Pan* the branch from the peroneal is absent, and the medial sural cutaneous supplies the sural region.

The common peroneal nerve exits the popliteal fossa on the deep surface of the biceps femoris and the superficial aspect of the lateral head of the gastrocnemius. Here it turns anteriorly between the fibular and tibial origins of the peroneus longus muscle and divides into its terminal branches, the superficial and deep peroneal nerves. The superficial peroneal descends through the anterior leg between the peroneal muscles and the extensor digitorum longus. It gives muscular branches to the peroneal muscles and then is sensory for the rest of its course (Plate 114). The deep peroneal passes through the proximal part of the extensor digitorum longus to the anterior compartment of the leg. It then descends to the ankle where it divides into terminal branches. It is accompanied by the anterior tibial artery for most of its course. The lateral sural cutaneous nerve leaves the common peroneal just before the latter disappears deep to the biceps femoris.

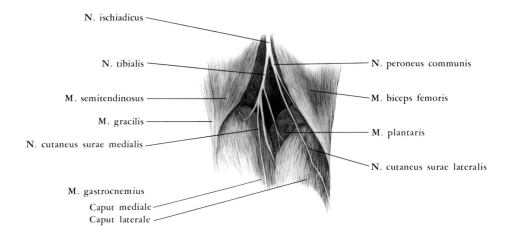

Papio

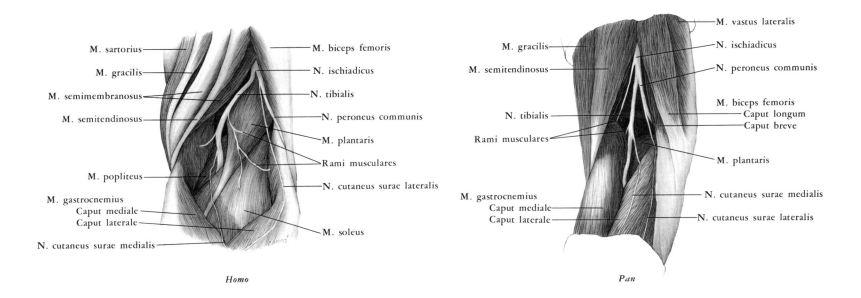

M. sartorius
M. gracilis
M. semimembranosus
M. semitendinosus

M. biceps femoris
N. ischiadicus
N. tibialis
N. peroneus communis
M. plantaris
Rami musculares

M. popliteus

M. gastrocnemius
Caput mediale
Caput laterale
N. cutaneus surae medialis

N. cutaneus surae lateralis

M. soleus

Homo

M. gracilis
M. semitendinosus

M. vastus lateralis
N. ischiadicus
N. peroneus communis

M. biceps femoris
Caput longum
Caput breve

N. tibialis
Rami musculares

M. plantaris

M. gastrocnemius
Caput mediale
Caput laterale

N. cutaneus surae medialis
N. cutaneus surae lateralis

Pan

PLATE 123

Popliteal Fossa II

In this view the medial and lateral heads of the gastrocnemius have been removed, exposing more of the deeper muscles, the soleus, popliteus, and plantaris. The popliteal artery is the deepest structure in the popliteal fossa as it passes through on its way to the leg. Although not shown, the popliteal vein lies dorsal to this artery throughout its course. The tibial nerve (cut) is the most superficial structure within the popliteal fossa.

The popliteal artery in *Homo* usually has five genicular arteries, which anastomose with each other around the knee (Plate 115). In *Papio* these arteries are quite variable, and only the superior medial and lateral genicular arteries are shown here (Plate 115). The other arteries depicted are small muscular branches. *Pan* usually has three to four genicular branches directly from the popliteal, although Sonntag (1923) reported a single genicular trunk dividing into three branches.

Near the distal border of the popliteus muscle the popliteal artery terminates by dividing into the anterior and posterior tibial arteries. The posterior tibial runs distally between the superficial and deep muscles within the posterior (flexor) compartment of the leg to reach the ankle, where it divides into the medial and lateral plantar arteries. This description holds for *Pan* and *Homo* but not for *Papio,* since the medial and lateral plantar arteries arise from the saphenous (Plate 115). Hill (1970), following Zuckerkandl (1895), states that there is no posterior tibial artery from the popliteal in *Papio.* A consistent, rather large artery descending from the popliteal within the posterior compartment is present in all *Papio* specimens dissected. This artery terminates near the ankle. On the other hand, Lineback (1933) and Berringer, Browning, and Schroeder (1968) found the posterior tibial from the popliteal giving rise to the medial and lateral plantar arteries in *Macaca mulatta.* The peroneal artery from the posterior tibial courses ventrally through the leg between the tibialis posterior muscle and the flexor digitorum fibularis (flexor hallucis longus in *Homo)* superficial to the lateral border of the calcaneus.

The anterior tibial artery begins at the distal border of the popliteus and passes anteriorly over the proximal border of the interosseous membrane to enter the anterior (extensor) compartment of the leg. It descends in this compartment to the ankle, where it continues as the dorsal pedal in *Homo.* In *Papio* and *Pan* the artery terminates just proximal to the ankle.

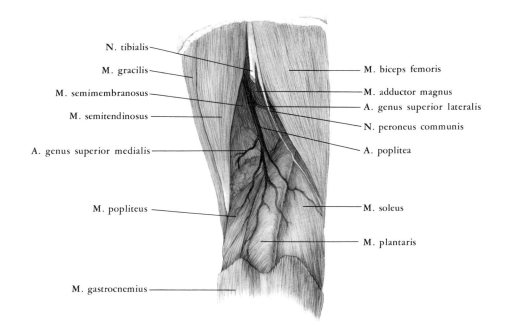

Papio

N. tibialis

M. gracilis

M. semimembranosus

M. semitendinosus

A. genus superior medialis

M. popliteus

M. gastrocnemius

M. biceps femoris

M. adductor magnus

A. genus superior lateralis

N. peroneus communis

A. poplitea

M. soleus

M. plantaris

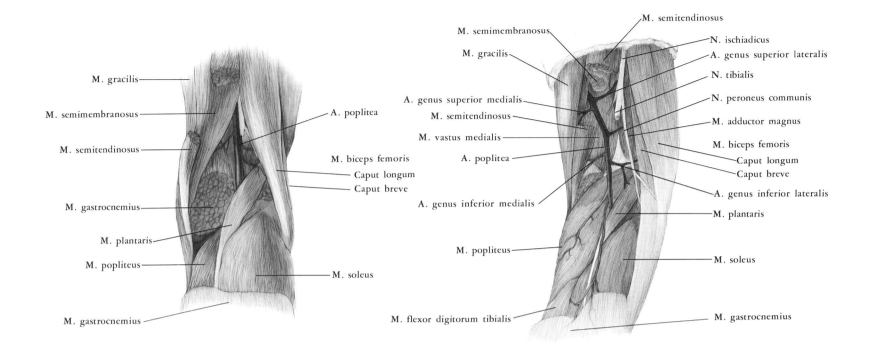

M. gracilis

M. semimembranosus

M. semitendinosus

M. gastrocnemius

M. plantaris

M. popliteus

M. gastrocnemius

A. poplitea

M. biceps femoris
Caput longum
Caput breve

M. soleus

Homo

M. semimembranosus

M. gracilis

A. genus superior medialis

M. semitendinosus

M. vastus medialis

A. poplitea

A. genus inferior medialis

M. popliteus

M. flexor digitorum tibialis

M. semitendinosus

N. ischiadicus

A. genus superior lateralis

N. tibialis

N. peroneus communis

M. adductor magnus

M. biceps femoris
Caput longum
Caput breve

A. genus inferior lateralis

M. plantaris

M. soleus

M. gastrocnemius

Pan

PLATE 124

Lateral Leg and Foot

The musculature of the leg arises from the distal end of the femur, as well as from the tibia and fibula. Distally, the muscles attach by tendons to the bones of the foot. There are three muscular compartments, anterior, lateral, and posterior. The lateral and anterior compartments are separated from each other by an intermuscular septum which in turn is separated from the posterior group by the interosseous membrane and a second intermuscular septum extending from the fibula to the crural fascia. The anterior and lateral groups are innervated by the peroneal nerve, and the posterior muscles by the tibial nerve.

The peroneus longus and brevis are present in the three animals and are similarly disposed. A third peroneal muscle, the peroneus digiti quinti, is normally present in *Papio* and *Pan* but absent in *Homo*. The peroneus tertius, which is actually a differentiated portion of the extensor digitorum longus, is present in *Homo* and absent in *Papio* and *Pan*. It has been reported in *Papio ursinus* (Wells 1935) and we have observed it in one *Macaca mulatta*.

The muscles of the anterior group are the tibialis anterior, extensor hallucis longus, and peroneus tertius. They are topographically similar in the three primates. Note that in *Papio* and *Pan* the extensor digitorum longus, after passing deep to the extensor retinaculum, is maintained by a separate trochlear arrangement of tough fibrous connective issue.

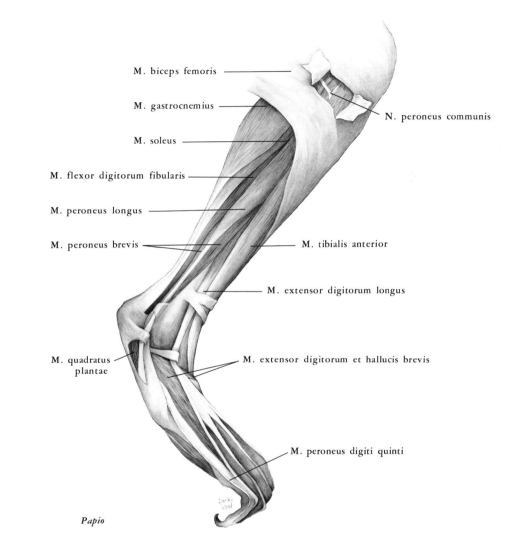

M. biceps femoris

M. gastrocnemius

M. soleus

M. flexor digitorum fibularis

M. peroneus longus

M. peroneus brevis

M. quadratus plantae

N. peroneus communis

M. tibialis anterior

M. extensor digitorum longus

M. extensor digitorum et hallucis brevis

M. peroneus digiti quinti

Papio

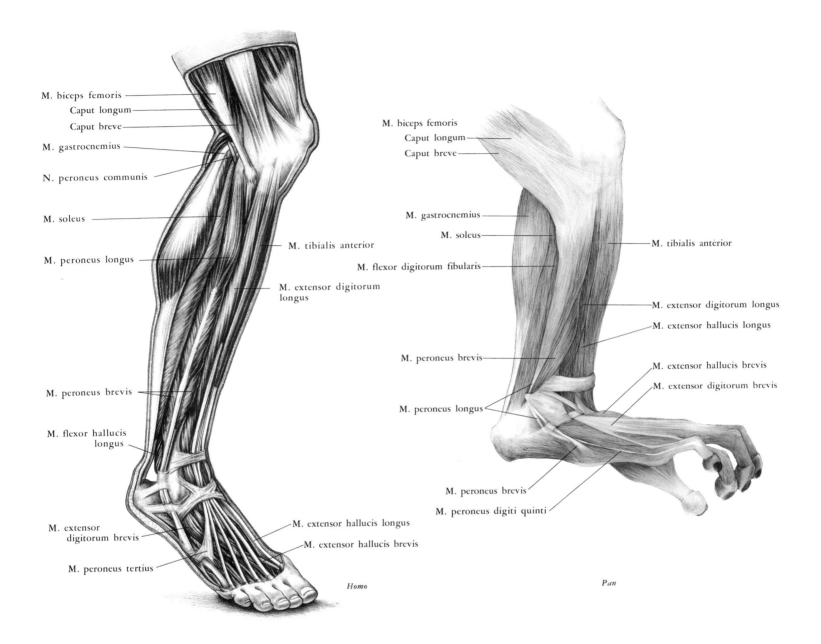

M. biceps femoris
Caput longum
Caput breve

M. gastrocnemius

N. peroneus communis

M. soleus

M. peroneus longus

M. tibialis anterior

M. extensor digitorum longus

M. peroneus brevis

M. flexor hallucis longus

M. extensor digitorum brevis

M. peroneus tertius

M. extensor hallucis longus

M. extensor hallucis brevis

Homo

M. biceps femoris
Caput longum
Caput breve

M. gastrocnemius

M. soleus

M. flexor digitorum fibularis

M. tibialis anterior

M. extensor digitorum longus

M. extensor hallucis longus

M. peroneus brevis

M. extensor hallucis brevis

M. extensor digitorum brevis

M. peroneus longus

M. peroneus brevis

M. peroneus digiti quinti

Pan

PLATE 125

Posterior Leg I

The gastrocnemius and soleus are often referred to as
the triceps surae. They extend through the posterior leg,
becoming tendinous some distance proximal to the heel.
The two tendons are fused together as the calcaneal
tendon. The soleus has a single head of origin from the
fibula in *Papio* and *Pan*. In *Homo* the muscle arises from
the tibia and the fibula. The gastrocnemius remains fleshy
for a much greater part of its length, and the medial belly
overlaps the lateral belly much more in *Pan* than in
the other species.

   In *Papio* the plantaris is large and its fleshy belly extends
farther distally than the fleshy portion of the gastrocnemius.
The tendon passes to the medial side of the calcaneal
tendon and passes over the tuber calcanei to continue
in the foot as the plantar aponeurosis. This is also the
arrangement of *Macaca mulatta* (Howell and Straus 1933b).
In *Pan* and *Homo* the tendon attaches to the medial side
of the calcaneus rather than continuing as the plantar
aponeurosis.

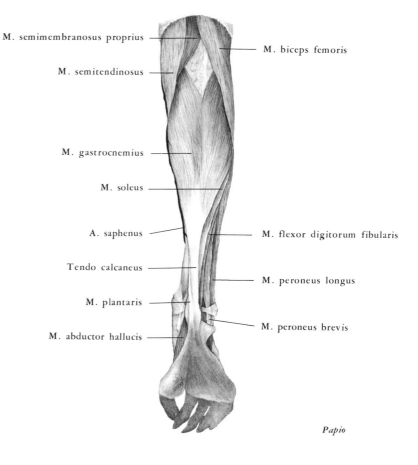

M. semimembranosus proprius

M. semitendinosus

M. gastrocnemius

M. soleus

A. saphenus

Tendo calcaneus

M. plantaris

M. abductor hallucis

M. biceps femoris

M. flexor digitorum fibularis

M. peroneus longus

M. peroneus brevis

Papio

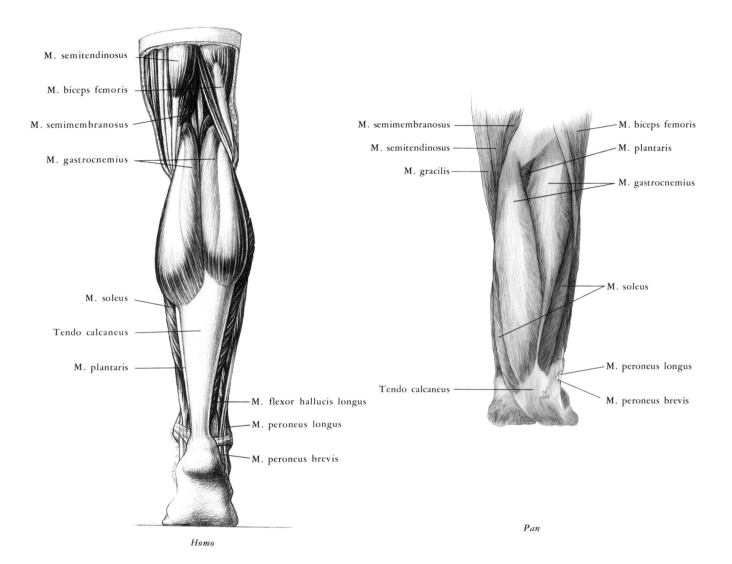

M. semitendinosus

M. biceps femoris

M. semimembranosus

M. gastrocnemius

M. soleus

Tendo calcaneus

M. plantaris

M. flexor hallucis longus

M. peroneus longus

M. peroneus brevis

Homo

M. semimembranosus

M. semitendinosus

M. gracilis

M. biceps femoris

M. plantaris

M. gastrocnemius

M. soleus

Tendo calcaneus

M. peroneus longus

M. peroneus brevis

Pan

PLATE 126

Posterior Leg II

The deep posterior muscles are the popliteus, flexor digitorum fibularis (flexor hallucis longus), flexor digitorum tibialis (flexor digitorum longus), and tibialis posterior. An additional muscle, the peroneotibialis, is present in *Papio*. They are separated from the superficial muscles by the transverse septum.

The popliteus is well developed in all three forms. The proximal part of the muscle runs horizontally, while its distal portion travels a much more oblique course, especially in *Papio*. The flexor digitorum tibialis arises from the posterior surface of the tibia. Its tendon passes posterior to the medial malleolus between the tendons of the tibialis posterior and flexor digitorum fibularis. The tendon divides in the foot to attach to digits II and V in *Papio* and *Pan*. In *Homo* the tendon separates into four slips, which attach to digits II, III, IV, and V (Plate 132). The flexor digitorum fibularis is a large muscle arising from the posterior surface of the fibula. Its tendon passes into the foot over the posterior surface of the talus, where in the sole it separates into three tendons supplying digits I, III, and IV in *Papio* and *Pan*. In *Homo* the tendon passes directly to the hallux. The tibialis posterior arises from the posterior surface of the tibia and the medial surface of the fibula. The muscle runs in a distomedial direction through the middle of the leg to the ankle where its tendon passes posterior to the medial malleolus and anterior to the tendon of the flexor digitorum tibialis. Its attachments in the foot are similar in the three primates. The peroneotibialis is usually present in *Papio* (see insert). It lies deep to the popliteus and passes between the proximal ends of the fibula and tibia. It probably represents a remnant of the old pronator stratum of lower vertebrates (Howell and Straus 1933b). It may occur in *Homo* and the anthropoids.

The tibial nerve and posterior tibial artery are shown coursing distally through the middle of the leg. The peroneal artery is shown in *Pan* and *Homo* arising from the posterior tibial at the distal border of the popliteus muscle. It then passes distally between the tibialis posterior and flexor hallucis longus. For most of its course through the leg, the tibial nerve lies along the lateral side of the artery. The posterior tibial artery is present in *Papio*, although, as mentioned earlier, it fails to reach the foot, terminating somewhat proximal to the ankle (Plate 115). An artery of comparable size and distribution was observed in all *Papio* dissections.

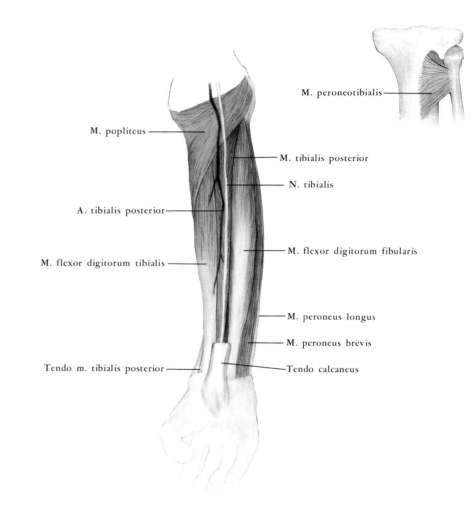

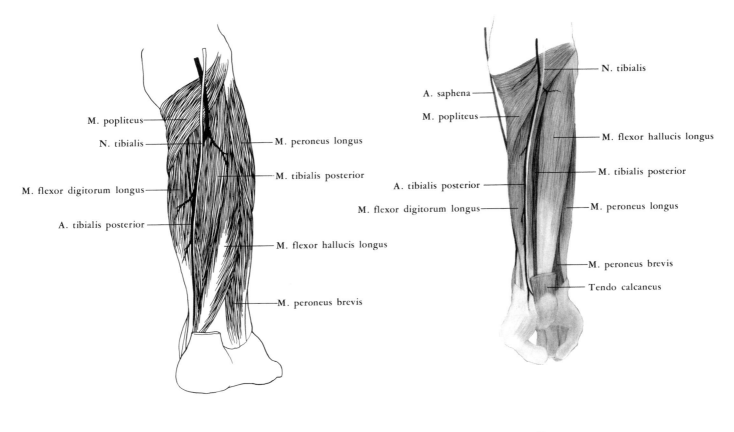

M. popliteus

N. tibialis

M. flexor digitorum longus

A. tibialis posterior

M. peroneus longus

M. tibialis posterior

M. flexor hallucis longus

M. peroneus brevis

Homo

A. saphena

M. popliteus

A. tibialis posterior

M. flexor digitorum longus

N. tibialis

M. flexor hallucis longus

M. tibialis posterior

M. peroneus longus

M. peroneus brevis

Tendo calcaneus

Pan

PLATE 127

Medial Ankle

The medial aspect of the ankle presents a number of important anatomical relations. There is a general similarity in pattern among the three primates, the major differences being terminological rather than anatomical.

The posterior division of the saphenous artery is shown coursing distally along the medial border of the calcaneal tendon in *Papio*. As the artery enters the sole of the foot, it divides into its terminal branches, the medial and lateral plantar arteries. In *Pan* and *Homo* the anatomical relations are similar, except that these terminal branches represent the division of the posterior tibial artery. Note that the posterior tibial artery, the posterior ramus and the saphenous artery, the tibial nerve and the tendons of the deep leg flexors all pass deep to the flexor retinaculum. The tibial nerve divides into the medial and lateral plantar nerves between the medial malleolus and the calcaneus. The superficial dorsal pedal artery, a branch of the anterior ramus of the saphenous, is visible on the anteromedial aspect of the ankle and foot in *Papio* and *Pan*. This artery is absent in *Homo*.

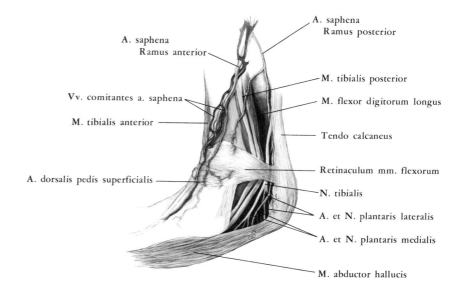

A. saphena
Ramus posterior

A. saphena
Ramus anterior

Vv. comitantes a. saphena

M. tibialis anterior

A. dorsalis pedis superficialis

M. tibialis posterior

M. flexor digitorum longus

Tendo calcaneus

Retinaculum mm. flexorum

N. tibialis

A. et N. plantaris lateralis

A. et N. plantaris medialis

M. abductor hallucis

Papio

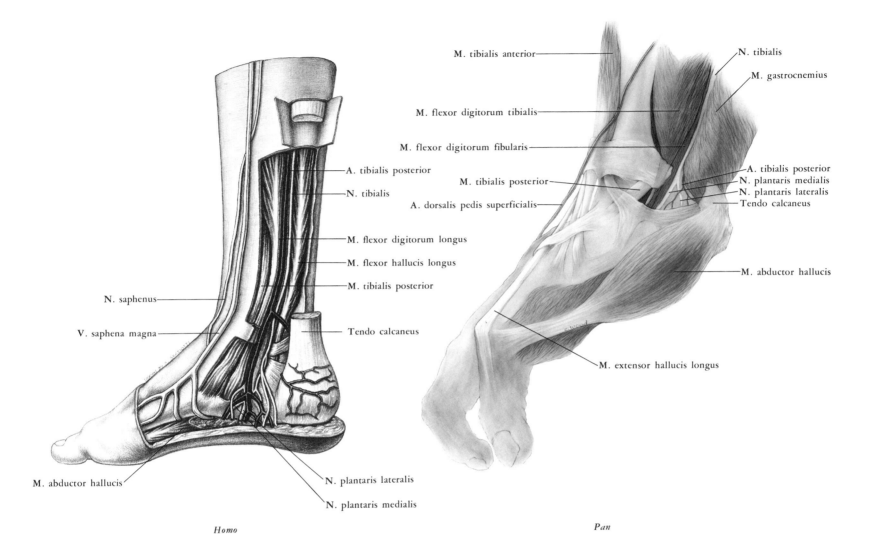

M. tibialis anterior⎯⎯⎯⎯⎯⎯⎯⎯⎯⎯⎯⎯⎯⎯

N. tibialis

M. gastrocnemius

M. flexor digitorum tibialis⎯⎯⎯⎯⎯⎯⎯⎯⎯

M. flexor digitorum fibularis⎯⎯⎯⎯⎯⎯⎯⎯⎯

A. tibialis posterior

M. tibialis posterior⎯⎯⎯⎯⎯

N. plantaris medialis

A. dorsalis pedis superficialis⎯⎯⎯⎯⎯⎯⎯

N. plantaris lateralis

Tendo calcaneus

A. tibialis posterior

N. tibialis

M. flexor digitorum longus

M. flexor hallucis longus

M. tibialis posterior

M. abductor hallucis

N. saphenus⎯⎯⎯⎯⎯⎯

V. saphena magna⎯⎯⎯⎯⎯

Tendo calcaneus

M. extensor hallucis longus

M. abductor hallucis⎯⎯⎯⎯⎯

N. plantaris lateralis

N. plantaris medialis

Homo

Pan

PLATE 128

Dorsal Foot

The extensor digitorum brevis is the only muscle intrinsic to the dorsum of the foot, although its tendon to the great toe is separately referred to as the extensor hallucis brevis. The muscle arises from the dorsal and lateral sides of the calcaneus. It divides into four muscle bellies whose tendons attach to the proximal phalanges of digits II, III, IV, and V, deep to the tendons of the extensor digitorum longus. In *Pan* and *Papio* the slip to the fifth toe is often wanting, as shown here.

The adductor hallucis and dorsal interossei belong to the plantar (flexor) group and will be discussed later.

In *Papio* and *Pan* observe the deep dorsal pedal artery passing onto the dorsum of the foot between the tendons of the tibialis anterior and extensor digitorum longus muscles. As it enters the foot, it courses deep to the belly of the extensor hallucis brevis before disappearing between the second and third metatarsals to anastomose with the lateral plantar, forming the plantar arterial arch. This is a branch of the anterior ramus of the saphenous artery and supplies much of the region supplied by the dorsal pedal in *Homo*.

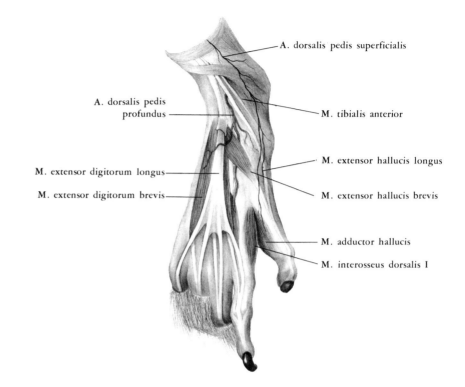

Papio

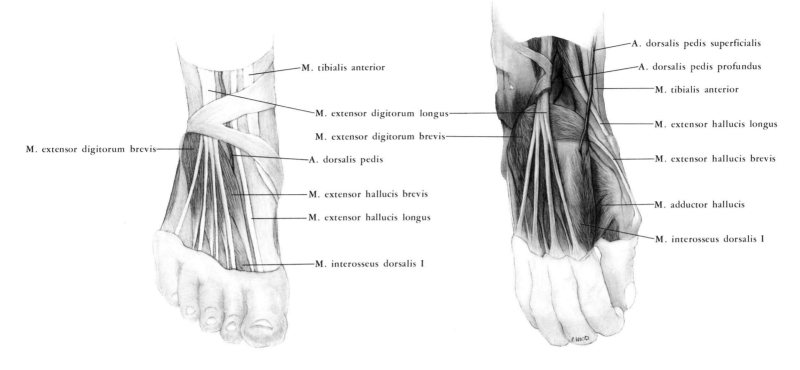

M. tibialis anterior

M. extensor digitorum longus

M. extensor digitorum brevis

A. dorsalis pedis

M. extensor hallucis brevis

M. extensor hallucis longus

M. interosseus dorsalis I

M. extensor digitorum brevis

Homo

A. dorsalis pedis superficialis

A. dorsalis pedis profundus

M. tibialis anterior

M. extensor hallucis longus

M. extensor digitorum longus

M. extensor digitorum brevis

M. extensor hallucis brevis

M. adductor hallucis

M. interosseus dorsalis I

Pan

PLATE 129

Topography of Foot

The topography of the plantar surface of the foot presents several interesting anatomical features. The plantar surface is devoid of hair, but presents a skin surface characterized by alternating ridges and sulci forming definite configurations, the dermatoglyphics (Plate 76). Specific patterns usually develop at elevations corresponding to the large, well-formed pads of lower mammals. These pads are usually more pronounced in Old World monkeys than they are in *Pan* and *Homo*. The morphological location of several plantar pattern sites are indicated in this plate.

The primitive phalangeal formula is 3 > 4 > 2 > 5 > 1, with the third digit forming the functional axis. In *Papio,* and usually in *Pan,* this is still the anatomical arrangement. In *Homo* the functional axis has migrated medially to the second digit, with a commensurate lengthening of the digit. The second toe is normally the longest, although as shown here, the great toe may assume this role (see Morton 1935).

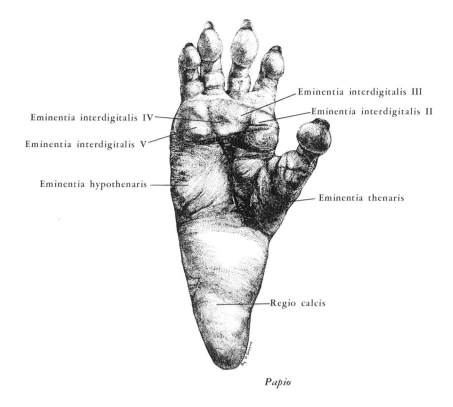

Papio

PLANTA PEDIS

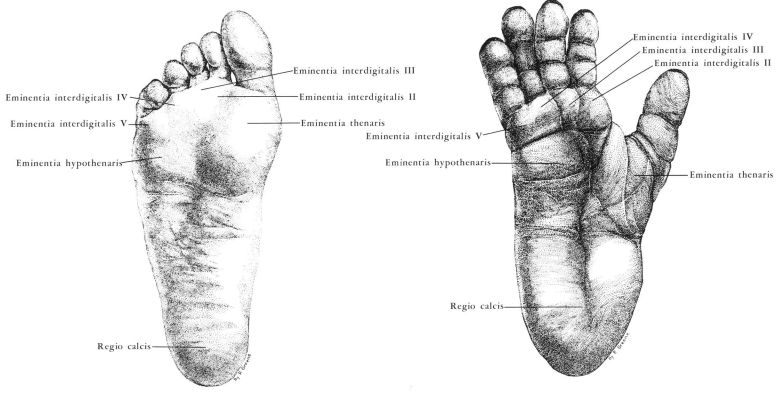

Eminentia interdigitalis III

Eminentia interdigitalis IV

Eminentia interdigitalis II

Eminentia interdigitalis V

Eminentia thenaris

Eminentia hypothenaris

Eminentia interdigitalis IV
Eminentia interdigitalis III
Eminentia interdigitalis II

Eminentia interdigitalis V

Eminentia hypothenaris

Eminentia thenaris

Regio calcis

Regio calcis

PLANTA PEDIS

Homo

Pan

PLATE 130

Plantar Foot I

The superficial fascia on the sole of the foot contains much
fat embedded in the dense fibrous tissue, deep to which
is the plantar aponeurosis. Three distinct regions may be
observed: a central, a lateral, and a medial. The central
region is thickened by bands of fibrous tissue that separate
toward the toes. This is the plantar aponeurosis and, in
Papio, represents the continuation of the tendon of the
plantaris muscle. Along the medial and lateral margins of
the foot the plantar fascia is thin and closely adherent
to the overlying skin. For a detailed discussion of the
plantar aponeurosis, see Loth 1907.

 The intrinsic muscles of the foot and associated
neurovascular structures are visible in this view as they
pass between separations of the aponeurosis.

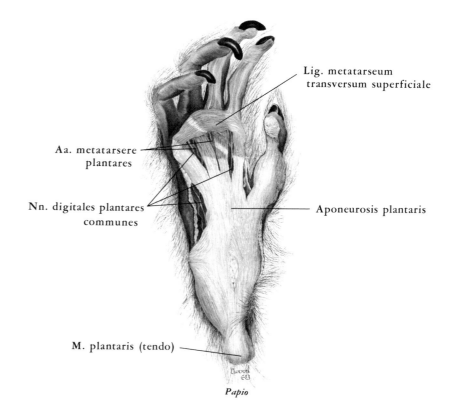

Lig. metatarseum
transversum superficiale

Aa. metatarsere
plantares

Nn. digitales plantares
communes

Aponeurosis plantaris

M. plantaris (tendo)

Papio

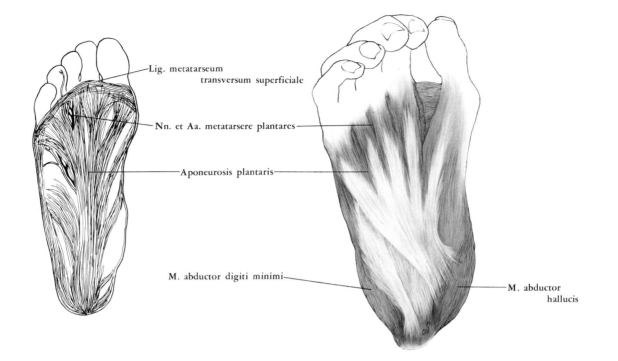

Lig. metatarseum
transversum superficiale

Nn. et Aa. metatarsere plantares

Aponeurosis plantaris

M. abductor digiti minimi

M. abductor
hallucis

Homo

Pan

PLATE 131

Plantar Foot II

The plantar aponeurosis is removed. The medial and lateral plantar arteries and nerves are clearly visible as they emerge from under cover of the flexor digitorum brevis. In *Homo* the lateral plantar artery is the larger of the two. In *Papio* and *Pan* they are about equal in caliber. The lateral plantar supplies metatarsal and digital arteries to the lateral two or three toes before passing deep to form an arterial arch by anastomosing with the perforating branch from the deep dorsal pedal in the second metatarsal space. The pattern is similar in the three primates except that the connection occurs in the first metatarsal space in *Homo* (Plate 115). In *Papio* and *Pan* the medial plantar usually supplies the medial three toes, whereas in *Homo* it is mainly responsible for the great toe. Occasionally in *Papio* there is a superficial plantar arch, formed by the two plantar arteries (Hill 1970).

The medial plantar nerve supplies the medial half of the sole of the foot plus the medial four and one-half toes, the lateral half of the foot and the lateral one and one-half toes being innervated by the lateral plantar nerve. This is the general pattern in these three primates, although there are certain minor differences in the actual distribution of the nerves.

The large flexor digitorum brevis muscle occupies a central position in this view. In *Papio* the muscle has two heads, a superficial and a deep. The former arises from the deep surface of the plantar aponeurosis and medial side of the calcaneus. It passes directly to the middle phalanx of the second toe. The latter head arises from the tendon of the flexor digitorum tibialis. It separates into three portions, which pass to digits III, IV, and V. In *Homo* there is a single head, which divides into four tendons supplying digits II, III, IV, and V. This probably corresponds to the superficial head of cercopithecids (Howell and Straus 1933b). *Pan* can have a single or double head, and the number of tendons is likewise variable. There are three tendons shown here (II, III, and IV); however, Sonntag (1923) reports only two (II and III).

Disposed to the medial and lateral sides of the flexor digitorum brevis are the intrinsic muscles of the great and little toes. These are discussed on the next plate.

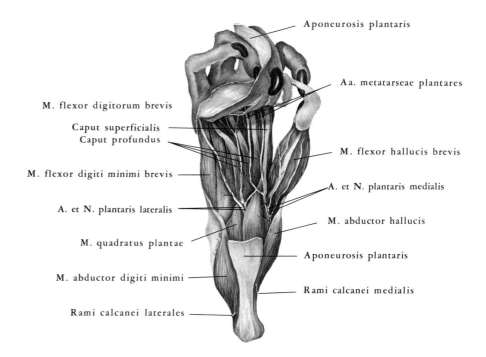

M. flexor digitorum brevis

Caput superficialis
Caput profundus

M. flexor digiti minimi brevis

A. et N. plantaris lateralis

M. quadratus plantae

M. abductor digiti minimi

Rami calcanei laterales

Aponeurosis plantaris

Aa. metatarseae plantares

M. flexor hallucis brevis

A. et N. plantaris medialis

M. abductor hallucis

Aponeurosis plantaris

Rami calcanei medialis

Papio

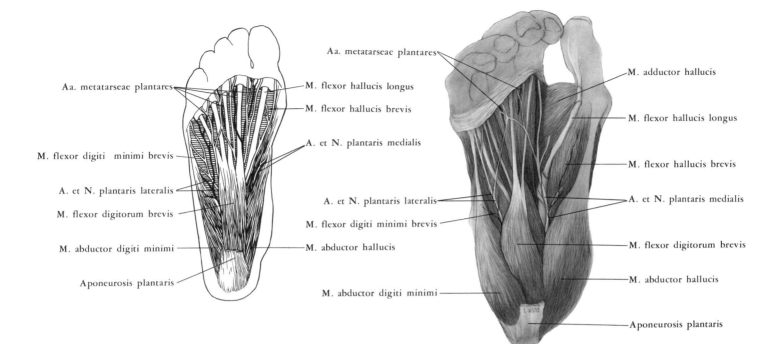

Aa. metatarseae plantares

M. flexor hallucis longus

M. flexor hallucis brevis

A. et N. plantaris medialis

M. flexor digiti minimi brevis

A. et N. plantaris lateralis

M. flexor digitorum brevis

M. abductor digiti minimi

Aponeurosis plantaris

Aa. metatarseae plantares

M. flexor digiti minimi brevis

A. et N. plantaris lateralis

M. flexor digitorum brevis

M. abductor hallucis

M. abductor digiti minimi

M. adductor hallucis

M. flexor hallucis longus

M. flexor hallucis brevis

A. et N. plantaris medialis

M. flexor digitorum brevis

M. abductor hallucis

Aponeurosis plantaris

Homo

Pan

PLATE 132

Plantar Foot III

The muscles of the great toe are the abductor hallucis, flexor hallucis brevis, and adductor hallucis. The opponens hallucis is not shown, but it may occur in all three primates. When present, it is derived from the medial portion of the flexor hallucis brevis. Hill (1970) reports it in his specimen of *Papio*. The flexor hallucis brevis and abductor hallucis muscles are arranged similarly in the three animals. The adductor hallucis has a transverse and oblique head of origin. In *Papio* and *Pan* the transverse portion arises from metatarsals II and III, whereas in *Homo* it usually arises from III, IV, and V. The oblique head arises from the long plantar ligament and passes to the lateral side of the great toe, where it joins the transverse head for insertion. Hill describes only a transverse head in *Papio*.

There are two muscles associated with the little toe in *Papio*, the abductor digiti minimi and flexor digiti minimi brevis. The opponens digiti minimi is normally absent. In *Pan* and *Homo* the opponens is a small, inconstant muscle which, if present, lies lateral to the short flexor.

The four lumbricales are small, slender, bipennate muscles. The three lateral ones arise from the adjacent sides of the tendons of the flexor digitorum tibialis; the first lumbrical arises from the medial margin of the tendon to the second toe. In *Papio* the first lumbrical is very small and may be absent (Hill 1970). In *Pan* the fourth lumbrical arises from the lateral side of the tendon to the fourth toe, as well as from the tendon to the little toe.

The quadratus plantae has a single head of origin, from the lateral border of the calcaneus in *Papio*. In *Homo* the muscle has two heads of origin. If the muscle is present in *Pan*, it is small and has a single, fleshy belly which is nonfunctional as a digital flexor (Straus 1949). In all three, the muscle attaches to the tendon of the long flexor.

Note that the tendons of the flexor digitorum brevis split to allow the tendons of the long flexors to pass through to the distal phalanges. Also, observe that in *Papio* and *Pan* the tendons of the flexor digitorum fibularis pass to digits I, III, and IV, and those of the flexor digitorum tibialis to II and V. In *Homo* the former supplies only the hallux, the latter being attached to the lateral four digits.

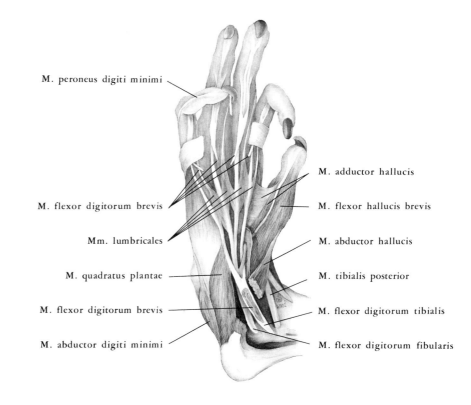

M. peroneus digiti minimi

M. flexor digitorum brevis

Mm. lumbricales

M. quadratus plantae

M. flexor digitorum brevis

M. abductor digiti minimi

M. adductor hallucis

M. flexor hallucis brevis

M. abductor hallucis

M. tibialis posterior

M. flexor digitorum tibialis

M. flexor digitorum fibularis

Papio

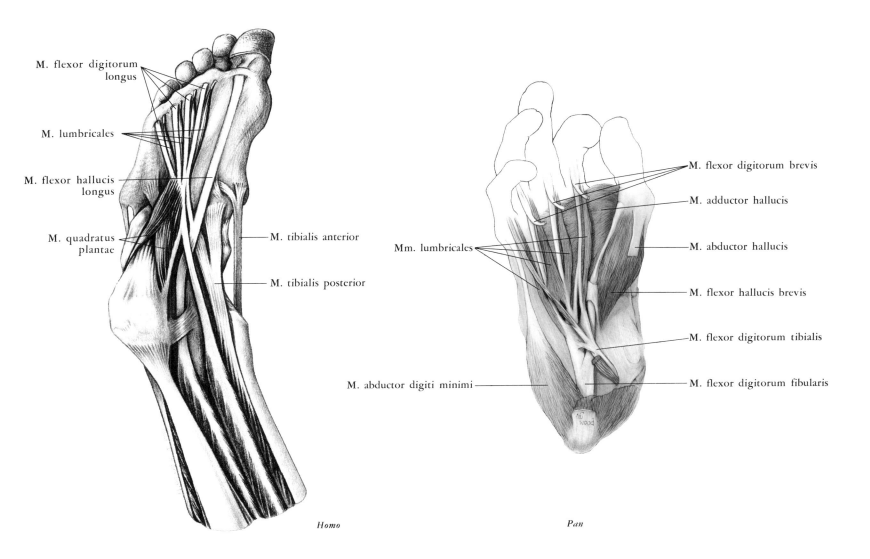

M. flexor digitorum
longus

M. lumbricales

M. flexor hallucis
longus

M. quadratus
plantae

M. tibialis anterior

M. tibialis posterior

Homo

M. flexor digitorum brevis

M. adductor hallucis

M. abductor hallucis

M. flexor hallucis brevis

M. flexor digitorum tibialis

Mm. lumbricales

M. abductor digiti minimi

M. flexor digitorum fibularis

Pan

PLATE 133

Plantar Foot IV

The long flexors and lumbricals have been removed to facilitate a clearer view of several muscles previously discussed. In addition, observe the three contrahentes muscles in *Papio*. This is the usual number in all cercopithecids. They represent the lateral continuation of the adductor hallucis muscle mass. The contrahentes are absent in *Pan* and *Homo*. These muscles are adductors toward an axis through digit III. Therefore, from their common aponeurotic origin the first passes to the lateral side of the proximal phalanx of digit II, and the second and third insert to the medial sides of digits IV and V. They are supplied by the deep branch of the lateral plantar nerve, which is shown passing between them and the underlying interosseous muscles.

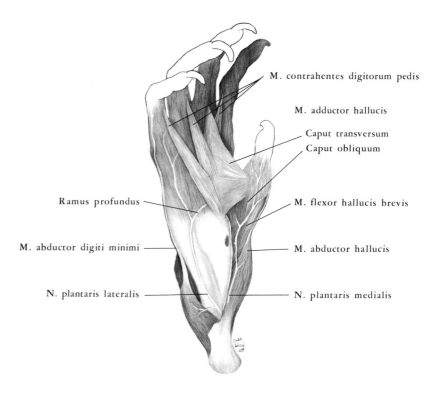

M. contrahentes digitorum pedis

M. adductor hallucis

Caput transversum
Caput obliquum

Ramus profundus

M. flexor hallucis brevis

M. abductor digiti minimi

M. abductor hallucis

N. plantaris lateralis

N. plantaris medialis

Papio

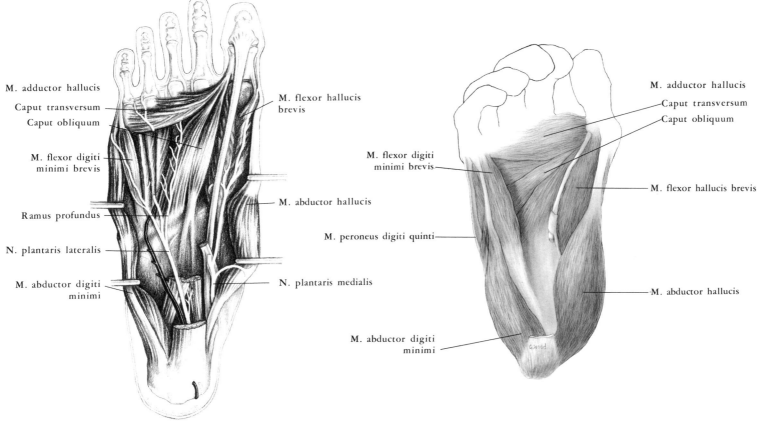

M. adductor hallucis

Caput transversum

Caput obliquum

M. flexor digiti
minimi brevis

Ramus profundus

N. plantaris lateralis

M. abductor digiti
minimi

M. flexor hallucis
brevis

M. abductor hallucis

N. plantaris medialis

Homo

M. adductor hallucis

Caput transversum

Caput obliquum

M. flexor digiti
minimi brevis

M. peroneus digiti quinti

M. abductor digiti
minimi

M. flexor hallucis brevis

M. abductor hallucis

Pan

PLATE 134

Plantar Foot V

The deepest intrinsic muscles of the foot are the interossei. These are primarily adductors and abductors of the toes, although because of their dorsal extension to the tendons of the extensor digitorum longus they assist in extension and flexion. In *Papio* and *Pan* the dorsal interossei abduct the second, third, and fourth toes to an axis through the middle toe, while the plantar interossei adduct the second, fourth, and fifth digits to this axis. In *Homo* the axis is through the second toe, and occasionally this relation is observed in *Pan*.

Note the abductor ossis metatarsi minimi present in *Papio* and *Pan*. This is an extremely variable muscle and simply represents a laterally detached portion of the abductor digiti minimi. It is normally absent in *Homo*.

One of the deepest structures in the foot is the tendon of the peroneus longus muscle. This tendon sweeps across the sole of the foot from lateral to medial to attach to the base of the metatarsal of the great toe.

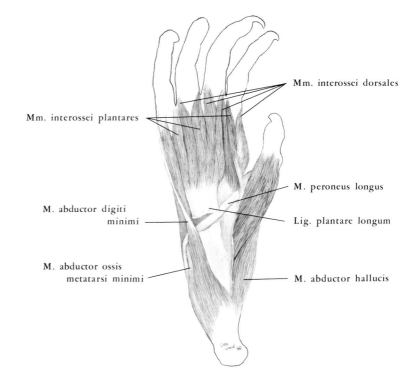

Mm. interossei dorsales

Mm. interossei plantares

M. peroneus longus

M. abductor digiti minimi

Lig. plantare longum

M. abductor ossis metatarsi minimi

M. abductor hallucis

Papio

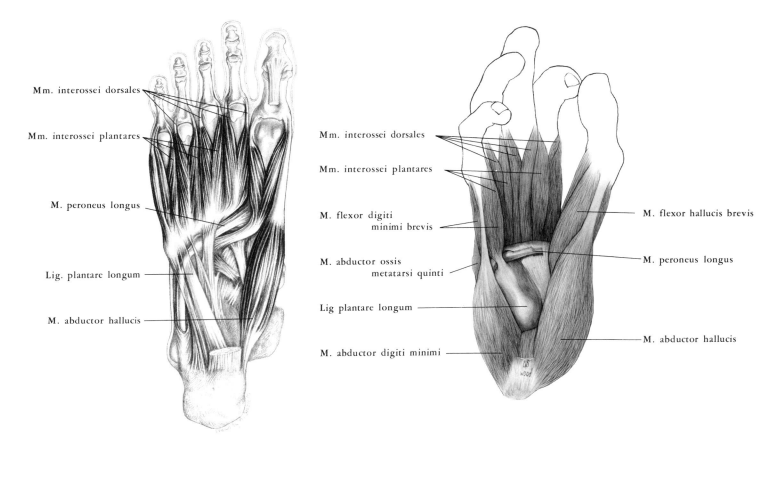

Mm. interossei dorsales

Mm. interossei plantares

M. peroneus longus

Lig. plantare longum

M. abductor hallucis

Homo

Mm. interossei dorsales

Mm. interossei plantares

M. flexor digiti minimi brevis

M. abductor ossis metatarsi quinti

Lig plantare longum

M. abductor digiti minimi

M. flexor hallucis brevis

M. peroneus longus

M. abductor hallucis

Pan

Part 9

MUSCLE-BONE MAPS

Muscles of Superior Member

1. M. omohyoideus
2. M. sternocleidomastoideus
3. M. trapezius
4. M. latissimus dorsi
5. M. rhomboideus major
6. M. rhomboideus minor
7. M. atlantoscapularis anterior
8. M. atlantoscapularis posterior
9. M. levator scapulae
10. M. pectoralis major
11. M. pectoralis minor
12. M. pectoralis abdominalis
13. M. panniculus carnosus
14. M. subclavius
15. M. serratus anterior
16. M. deltoideus
17. M. subscapularis
18. M. supraspinatus
19. M. infraspinatus
20. M. teres major
21. M. teres minor
22. M. biceps brachii caput longum
23. M. biceps brachii caput breve
24. M. coracobrachialis caput profundus
25. M. coracobrachialis caput medius
26. M. brachialis
27. M. triceps brachii caput longum
28. M. triceps brachii caput laterale
29. M. triceps brachii caput mediale
30. M. dorsoepitrochlearis
31. Mm. flexores
32. M. pronator teres
33. M. flexor carpi radialis
34. M. palmaris longus
35. M. flexor carpi ulnaris
36. M. epitrochleoanconeus
37. M. flexor digitorum superficialis
38. M. flexor digitorum profundus
39. M. flexor pollicis longus
40. M. pronator quadratus
41. M. brachioradialis
42. Mm. extensores
43. M. extensor carpi radialis longus
44. M. extensor carpi radialis brevis
45. M. extensor digitorum
46. M. extensor digiti anularis
47. M. extensor digiti minimi
48. M. extensor carpi ulnaris
49. M. anconeus
50. M. supinator
51. M. abductor pollicis longus
52. M. extensor pollicis brevis
53. M. extensor pollicis longus
54. M. extensor digiti indicis
55. M. extensor digiti medius
56. M. abductor pollicis brevis
57. M. opponens pollicis
58. M. flexor pollicis brevis
59. M. adductor pollicis
60. M. palmaris brevis
61. M. abductor digiti minimi
62. M. flexor digiti minimi brevis
63. M. opponens digiti minimi
64. Mm. lumbricales manus
65. Mm. contrahentes manus
66. Mm. interossei palmares
67. Mm. interossei dorsales

Muscles of Inferior Member

1. M. erector spinae
2. M. quadratus lumborum
3. M. latissimus dorsi
4. M. obliquus externus abdominis
5. M. obliquus internus abdominis
6. M. transversus abdominis
7. M. rectus abdominis
8. M. iliocaudalis
9. M. pubocaudalis
10. M. levator ani
11. M. ischiocaudalis
12. M. coccygeus
13. M. flexor caudae longus
14. M. abductor caudae lateralis
15. Aponeurosis margo acetabuli
16. M. psoas minor
17. M. psoas major
18. M. iliacus
19. M. iliopsoas
20. M. sartorius
21. Lig. patellae
22. M. rectus femoris
23. M. vastus medialis
24. M. vastus lateralis
25. M. vastus intermedius
26. M. articularis genus
27. M. obturatorius externus
28. M. gracilis
29. M. pectineus
30. M. adductor longus
31. M. adductor brevis
32. M. adductor magnus
33. M. gluteus maximus
34. M. tensor fasciae latae
35. M. gluteus medius
36. M. piriformis
37. M. gluteus minimus
38. M. obturatorius internus
39. M. gemellus superior
40. M. gemellus inferior
41. M. quadratus femoris
42. M. biceps femoris caput longum
43. M. biceps femoris caput breve
44. M. semimembranosus pars proprius
45. M. semimembranosus pars accessorius
46. M. semitendinosus
47. M. tibialis anterior
48. M. extensor digitorum longus
49. M. peroneus tertius
50. M. extensor hallucis longus
51. M. extensor digitorum brevis
52. M. peroneus longus
53. M. peroneus brevis
54. M. peroneus digiti quinti
55. M. gastrocnemius caput mediale
56. M. gastrocnemius caput laterale
57. M. soleus
58. Tendo calcaneus
59. M. plantaris
60. M. popliteus
61. M. peroneotibialis
62. M. flexor digitorum tibialis
63. M. flexor digitorum longus
64. M. flexor digitorum fibularis
65. M. flexor hallucis longus
66. M. tibialis posterior
67. M. flexor digitorum brevis
68. M. abductor hallucis
69. M. abductor digiti quinti
70. M. quadratus plantae
71. M. flexor hallucis brevis caput laterale
72. M. flexor hallucis brevis caput mediale
73. M. flexor digiti quinti
74. M. adductor hallucis caput obliquum
75. M. adductor hallucis caput transversum
76. Mm. contrahentes pedis
77. Mm. interossei plantares
78. Mm. interossei dorsales

PLATE 135

Right Clavicle

2. M. sternocleidomastoideus
3. M. trapezius
10. M. pectoralis major
16. M. deltoideus

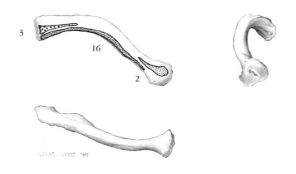

Papio

288

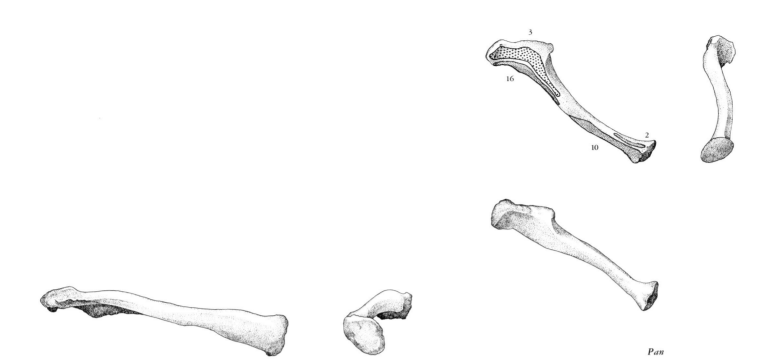

Pan

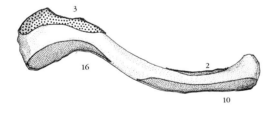

Homo

PLATE 136

Right Scapula

1. M. omohyoideus
3. M. trapezius
4. M. latissimus dorsi
5. M. rhomboideus major
6. M. rhomboideus minor
7. M. atlantoscapularis anterior
8. M. atlantoscapularis posterior
9. M. levator scapulae
11. M. pectoralis minor
15. M. serratus anterior
16. M. deltoideus
17. M. subscapularis
18. M. supraspinatus
19. M. infraspinatus
20. M. teres major
21. M. teres minor
22. M. biceps brachii caput longum
23. M. biceps brachii caput breve
25. M. coracobrachialis caput medius
27. M. triceps brachii caput longum

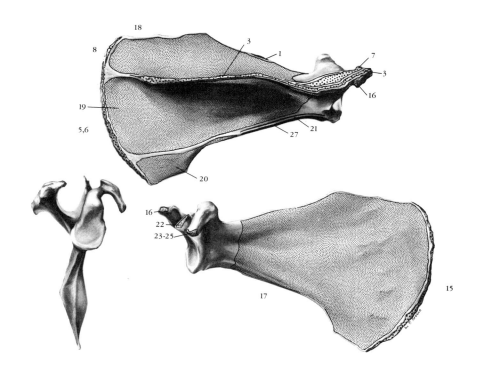

Papio

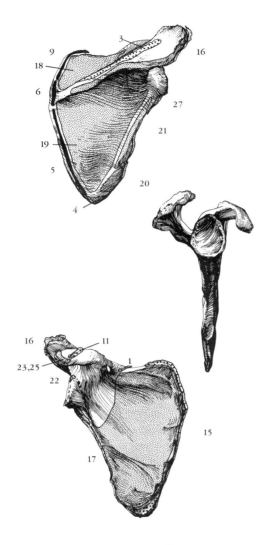

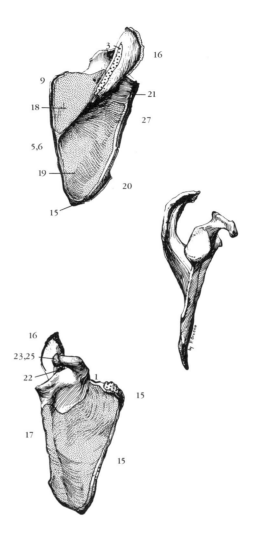

Homo

Pan

PLATE 137

Right Humerus

4. M. latissimus dorsi
10. M. pectoralis major
13. M. panniculus carnosus
16. M. deltoideus
17. M. subscapularis
18. M. supraspinatus
19. M. infraspinatus
20. M. teres major
21. M. teres minor
24. M. coracobrachialis caput profundus
25. M. coracobrachialis caput medius
26. M. brachialis
28. M. triceps brachii caput laterale
29. M. triceps brachii caput mediale
30. M. dorsoepitrochlearis
31. Mm. flexores
36. M. epitrochleoanconeus
41. M. brachioradialis
42. Mm. extensores
43. M. extensor carpi radialis longus
44. M. extensor carpi radialis brevis
49. M. anconeus

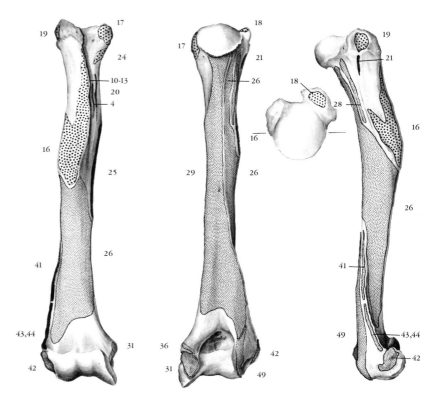

Papio

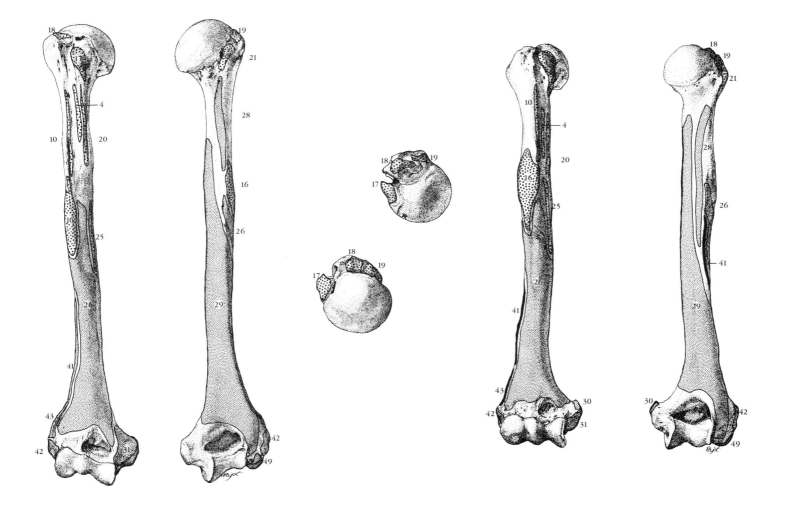

Homo

Pan

PLATE 138

Right Ulna

26. M. brachialis
27. M. triceps brachii caput longum
32. M. pronator teres
35. M. flexor carpi ulnaris
36. M. epitrochleoanconeus
37. M. flexor digitorum superficialis
38. M. flexor digitorum profundus
40. M. pronator quadratus
48. M. extensor carpi ulnaris
49. M. anconeus
50. M. supinator
51. M. abductor pollicis longus
53. M. extensor pollicis longus
54. M. extensor digiti indicus
55. M. extensor digiti medius

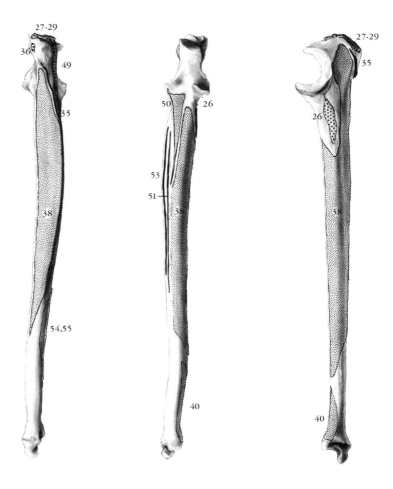

Papio

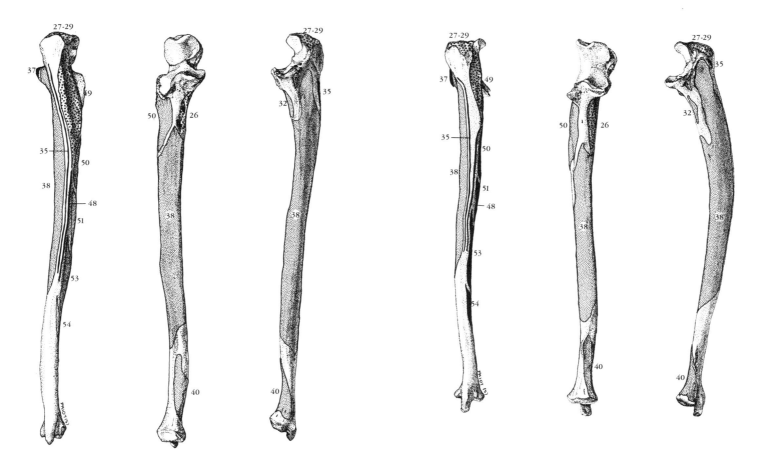

Homo

Pan

PLATE 139

Right Radius

22. M. biceps brachii caput longum
23. M. biceps brachii caput breve
32. M. pronator teres
33. M. flexor carpi radialis
37. M. flexor digitorum superficialis
39. M. flexor pollicis longus
40. M. pronator quadratus
41. M. brachioradialis
50. M. supinator
51. M. abductor pollicis longus
52. M. extensor pollicis brevis

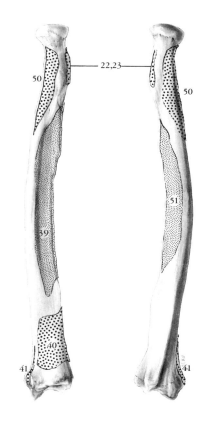

Papio

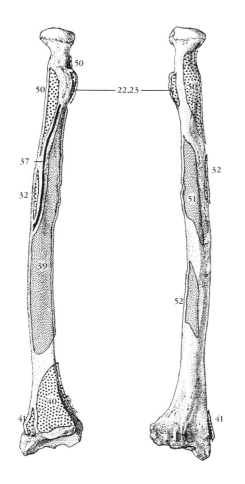

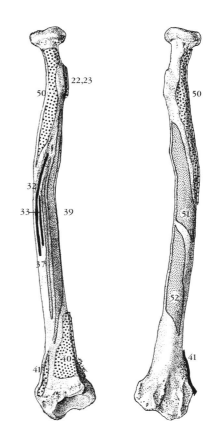

Homo

Pan

PLATE 140

Right Dorsal Hand

43. M. extensor carpi radialis longus
44. M. extensor carpi radialis brevis
45. M. extensor digitorum
46. M. extensor digiti anularis
47. M. extensor digiti minimi
48. M. extensor carpi ulnaris
51. M. abductor pollicis longus
52. M. extensor pollicis brevis
53. M. extensor pollicis longus
54. M. extensor digiti indicis
55. M. extensor digiti medius
59. M. adductor pollicis
61. M. abductor digiti minimi
67. Mm. interossei dorsales

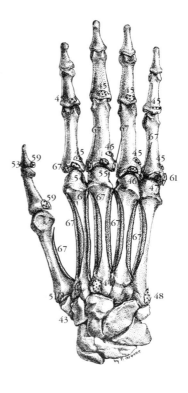

Papio

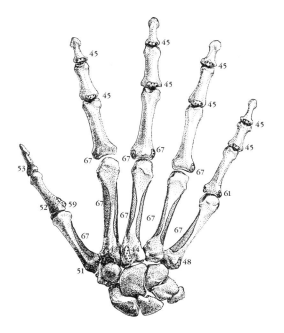

Homo

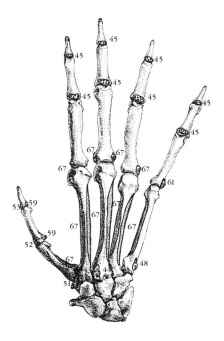

Pan

PLATE 141

Right Ventral Hand

33. M. flexor carpi radialis
35. M. flexor carpi ulnaris
37. M. flexor digitorum superficialis
38. M. flexor digitorum profundus
39. M. flexor pollicis longus
48. M. extensor carpi ulnaris
51. M. abductor pollicis longus
56. M. abductor pollicis brevis
57. M. opponens pollicis
58. M. flexor pollicis brevis
59. M. adductor pollicis
61. M. abductor digiti minimi
62. M. flexor digiti minimi brevis
63. M. opponens digiti minimi
64. Mm. lumbricales
65. Mm. contrahentes manus
66. Mm. interossei palmares

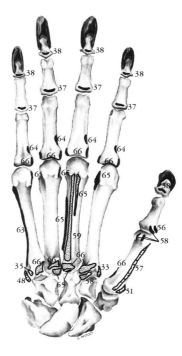

Papio

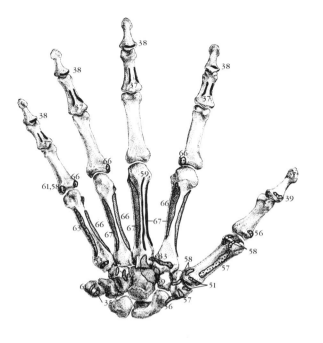

Homo

Pan

PLATE 142

Right Lateral Hip Bone

1. M. erector spinae
2. M. quadratus lumborum
3. M. latissimus dorsi
4. M. obliquus externus abdominis
5. M. obliquus internus abdominis
6. M. transversus abdominis
7. M. rectus abdominis
14. M. abductor caudae lateralis
15. Aponeurosis margo acetabuli
20. M. sartorius
22. M. rectus femoris
27. M. obturatorius externus
28. M. gracilis
29. M. pectineus
30. M. adductor longus
31. M. adductor brevis
32. M. adductor magnus
33. M. gluteus maximus
34. M. tensor fasciae latae
35. M. gluteus medius
36. M. piriformis
37. M. gluteus minimus
39. M. gemellus superior
40. M. gemellus inferior
41. M. quadratus femoris
42. M. biceps femoris caput longum
44. M. semimembranosus pars proprius
45. M. semimembranosus pars accessorius
46. M. semitendinosus

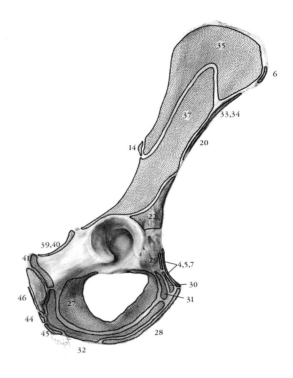

Papio

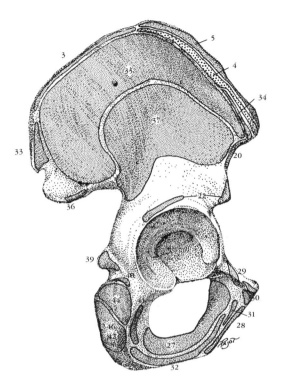

Homo

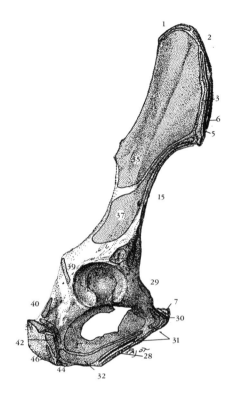

Pan

PLATE 143

Right Medial Hip Bone

1. M. erector spinae
2. M. quadratus lumborum
4. M. obliquus externus abdominis
5. M. obliquus internus abdominis
6. M. transversus abdominis
7. M. rectus abdominis
8. M. iliocaudalis
9. M. pubocaudalis
10. M. levator ani
11. M. ischiocaudalis
12. M. coccygeus
15. Aponeurosis margo acetabuli
16. M. psoas minor
18. M. iliacus
20. M. sartorius
22. M. rectus femoris
29. M. pectineus
38. M. obturatorius internus
40. M. gemellus inferior

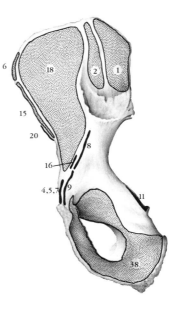

Papio

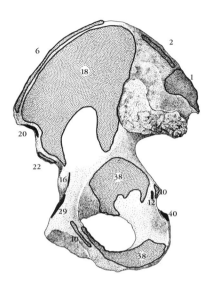

Homo

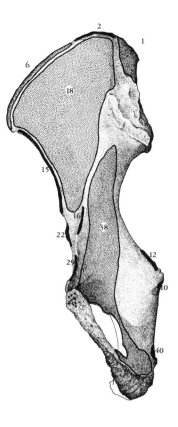

Pan

PLATE 144

Ventral Pelvis

1. M. erector spinae
2. M. quadratus lumborum
4. M. obliquus externus abdominis
5. M. obliquus internus abdominis
6. M. transversus abdominis
7. M. rectus abdominis
13. M. flexor caudae longus
15. Aponeurosis margo acetabuli
16. M. psoas minor
17. M. psoas major
18. M. iliacus
20. M. sartorius
22. M. rectus femoris
27. M. obturatorius externus
28. M. gracilis
29. M. pectineus
30. M. adductor longus
31. M. adductor brevis
32. M. adductor magnus
33. M. gluteus maximus
36. M. piriformis
41. M. quadratus femoris
42. M. biceps femoris caput longum
44. M. semimembranosus pars proprius
45. M. semimembranosus pars accessorius
46. M. semitendinosus

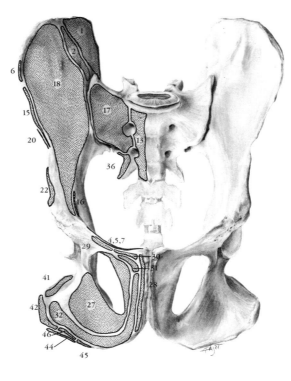

Papio

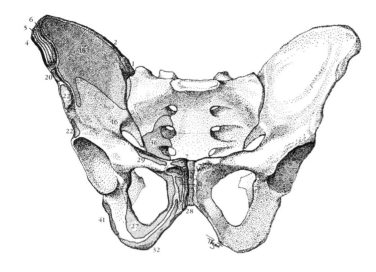

Homo

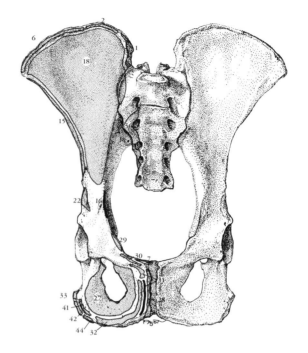

Pan

PLATE 145

Right Femur

19. M. iliopsoas
23. M. vastus medialis
24. M. vastus lateralis
25. M. vastus intermedius
26. M. articularis genus
27. M. obturatorius externus
29. M. pectineus
30. M. adductor longus
31. M. adductor brevis
32. M. adductor magnus
33. M. gluteus maximus
35. M. gluteus medius
36. M. piriformis
37. M. gluteus minimus
38. M. obturatorius internus
41. M. quadratus femoris
43. M. biceps femoris caput breve
45. M. semimembranosus pars accessorius
55. M. gastrocnemius caput mediale
56. M. gastrocnemius caput laterale
59. M. plantaris
60. M. popliteus

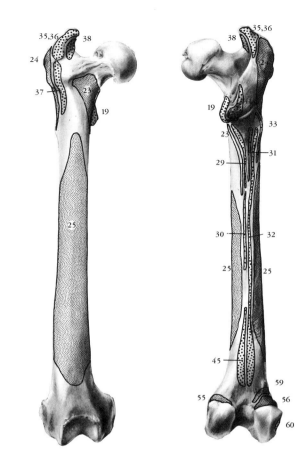

Papio

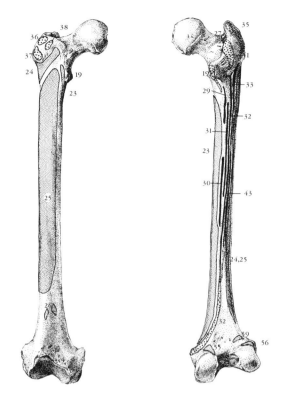

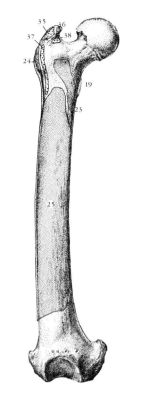

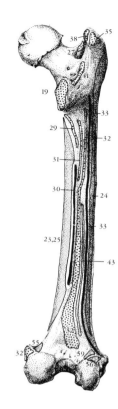

Homo   Pan

PLATE 146

Right Tibia

20. M. sartorius
21. Lig. patellae
28. M. gracilis
42. M. biceps femoris caput longum
44. M. semimembranosus pars proprius
46. M. semitendinosus
47. M. tibialis anterior
48. M. extensor digitorum longus
52. M. peroneus longus
57. M. soleus
60. M. popliteus
61. M. peroneotibialis
62. M. flexor digitorum tibialis
63. M. flexor digitorum longus
64. M. flexor digitorum fibularis
66. M. tibialis posterior

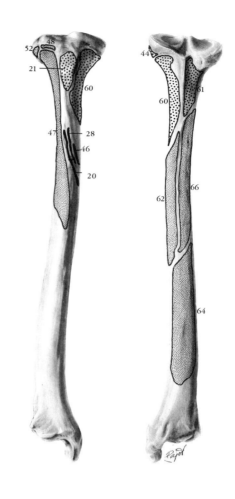

Papio

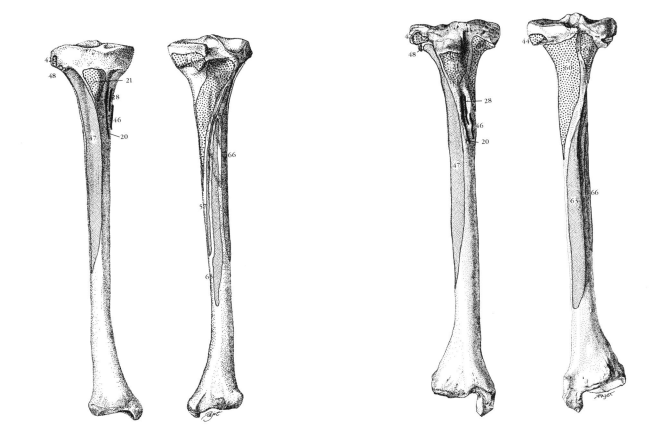

Homo

Pan

PLATE 147

Right Fibula

42. M. biceps femoris caput longum
43. M. biceps femoris caput breve
48. M. extensor digitorum longus
49. M. peroneus tertius
50. M. extensor hallucis longus
52. M. peroneus longus
53. M. peroneus brevis
54. M. peroneus digiti quinti
57. M. soleus
61. M. peroneotibialis
64. M. flexor digitorum fibularis
65. M. flexor hallucis longus
66. M. tibialis posterior

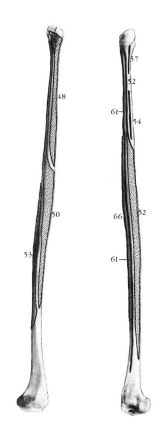

Papio

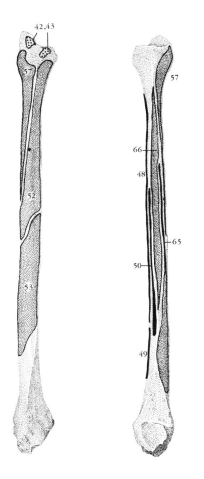

Homo

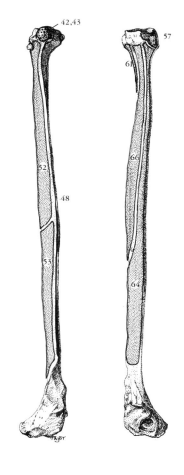

Pan

PLATE 148

Right Dorsal Foot

48. M. extensor digitorum longus
49. M. peroneus tertius
50. M. extensor hallucis longus
51. M. extensor digitorum brevis
53. M. peroneus brevis
54. M. peroneus digiti quinti
58. Tendo calcaneus
69. M. abductor digiti quinti
71. M. flexor hallucis brevis caput laterale
73. M. flexor digiti quinti
74. M. adductor hallucis caput obliquum
75. M. adductor hallucis caput transversum
78. Mm. interossei dorsales

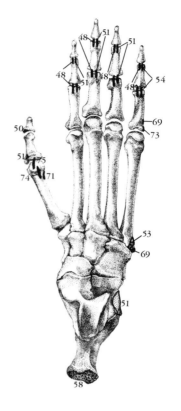

Papio

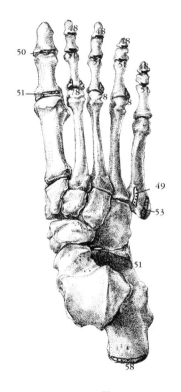

Homo

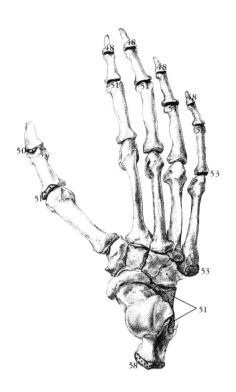

Pan

PLATE 149

Right Ventral Foot

47. M. tibialis anterior
52. M. peroneus longus
53. M. peroneus brevis
54. M. peroneus digiti quinti
62. M. flexor digitorum tibialis
63. M. flexor digitorum longus
64. M. flexor digitorum fibularis
65. M. flexor hallucis longus
66. M. tibialis posterior
67. M. flexor digitorum brevis
68. M. abductor hallucis
69. M. abductor digiti quinti
70. M. quadratus plantae
71. M. flexor hallucis brevis caput laterale
72. M. flexor hallucis brevis caput mediale
73. M. flexor digiti quinti
74. M. adductor hallucis caput obliquum
75. M. adductor hallucis caput transversum
76. Mm. contrahentes pedis
77. Mm. interossei plantares
78. Mm. interossei dorsales

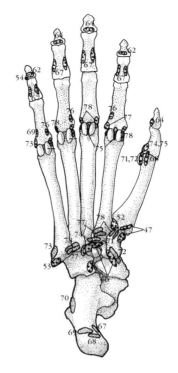

Papio

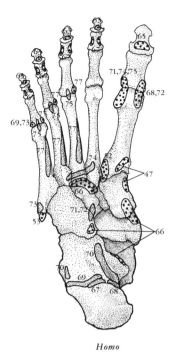

Homo

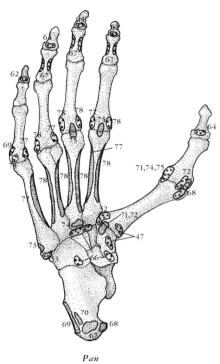

Pan

Part 10

MUSCLE CHARTS

ORIGIN

INSERTION

INNERVATION

TRAPEZIUS

	PAPIO	*HOMO*	*PAN*
Origin	External occipital protuberance; medial ⅓ superior nuchal line; nuchal ligament and spinous processes of C7-T10	Similar to *Papio*	Similar to *Papio* (no nuchal ligament)
Insertion	Lateral end cranial surface of clavicle, cranial margin of acromion and scapula spine	Similar to *Papio*	Similar to *Papio*
Nerve	Spinal accessory	Spinal accessory	Spinal accessory

LATISSIMUS DORSI

	PAPIO	*HOMO*	*PAN*
Origin	Spinous processes of lower 6 thoracic and lumbar vertebrae via the lumbar aponeurosis	Spinous processes of the lower 6 thoracic, lumbar, and sacral vertebrae via the lumbar aponeurosis; the posterior part of the external lip of the iliac crest; caudal 3 or 4 ribs and inferior angle of the scapula	Similar to *Homo* (no attachment to scapula)
Insertion	Floor of intertubercular groove of humerus	Similar to *Papio*	Similar to *Papio*
Nerve	Thoracodorsal	Thoracodorsal	Thoracodorsal

RHOMBOIDEI

	PAPIO	*HOMO*	*PAN*
Origin	Pars capitis; median part of superior nuchal line of the occipital bone Pars cervicis: ligamentum nuchae Pars thoracis: spinous processes of C7-T7	Major: spinous processes of T2-5 Minor: ligamentum nuchae and spinous processes of C7-T1	Single undivided rhomboideus: spinous processes of C6-T4
Insertion	Pars capitis: vertebral border of scapula opposite spine Pars cervicis: vertebral border of scapula below spine Pars thoracis: vertebral border of scapula between spine and inferior angle	Major: medial border of scapula between spine and inferior angle Minor: root of the scapula spine	Lower ¾ of vertebral border of scapula (slightly overlapping the levator scapulae cranially)
Nerve	Dorsal scapula	Dorsal scapula	Dorsal scapula

ATLANTOSCAPULARIS/LEVATOR SCAPULAE

	PAPIO	*HOMO*	*PAN*
Origin	Anterior atlantoscapularis: ventral part of transverse process of atlas Posterior atlantoscapularis: dorsal part of transverse process of atlas	Levator scapulae: transverse processes of C1-4	Similar to *Homo*
Insertion	Anterior: cranial margin of acromion Posterior: vertebral border of scapula between spine and superior angle	Medial border of scapula between spine and superior angle	Similar to *Homo*
Nerve	Anterior: C3-4 Posterior: C4	C3-4	C3-4

PECTORALIS MAJOR

Origin	Claviculomanubrial joint capsule and entire length of lateral sternum	Medial ½ anterior border of clavicle, lateral sternum to 7th rib, and aponeurosis of m. external abdominal oblique	Pars thoracis: similar to *Homo* Pars abdominalis: fascia over the m. external oblique, and lower borders of costal cartilages 5-7
Insertion	Lateral lip of the intertubercular groove of the humerus	Similar to *Papio*	Similar to *Papio*
Nerve	Medial pectoral and lateral pectoral	Medial pectoral and lateral pectoral	Medial pectoral and lateral pectoral

PECTORALIS MINOR

Origin	Middle ⅓ body of sternum	Outer surfaces of ribs 3-5 near the costochondral junction	Similar to *Homo*
Insertion	Capsule of shoulder joint via deep pectoral aponeurosis	Coracoid process of scapula	Capsule of shoulder joint (and occasionally the coracoid process of the scapula, or both)
Nerve	Medial pectoral	Medial pectoral	Medial pectoral

PECTORALIS ABDOMINALIS

	PAPIO	*HOMO*	*PAN*
Origin	Sheath of m. rectus abdominis lateral to the linea alba	Absent	Absent
Insertion	Proximal ½ lateral lip of inter-tubercular groove of humerus via deep pectoral aponeurosis		
Nerve	Medial pectoral		

SUBCLAVIUS

	PAPIO	*HOMO*	*PAN*
Origin	First rib at the costochondral junction	Similar to *Papio*	Similar to *Papio*
Insertion	Subclavian groove of clavicle	Similar to *Papio*	Similar to *Papio*
Nerve	N. to subclavius	N. to subclavius	N. to subclavius

PANNICULUS CARNOSUS

	PAPIO	*HOMO*	*PAN*
Origin	Superficial fascia over anterior surface of thigh, gluteal and lateral thoracic regions	Absent	Absent
Insertion	Distal ½ lateral lip of inter-tubercular groove of humerus via the deep pectoral aponeurosis		
Nerve	Medial pectoral		

SERRATUS ANTERIOR

	PAPIO	*HOMO*	*PAN*
Origin	Pars cervicis: transverse processes of the last 6 cervical vertebrae Pars thoracis: outer surfaces upper 9 or 10 ribs near their costochondral junction	Upper 8 or 9 ribs about midway between their angles and cartilages	Similar to *Homo*
Insertion	Costal surface of entire vertebral border of scapula	Similar to *Papio*	Similar to *Papio*
Nerve	Long thoracic	Long thoracic	Long thoracic

DELTOIDEUS

	PAPIO	*HOMO*	*PAN*
Origin	Entire anterior border of clavicle, caudal border of acromion and scapular spine	Lateral ⅓ anterior border of clavicle, caudal border of acromion and scapular spine	Similar to *Homo*
Insertion	Deltoid tuberosity of humerus	Similar to *Papio*	Similar to *Papio*
Nerve	Axillary	Axillary	Axillary

SUBSCAPULARIS

	PAPIO	*HOMO*	*PAN*
Origin	Subscapular fossa of scapula	Similar to *Papio*	Similar to *Papio*
Insertion	Lesser tuberosity of humerus	Similar to *Papio*	Similar to *Papio*
Nerve	Subscapulars (up to 5)	Subscapulars (usually 2)	Subscapulars (usually 2)

SUPRASPINATUS

	PAPIO	*HOMO*	*PAN*
Origin	Supraspinous fossa of scapula	Similar to *Papio*	Similar to *Papio*
Insertion	Superior facet of greater tuberosity of humerus	Similar to *Papio*	Similar to *Papio*
Nerve	Suprascapular	Suprascapular	Suprascapular

INFRASPINATUS

	PAPIO	*HOMO*	*PAN*
Origin	Infraspinous fossa of scapula	Similar to *Papio*	Similar to *Papio*
Insertion	Middle facet of greater tuberosity of the humerus	Similar to *Papio*	Similar to *Papio*
Nerve	Suprascapular	Suprascapular	Suprascapular

TERES MAJOR

	PAPIO	*HOMO*	*PAN*
Origin	Dorsal surface of the expanded inferior angle of the scapula	Similar to *Papio*	Similar to *Papio*
Insertion	Medial lip of intertubercular groove of humerus	Similar to *Papio*	Similar to *Papio*
Nerve	Lower subscapular	Lower subscapular	Lower subscapular

TERES MINOR

	PAPIO	*HOMO*	*PAN*
Origin	Glenoidal ½ axillary border of scapula	Similar to *Papio*	Similar to *Papio*
Insertion	Lowest facet of the greater tuberosity of the humerus and adjacent shaft just below the anatomical neck	Similar to *Papio*	Similar to *Papio*
Nerve	Axillary	Axillary	Axillary

324

BICEPS BRACHII

	PAPIO	HOMO	PAN
Origin	Short head: coracoid process of scapula (from common coracoid tendon with m. coracobrachialis) Long head: supraglenoid tuberosity of scapula	Similar to *Papio*	Similar to *Papio*
Insertion	Radial tuberosity of radius	Similar to *Papio*	Similar to *Papio*
Nerve	Musculocutaneus	Musculocutaneus	Musculocutaneus

CORACOBRACHIALIS

Origin	Coracoid process of scapula from the common coracoid tendon	Similar to *Papio*	Similar to *Papio*
Insertion	Profundus: surgical neck of humerus Medius: medial surface and border of the humeral shaft	Medial surface and border of the humeral shaft	Similar to *Homo*
Nerve	Musculocutaneus	Musculocutaneus	Musculocutaneus

BRACHIALIS

Origin	Lower ⅔ anterior surface of humerus	Similar to *Papio*	Similar to *Papio*
Insertion	Coronoid process and tuberosity of ulna	Similar to *Papio*	Similar to *Papio*
Nerve	Musculocutaneus	Musculocutaneus	Musculocutaneus

TRICEPS BRACHII

	PAPIO	HOMO	PAN
Origin	Long head: glenoidal ½ axillary border of scapula Lateral head: upper posterior and lateral surface of humeral shaft to capsule of shoulder joint Medial head: entire posterior surface of humeral shaft from capsule of shoulder joint to olecranon fossa	Long head: infraglenoid tuberosity of scapula Lateral head: upper posterior and lateral surface of humeral shaft Medial head: distal ⅓ posterior surface of humeral shaft	Long head: similar to *Papio* Lateral head: proximal ½ posterior and lateral surface of humeral shaft Medial head: distal ¾ posterior surface of humeral shaft
Insertion	Olecranon process of the ulna	Similar to *Papio*	Similar to *Papio*
Nerve	Radial	Radial	Radial

DORSOEPITROCHLEARIS

Origin	Tendon of m. latissimus dorsi	Rare	Similar to *Papio*
Insertion	By a broad aponeurosis into the medial and long heads of the m. triceps brachii to the olecranon process of the ulna, and by a fascial extension to the medial condyle of the humerus	Rare	Medial condyle of the humerus by a broad aponeurosis
Nerve	Radial	Radial	Radial

PRONATOR TERES

Origin	Medial epicondylar ridge of the humerus (no ulnar head)	Humeral head: medial epicondylar ridge of humerus Ulnar head: medial side of the coronoid process of the ulna	Similar to *Homo*
Insertion	Middle ⅓ of the lateral surface of the radius	Similar to *Papio*	Similar to *Papio*
Nerve	Median	Median	Median

FLEXOR CARPI RADIALIS

	PAPIO	*HOMO*	*PAN*
Origin	Medial epicondyle of the humerus	Similar to *Papio*	Medial epicondyle of the humerus; lateral border of the radius just medial to the attachment of the m. pronator teres
Insertion	Bases of metacarpals II and III	Similar to *Papio*	Similar to *Papio*
Nerve	Median	Median	Median

PALMARIS LONGUS

Origin	Medial epicondyle of the humerus	Similar to *Papio* (frequently absent)	Similar to *Papio* (frequently absent)
Insertion	Tendon disperses in palm as the palmar aponeurosis	Similar to *Papio*	Similar to *Papio*
Nerve	Median	Median	Median

FLEXOR CARPI ULNARIS

Origin	Humeral head: medial epicondyle of the humerus Ulnar head: olecranon and dorsal border of the ulna	Similar to *Papio*	Similar to *Papio*
Insertion	Pisiform bone	Similar to *Papio*	Similar to *Papio*
Nerve	Ulnar	Ulnar	Ulnar

EPITROCHLEO-ANCONEUS

Origin	Medial epicondyle of humerus	Absent	Absent
Insertion	Olecranon of ulna		
Nerve	Ulnar		

FLEXOR DIGITORUM SUPERFICIALIS

	PAPIO	*HOMO*	*PAN*
Origin	Medial epicondyle of humerus (no ulnar or radial heads)	Humeral head: medial epicondyle of humerus Ulnar head: coronoid process of ulna Radial head: oblique line of radius	Similar to *Homo* (radial head extends farther distally)
Insertion	Volar surfaces of the middle phalanges of digits II-V; an additional stout bundle of fibers connects this muscle with the m. flexor digitorum profundus in the middle of the forearm	Similar to *Papio*	Similar to *Papio*
Nerve	Median	Median	Median

FLEXOR DIGITORUM PROFUNDUS

Origin	Medial and volar surfaces of the radius; interosseus membrane; volar and lateral surfaces of the ulna	Medial and volar surfaces of the ulna; interosseus membrane	Similar to *Homo*
Insertion	Volar surfaces of the distal phalanges of digits I-V (this muscle supplies the long pollical tendon)	Volar surfaces of the distal phalanges of digits II-V	Volar surfaces of the distal phalanges of digits III-V
Nerve	Median	Median and ulnar	Median and ulnar

BRACHIORADIALIS

Origin	Proximal ½ lateral supracondylar ridge of humerus	Proximal ⅔ lateral supracondylar ridge of humerus	Lateral supracondylar ridge as high as the deltoid tuberosity
Insertion	Lateral side of the styloid process of the radius	Similar to *Papio*	Similar to *Papio*
Nerve	Radial	Radial	Radial

EXTENSOR CARPI RADIALIS LONGUS

	PAPIO	*HOMO*	*PAN*
Origin	Distal ½ lateral supracondylar ridge of humerus	Distal ⅓ lateral supracondylar ridge of humerus	Similar to *Homo*
Insertion	Dorsal surface of the base of metacarpal II	Similar to *Papio*	Similar to *Papio*
Nerve	Radial	Radial	Radial

EXTENSOR CARPI RADIALIS BREVIS

Origin	Lateral epicondyle of the humerus	Similar to *Papio*	Similar to *Papio*
Insertion	Dorsal surface of the base of metacarpal III	Similar to *Papio*	Similar to *Papio*
Nerve	Radial	Radial	Radial

EXTENSOR DIGITORUM

Origin	Lateral epicondyle of the humerus intermuscular septum	Similar to *Papio*	Similar to *Papio*
Insertion	Sides of the proximal phalanges and bases of the middle phalanges of the medial four digits	By tendinous slips into the dorsal surfaces of all three phalanges of the medial four digits	Similar to *Homo*
Nerve	Radial	Radial	Radial

EXTENSOR DIGITI ANULARIS

	PAPIO	HOMO	PAN
Origin	Lateral epicondyle of the humerus in common with the m. extensor digiti minimi	Absent	Absent
Insertion	Ulnar side of the dorsal surface of the proximal phalanx of digit IV		
Nerve	Radial		

EXTENSOR DIGITI MINIMI

	PAPIO	HOMO	PAN
Origin	Lateral epicondyle of the humerus	Common extensor tendon and intermuscular septum	Similar to Papio
Insertion	Ulnar side of the dorsal surface of the proximal phalanx of digit V	Similar to Papio	Similar to Papio
Nerve	Radial	Radial	Radial

EXTENSOR CARPI ULNARIS

	PAPIO	HOMO	PAN
Origin	Lateral epicondyle of the humerus	Lateral epicondyle of the humerus, and posterior border of the ulna	Similar to Homo
Insertion	Dorsal surface of the base of metacarpal V	Similar to Papio	Similar to Papio
Nerve	Radial	Radial	Radial

ANCONEUS

	PAPIO	HOMO	PAN
Origin	Posterolateral surface of the capsule of the elbow joint	Lateral epicondyle of the humerus	Similar to Homo
Insertion	Posterior border of the ulna just distal to the elbow joint	Lateral side of the olecranon and posterior border of the ulna	Similar to Homo
Nerve	Radial	Radial	Radial

SUPINATOR

	PAPIO	*HOMO*	*PAN*
Origin	Lateral epicondyle of the humerus and lateral border of the proximal ¼ of the ulna	Similar to *Papio*	Similar to *Papio*
Insertion	Lateral and volar surfaces of the proximal ⅓ of the radius	Similar to *Papio*	Similar to *Papio*
Nerve	Radial	Radial	Radial

ABDUCTOR POLLICIS LONGUS

Origin	Dorsal surface of the ulna; interosseous membrane; middle two quarters of the dorsal surface of the radius	Similar to *Papio*	Similar to *Papio* (ulna attachment variable)
Insertion	Radial side of metacarpal I; sesamoid bone (prepollex)	Radial side of metacarpal I	Radial surface of the trapezium; sesamoid bone (prepollex)
Nerve	Radial	Radial	Radial

EXTENSOR DIGITI INDICIS

Origin	Distal aspect of the dorsal surface of the ulna in common with the m. extensor digiti medius; interosseous membrane	Distal aspect of the dorsal surface of the ulna; interosseous membrane	Similar to *Homo*
Insertion	Dorsum of the proximal phalanx of digit II	Similar to *Papio*	Similar to *Papio* (quite variable)
Nerve	Radial	Radial	Radial

EXTENSOR DIGITI MEDIUS

	PAPIO	HOMO	PAN
Origin	Distal aspect of the dorsal surface of the ulna in common with the m. extensor digiti indicis	Absent	Absent
Insertion	Dorsum of the proximal phalanx of digit III		
Nerve	Radial		

ABDUCTOR POLLICIS BREVIS

	PAPIO	HOMO	PAN
Origin	Volar transverse carpal ligament; navicular and sesamoid bone of the m. abductor pollicis longus	Volar transverse carpal ligament; navicular and trapezium	Volar transverse carpal ligament; trapezium and sesamoid bone of the m. abductor pollicis longus
Insertion	Radial side of the base of the proximal phalanx of the pollex	Similar to *Papio*	Similar to *Papio*
Nerve	Median	Median	Median

OPPONENS POLLICIS

	PAPIO	HOMO	PAN
Origin	Volar transverse carpal ligament; trapezium	Similar to *Papio*	Similar to *Papio*
Insertion	Radial border of metacarpal I	Similar to *Papio*	Similar to *Papio*
Nerve	Median	Median	Median

FLEXOR POLLICIS BREVIS

	PAPIO	*HOMO*	*PAN*
Origin	Superficial head: volar transverse carpal ligament Deep head: ulnar side of the II; trapezoid and base of metacarpal II	Superficial head: volar transverse carpal ligament and trapezium Deep head: trapezoid and capitate	Superficialhead: similar to *Homo* Deep head: absent
Insertion	Superficial head: radial side of the base of the first pollical phalanx (into sesamoid) Deep head: ulnar side of the base of the first pollical phalanx (into sesamoid)	Similar to *Papio*	Superficial head: similar to *Papio*
Nerve	Superficial head: median Deep head: ulnar	Superficial head: median Deep head: ulnar	Median

ADDUCTOR POLLICIS

	PAPIO	*HOMO*	*PAN*
Origin	Bases of metacarpals II and III; contrahentes tendons; metacarpophalangeal joint capsules II and III	Oblique head: capitate bone; bases of metacarpals II and III Transverse head: volar surface of metacarpal III	Similar to *Homo*
Insertion	Ulnar side of the base of the first pollical phalanx and ulna sesamoid, and into the ulnar side of the distal pollical phalanx	Ulnar side of the base of the first pollical phalanx and ulna sesamoid	Similar to *Homo* (the oblique head sends a fine tendon along the ulnar side of the pollex which terminates on the distal phalanx)
Nerve	Ulnar	Ulnar	Ulnar

PALMARIS BREVIS

	PAPIO	*HOMO*	*PAN*
Origin	Ulnar side of the palmar aponeurosis	Similar to *Papio*	Similar to *Papio*
Insertion	Skin over the hypothenar eminence	Similar to *Papio*	Similar to *Papio*
Nerve	Ulnar	Ulnar	Ulnar

ABDUCTOR DIGITI MINIMI

	PAPIO	*HOMO*	*PAN*
Origin	Volar transverse carpal ligament; pisiform bone	Volar transverse carpal ligament; pisiform bone and hook of the hamate (occasionally)	Similar to *Homo*
Insertion	Ulnar side of the base of the proximal phalanx of digit V	Similar to *Papio*	Similar to *Papio*
Nerve	Ulnar	Ulnar	Ulnar

FLEXOR DIGITI MINIMI BREVIS

Origin	Volar transverse carpal ligament; hamulus of the hamate	Similar to *Papio*	Similar to *Papio*
Insertion	Ulnar side of the proximal phalanx of digit V with an extension of the dorsal aponeurosis	Similar to *Papio*	Similar to *Papio*
Nerve	Ulnar	Ulnar	Ulnar

OPPONENS DIGITI MINIMI

Origin	Volar transverse carpal ligament; hamulus of the hamate bone	Similar to *Papio*	Similar to *Papio*
Insertion	Ulnar border of metacarpal V	Similar to *Papio*	Similar to *Papio*
Nerve	Ulnar	Ulnar	Ulnar

Mm. LUMBRICALES

	PAPIO	*HOMO*	*PAN*
Origin	All four arise in the palm from the tendons of the m. flexor digitorum profundus 1st: tendon to digit II 2nd: adjacent sides of tendons to digits II and III 3rd: adjacent sides of tendons to digits III and IV 4th: adjacent sides of tendons to digits IV and V	Similar to *Papio*	Similar to *Papio*
Insertion	Radial sides of the proximal phalanges of digits II-V with dorsal extensions into the extensor aponeurosis	Similar to *Papio*	Similar to *Papio*
Nerve	Median (1st and 2nd lumbricals); ulnar (3rd and 4th lumbricals)	Median (1st and 2nd lumbricals); ulnar (3rd and 4th lumbricals)	Median (1st and 2nd lumbricals); ulnar (3rd and 4th lumbricals)

Mm. CONTRAHENTES MANUS

Origin	All three from the contrahens tendon (extending from the bases of metacarpals II and III to the head of metacarpal III)	Absent	Reduced and aponeurotic
Insertion	1st: ulna side of the proximal phalanx of digit II 2nd: radial side of the proximal phalanx of digit IV 3rd: radial side of the proximal phalanx of digit V		Reduced and aponeurotic
Nerve	Ulnar		

Mm. INTEROSSEI PALMARES

	PAPIO	HOMO	PAN
Origin	Variable in number; usually only three distinct muscles 1st: bases of metacarpals II and III 2nd: bases of metacarpals III and IV 3rd: bases of metacarpals IV and V	1st: from the ulnar side of metacarpal II 2nd: from the radial side of metacarpal IV 3rd: from the radial side of metacarpal V	Similar to *Homo*
Insertion	All three are inserted to the proximal phalanges of their corresponding digits with dorsal extensions to the extensor aponeuroses. 1st: to the ulnar side of digit II 2nd: to the radial side of digit IV 3rd: to the radial side of digit V	Similar to *Papio*	Similar to *Papio*
Nerve	Ulnar	Ulnar	Ulnar

Mm. INTEROSSEI DORSALES

	PAPIO	HOMO	PAN
Origin	1st: adjacent sides of metacarpals I and II 2nd: adjacent sides of metacarpals II and III 3rd: adjacent sides of metacarpals III and IV 4th: adjacent sides of metacarpals IV and V	Similar to *Papio*	Similar to *Papio*
Insertion	All four are inserted to the proximal phalanges of their corresponding digits with dorsal extensions to the extensor aponeuroses. 1st: radial side of the proximal phalanx of digit II 2nd: radial side of the proximal phalanx of digit III 3rd: ulnar side of the proximal phalanx of digit III 4th: ulnar side of proximal phalanx of digit IV	Similar to *Papio*	Similar to *Papio*
Nerve	Ulnar	Ulnar	Ulnar

PSOAS MAJOR

	PAPIO	*HOMO*	*PAN*
Origin	Vertebral bodies; discs; and transverse processes of L1-7	Vertebral bodies; discs; and transverse processes of T12-L5	Vertebral bodies; discs; and transverse processes of T13-L4 and last rib
Insertion	Lesser trochanter of femur	Similar to *Papio*	Similar to *Papio*
Nerve	Femoral	Femoral	Femoral

PSOAS MINOR

Origin	Vertebral bodies and discs of L1-4	Vertebral bodies and discs of T12-L1	Vertebral bodies and discs of T13-L1
Insertion	Iliopectineal line of innominate	Similar to *Papio*	Similar to *Papio*
Nerve	Femoral	Femoral	Femoral

ILIACUS

Origin	Iliac crest and upper iliac fossa of innominate; anterior sacroiliac ligament	Similar to *Papio*	Similar to *Papio*
Insertion	Lesser trochanter of femur	Similar to *Papio*	Similar to *Papio*
Nerve	Femoral	Femoral	Femoral

SARTORIUS

Origin	Middle ⅓ of margo acetabuli of ilium (see Benton and Gavan 1960)	Anterior superior iliac spine, and upper ½ of iliac notch	Via aponeurosis of entire length of margo acetabuli of ilium (see Benton and Gavan 1960)
Insertion	Proximomedial tibia	Similar to *Papio*	Similar to *Papio*
Nerve	Femoral	Femoral	Femoral

RECTUS FEMORIS

	PAPIO	HOMO	PAN
Origin	Ante-acetabular process of ilium (heads not completely separate)	Straight head: anterior inferior iliac spine of ilium Reflected head: cranial margin of acetabulum	Similar to Papio
Insertion	Base of patella	Similar to Papio	Similar to Papio
Nerve	Femoral	Femoral	Femoral

VASTUS MEDIALIS

Origin	Intertrochanteric line and medial lip of linea aspera for proximal ⅓ of femoral shaft	Intertrochanteric line and medial lip of linea aspera for entire length of femoral shaft to medial supracondylar line	Similar to Homo
Insertion	Medial patella	Similar to Papio	Similar to Papio
Nerve	Femoral	Femoral	Femoral

VASTUS LATERALIS

Origin	Lateral aspect of greater trochanter of femur	Anterior inferior border of greater trochanter; intertrochanteric line; gluteal tuberosity and entire lateral lip of linea aspera of femur	Similar to Homo
Insertion	Lateral patella	Similar to Papio	Similar to Papio
Nerve	Femoral	Femoral	Femoral

VASTUS INTERMEDIUS

Origin	Anterior surface of femoral shaft (m. articularis genus absent)	Anterior surface of femoral shaft (m. articularis genus present)	Similar to Paplo
Insertion	Base of patella	Similar to Papio	Similar to Papio
Nerve	Femoral	Femoral	Femoral

OBTURATORIUS EXTERNUS

	PAPIO	*HOMO*	*PAN*
Origin	Outer margin of obturator foramen of innominate; outer surface of obturator foramen	Similar to *Papio*	Similar to *Papio*
Insertion	Trochanteric fossa of femur	Similar to *Papio*	Similar to *Papio*
Nerve	Obturator	Obturator	Obturator

GRACILIS

Origin	Medial margin of inferior ramus of pubis and upper margin of inferior ramus of ischium	Medial margin of inferior ramus of pubis	Similar to *Homo*
Insertion	Proximomedial tibia	Similar to *Papio*	Similar to *Papio*
Nerve	Obturator	Obturator	Obturator

PECTINEUS

Origin	Pectineal line of pubis	Similar to *Papio*	Similar to *Papio*
Insertion	Pectineal line of femur	Similar to *Papio*	Similar to *Papio*
Nerve	Femoral	Femoral and obturator	Femoral and obturator

ADDUCTOR LONGUS

Origin	Superior ramus of pubis	Pubic angle between crest and symphysis	Similar to *Papio*
Insertion	Middle ⅓ of medial lip of linea aspera of femur	Similar to *Papio*	Similar to *Papio*
Nerve	Obturator	Obturator	Obturator

ADDUCTOR BREVIS

	PAPIO	*HOMO*	*PAN*
Origin	Pubic angle and superior ramus of pubis	Inferior ramus of pubis	Two heads (occasionally three) from the pubic angle and inferior ramus of pubis
Insertion	Pectineal line and proximal ⅓ of medial lip of linea aspera of femur	Similar to *Papio*	Similar to *Papio*
Nerve	Obturator	Obturator	Obturator

ADDUCTOR MAGNUS

Origin	Inferior ischiopubic ramus and ischial tuberosity of ischium	Similar to *Papio*	Similar to *Papio*
Insertion	Gluteal tuberosity; linea aspera; and popliteal surface of femur	Gluteal tuberosity; linea aspera; medial supracondylar line; and adductor tubercle of femur	Gluteal tuberosity; linea aspera; popliteal surface; and adductor tubercle of femur
Nerve	Obturator	Obturator and sciatic	Obturator and sciatic

GLUTEUS MAXIMUS

Origin	Transverse processes of the cranial one or two caudal vertebrae	Gluteal surface behind the posterior gluteal line; dorsal surface of the sacrum and coccyx; sacrotuberous ligament	Dorsal surface of the sacrum and coccyx; sacrotuberous ligament; ischial tuberosity of ischium
Insertion	Gluteal tuberosity and proximal ¼ lateral lip of linea aspera of femur	Similar to *Papio*	Gluteal tuberosity and entire lateral lip of linea aspera to lateral condyle of femur
Nerve	Inferior gluteal	Inferior gluteal	Inferior gluteal

TENSOR FASCIAE LATAE

	PAPIO	*HOMO*	*PAN*
Origin	Upper ½ of margo acetabuli of ilium	External lip of iliac crest and margo acetabuli of ilium	Aponeurosis of margo acetabuli of ilium
Insertion	Iliotibial tract to femoral shaft, patella, fascia of upper leg	Similar to *Papio*	Similar to *Papio*
Nerve	Superior gluteal	Superior gluteal	Superior gluteal

GLUTEUS MEDIUS

Origin	Upper gluteal surface of ilium	Similar to *Papio*	Similar to *Papio*
Insertion	Greater trochanter of femur	Similar to *Papio*	Similar to *Papio*
Nerve	Superior gluteal	Superior gluteal	Superior gluteal

PIRIFORMIS

Origin	Transverse processes of S2-3	Pelvic surface of sacrum between anterior sacral foramina; margin of greater sciatic foramen of innominate; sacrotuberous ligament	Similar to *Homo*
Insertion	Greater trochanter of femur	Similar to *Papio*	Similar to *Papio*
Nerve	N. to piriformis	N. to piriformis	N. to piriformis

GLUTEUS MINIMUS

Origin	Caudal ½ of gluteal surface of ilium from margo acetabuli to margin of greater sciatic notch	Similar to *Papio*	Caudal ¼ gluteal surface of ilium from margo acetabuli to margin of greater sciatic notch
Insertion	Anterior surface of greater trochanter of femur	Similar to *Papio*	Similar to *Papio*
Nerve	Superior gluteal	Superior gluteal	Superior gluteal

SCANSORIUS

	PAPIO	HOMO	PAN
Origin	Inconstant (the more ventral fibers of m. gluteus minimus may form a separate head, which is then called m. scansorius)	Absent	Absent (see Sigmon 1969)
Insertion	Anterior surface of greater trochanter of femur		
Nerve	Superior gluteal		

OBTURATORIUS INTERNUS

	PAPIO	HOMO	PAN
Origin	Inner obturator membrane; pelvic surface superior pubic and ischiopubic rami of innominate	Similar to Papio	Similar to Papio
Insertion	Medial surface of greater trochanter of femur	Similar to Papio	Similar to Papio
Nerve	N. to obturator internus (n. puboischiofemoralis)	N. to obturator internus(and superior gemellus)	N. to obturator internus (and superior gemellus)

Mm. GEMELLI

	PAPIO	HOMO	PAN
Origin	Not differentiated, ischial ramus and tuberosity of ischium	Superior: ischial spine Inferior: ischial spine	Similar to Homo
Insertion	Tendon of m. obturator internus	Similar to Papio	Similar to Papio
Nerve	N. to gemelli (n. puboischiofemoralis)	Superior: n. to obturator internus Inferior: n. to quadratus femoris	Superior: n. to obturator internus Inferior: n. to quadratus femoris

QUADRATUS FEMORIS

	PAPIO	*HOMO*	*PAN*
Origin	Ischial tuberosity of ischium	Similar to *Papio*	Similar to *Papio*
Insertion	Lower intertrochanteric crest and lesser trochanter of femur	Linea quadrata of femur	Similar to *Papio*
Nerve	N. to quadratus femoris (n. puboischiofemoralis)	N. to quadratus femoris (and inferior gemellus)	N. to quadratus femoris (and inferior gemellus)

BICEPS FEMORIS

	PAPIO	*HOMO*	*PAN*
Origin	Long head: ischial tuberosity of ischium	Long head: similar to *Papio*	Long head: similar to *Papio*
	Short head: absent	Short head: middle ⅓ lateral lip of linea aspera of femur	Short head: lower ⅓ lateral lip of linea aspera of femur
Insertion	Fascia lata; aponeurosis to anterior border of proximal ½ of tibia	Long head: head of fibula; lateral condyle of tibia	Long head: similar to *Homo*
		Short head: lateral condyle of tibia	Short head: head and proximal inch of fibular shaft
Nerve	N. to hamstrings (n. flexores femoris)	Long head: n. to hamstrings (tibial division of sciatic) Short head: common peroneal division of sciatic	Long head: n. to hamstrings (n. flexores femoris) Short head: common peroneal division of sciatic

SEMIMEMBRANOSUS

	PAPIO	*HOMO*	*PAN*
Origin	Two heads from ischial tuberosity of ischium	Single head from ischial tuberosity	Similar to *Homo*
Insertion	Proprius: medial condyle of tibia	Posteromedial condyle of tibia	Similar to *Homo*
	Accessorius: linea aspera to popliteal surface of femur		
Nerve	Flexores femoris	N. to hamstrings (from tibial division of sciatic)	Flexores femoris

SEMITENDINOSUS

	PAPIO	*HOMO*	*PAN*
Origin	Ischial tuberosity of ischium	Similar to *Papio*	Similar to *Papio*
Insertion	Proximomedial tibia	Similar to *Papio*	Similar to *Papio*
Nerve	Flexores femoris	N. to hamstrings (from tibial division of sciatic)	Flexores femoris

TIBIALIS ANTERIOR

	PAPIO	*HOMO*	*PAN*
Origin	Lateral condyle and proximolateral shaft of tibia; interosseous membrane	Similar to *Papio*	Similar to *Papio*
Insertion	Base of medial cuneiform; base of hallucal metatarsal (the muscle belly is usually divided, and the lateral part is then called m. abductor hallucis longus)	Similar to *Papio* (muscle belly rarely divided)	Similar to *Papio* (muscle belly usually divided)
Nerve	Deep peroneal	Deep peroneal	Deep peroneal

EXTENSOR DIGITORUM LONGUS

	PAPIO	*HOMO*	*PAN*
Origin	Lateral condyle of tibia; head and anterior surface of fibula; interosseous membrane	Similar to *Papio*	Similar to *Papio*
Insertion	Dorsal bases of middle and distal phalanges of lateral four digits	Similar to *Papio*	Similar to *Papio*
Nerve	Deep peroneal	Deep peroneal	Deep peroneal

PERONEUS TERTIUS

	PAPIO	HOMO	PAN
Origin	Absent	Distal fibula; interosseous membrane	Absent
Insertion		Dorsal base of metatarsal V	
Nerve		Deep peroneal	

EXTENSOR HALLUCIS LONGUS

	PAPIO	HOMO	PAN
Origin	Middle ⅓ of anteromedial surface of fibula; interosseous membrane	Similar to *Papio*	Similar to *Papio*
Insertion	Bases of both hallucal phalanges	Bases of distal phalanx of hallux	Similar to *Homo*
Nerve	Deep peroneal	Deep peroneal	Deep peroneal

EXTENSOR DIGITORUM BREVIS

	PAPIO	HOMO	PAN
Origin	Superolateral surface of calcaneus	Similar to *Papio*	Similar to *Papio*
Insertion	Dorsal surface of base of proximal hallucal phalanx (m. extensor hallucis brevis); lateral sides of middle and distal phalanges of digits II-IV	Dorsal surface of base of proximal hallucal phalanx (m. extensor hallucis brevis); lateral sides of tendons of m. extensor digitorum longus to middle and distal phalanges of digits II-IV	Similar to *Papio*
Nerve	Deep peroneal	Deep peroneal	Deep peroneal

PERONEUS LONGUS

	PAPIO	HOMO	PAN
Origin	Lateral tibial condyle; lateral fibular head and shaft	Lateral fibular head and shaft	Similar to *Homo*
Insertion	Base of hallucal metatarsal (accessory slips may attach to base of metatarsal V and cuboid)	Base of hallucal metatarsal; lateral surface of cuneiform I	Similar to *Homo*
Nerve	Superficial peroneal	Superficial peroneal	Superficial peroneal

PERONEUS BREVIS

	PAPIO	HOMO	PAN
Origin	Distolateral surface of fibula	Similar to Papio	Similar to Papio
Insertion	Tuberosity of metatarsal V	Similar to Papio	Similar to Papio (may send slip to dorsal expansion over proximal phalanx of digit V)
Nerve	Superficial peroneal	Superficial peroneal	Superficial peroneal

PERONEUS DIGITI QUINTI

Origin	Upper posterolateral edge of fibular shaft	Absent	(The slip from the peroneus brevis is a remnant of this muscle.)
Insertion	Lateral side of distal phalanx of digit V		
Nerve	Superficial peroneal		

GASTROCNEMIUS

Origin	Medial head: upper posteromedial condyle of femur	Similar to Papio	Similiar to Papio
	Lateral head: upper posterolateral femoral condyle		
Insertion	Calcaneal tuberosity	Similar to Papio	Similar to Papio
Nerve	Tibial	Tibial	Tibial

SOLEUS

	PAPIO	*HOMO*	*PAN*
Origin	Posterior head of fibula	Posterior head of fibula; popliteal line of tibia	Similar to *Papio*
Insertion	Calcaneal tuberosity	Similar to *Papio*	Similar to *Papio*
Nerve	Tibial	Tibial	Tibial

PLANTARIS

Origin	Posterolateral surface of lateral femoral condyle	Similar to *Papio*	Similar to *Papio* (frequently absent)
Insertion	Passes dorsal to calcaneal tuberosity and into sole of foot as plantar aponeurosis	Posteromedial surface of calcaneus	Expanded insertion into calcaneal tendon
Nerve	Tibial	Tibial	Tibial

POPLITEUS

Origin	Lateral epicondyle of femur	Similar to *Papio*	Similar to *Papio*
Insertion	Medial condyle of tibia and posteromedial tibial shaft	Posterior tibia above popliteal line	Similar to *Papio*
Nerve	Tibial	Tibial	Tibial

PERONEOTIBIALIS

Origin	Anteromedial head of fibula	Absent	Similar to *Papio* (infrequent)
Insertion	Proximal ⅓ posterolateral surface of tibia		Similar to *Papio* (infrequent)
Nerve	Tibial		Tibial

FLEXOR DIGITORUM LONGUS (FLEXOR DIGITORUM TIBIALIS)

	PAPIO	HOMO	PAN
Origin	Posteromedial ⅓ of tibial shaft	Similar to Papio	Similar to Papio
Insertion	Plantar surface of bases of distal phalanges of digits II and V, with smaller tendons to digits I, III, and IV	Plantar surface of bases of distal phalanges of digits II-V	Similar to Papio
Nerve	Tibial	Tibial	Tibial

FLEXOR HALLUCIS LONGUS (FLEXOR DIGITORUM FIBULARIS)

Origin	Posterior head and shaft of fibula; posterior surface of distal ½ of tibial shaft, interosseous membrane	Distal ⅔ of posterior fibular shaft; interosseous membrane	Posterior head and shaft of fibula; interosseous membrane
Insertion	Plantar surface of bases of distal phalanges of digits I, II, and IV	Plantar surface of base of distal phalanx of hallux	Similar to Papio
Nerve	Tibial	Tibial	Tibial

TIBIALIS POSTERIOR

Origin	Proximal ½ posterolateral surface of tibia; head and proximal ½ posteromedial surface of fibula	Similar to Papio (no attachment to fibula head)	Similar to Papio
Insertion	Navicular, cuneiforms I, II, and III; cuboid, plantar surface of bases of metatarsals II, III, and IV	Similar to Papio	Similar to Papio
Nerve	Tibial	Tibial	Tibial

FLEXOR DIGITORUM BREVIS

	PAPIO	*HOMO*	*PAN*
Origin	Superficial head: deep surface of plantar aponeurosis; medial process of calcaneus Deep head: undivided tendon of m. flexor digitorum tibialis	Superficial head only	Similar to *Homo*
Insertion	Superficial head: plantar surface of middle phalanx of digit II Deep head: plantar surface of middle phalanges of digits III, IV, and V	Middle phalanges of digits II, III, IV, and V	Similar to *Homo* (tendon to digit V is vestigial)
Nerve	Medial plantar	Medial plantar	Medial plantar

ABDUCTOR HALLUCIS BREVIS

	PAPIO	*HOMO*	*PAN*
Origin	Medial process of calcaneous	Similar to *Papio*	Similar to *Papio*
Insertion	Medial side of metatarsophalangeal joint capsule, with extension to base of proximal hallucal phalanx	Similar to *Papio*	Similar to *Papio*
Nerve	Medial plantar	Medial plantar	Medial plantar

ABDUCTOR DIGITI QUINTI

	PAPIO	*HOMO*	*PAN*
Origin	Lateral process of calcaneus; deep surface of plantar aponeurosis	Lateral and medial processes of calcaneus; deep surface of plantar aponeurosis	Similar to *Papio*
Insertion	Lateral surface of proximal phalanx of digit V (those fibers attaching to the tuberosity of metatarsal V and the m. abductor ossis metatarsi quinti)	Similar to *Papio*	Similar to *Papio*
Nerve	Lateral plantar	Lateral plantar	Lateral plantar

QUADRATUS PLANTAE

	PAPIO	HOMO	PAN
Origin	Single head from lateral side of calcaneus	Lateral head: lateral side of calcaneus Medial head: medial side of calcaneus	Similar to *Papio* (frequently absent)
Insertion	Lateral side of long flexor tendon to digit V, with additional slips to tendons of medial four digits (III and IV may be missing)	Lateral border of undivided tendon of flexor digitorum longus	Similar to *Papio* (frequently absent)
Nerve	Lateral plantar	Lateral plantar	Lateral plantar

FLEXOR HALLUCIS BREVIS

	PAPIO	HOMO	PAN
Origin	Medial head: navicular and medial cuneiform Lateral head: medial cuneiform	Single head from medial plantar surface of cuboid; lateral cuneiform and tendon of m. tibialis posterior	Medial head: medial cuneiform; plantar base of hallucal metatarsal Lateral head: sheath of m. peroneus longus; long plantar ligament
Insertion	Medial head: medial side of base of proximal phalanx of hallux and hallucal metatarsophalangeal joint capsule Lateral head: lateral side of base of proximal phalanx of hallux and hallucal metatarsophalangeal joint capsule	Similar to *Papio*	Similar to *Papio*
Nerve	Medial plantar	Medial plantar	Medial plantar

FLEXOR DIGITI QUINTI BREVIS

	PAPIO	HOMO	PAN
Origin	Base of metatarsal V; sheath of peroneus longus tendon	Similar to *Papio*	Similar to *Papio*
Insertion	Lateral side of base of proximal phalanx of digit V	Similar to *Papio*	Similar to *Papio*
Nerve	Lateral plantar	Lateral plantar	Lateral plantar

ADDUCTOR HALLUCIS

	PAPIO	*HOMO*	*PAN*
Origin	Transverse head: head and joint capsules of metatarsals II and III; contrahentes of II and IV Oblique head: bases of metatarsals II and III	Transverse head: heads and joint capsules of metatarsals III, IV, and V Oblique head: bases of metatarsals II, III, and IV	Transverse head: heads and joint capsules of metatarsals II and III Oblique head: base of metatarsal III
Insertion	Lateral side of base of proximal hallucal phalanx	Similar to *Papio*	Similar to *Papio*
Nerve	Lateral plantar	Lateral plantar	Lateral plantar

Mm. CONTRAHENTES

Origin	Three muscles from a common aponeurotic tendon attached to sheath of m. peroneus longus tendon	Absent	Absent
Insertion	Proximal phalanges of digits II (laterally) and IV and V (medially)		
Nerve	Lateral plantar		

Mm. LUMBRICALES

Origin	Four muscles from sides of long flexor tendons: 1. Medial side of tendon to digit II 2. Lateral side of tendon to digit II; medial side of tendon to digit III 3. Lateral side of tendon to digit III; medial side of tendon to digit IV 4. Lateral side of tendon to digit IV; medial side of tendon to digit V	Similar to *Papio*	Similar to *Papio*
Insertion	Dorsal expansions of extensor tendons over proximal phalanges of lateral four digits	Similar to *Papio*	Similar to *Papio*
Nerve	II: Medial plantar V: Lateral plantar III: Variable IV: Variable	Same as *Papio*	Same as *Papio*

Mm. INTEROSSEI DORSALES

	PAPIO	HOMO	PAN
Origin	First and second dorsals from base of metatarsal II and sheath of m. peroneus longus; third and fourth dorsals from bases of metatarsals IV and V and sheath of m. peroneus longus	Sides and bases of metatarsals I-V	Similar to *Homo*
Insertion	Sides of proximal phalanges of lateral four digits: First dorsal to digit II, medially Second dorsal to digit III, medially Third dorsal to digit III, laterally Fourth dorsal to digit IV, laterally	Sides of proximal phalanges of lateral four digits: First dorsal to digit II, medially Second dorsal to digit II, laterally Third dorsal to digit III, laterally Fourth dorsal to digit IV, laterally	Similar to *Papio*
Nerve	Lateral plantar	Lateral plantar	Lateral plantar

Mm. INTEROSSEI PLANTARES

	PAPIO	HOMO	PAN
Origin	First plantar from base of metatarsal II and sheath of m. peroneus longus; second and third plantars from base of metatarsals IV and V and sheath of m. peroneus longus	Bases of metatarsals III-V	First plantar from shaft of metatarsal II, laterally Second plantar from shaft of metatarsal IV, medially Third plantar from base of metatarsal IV, medially
Insertion	Sides of proximal phalanges of lateral digits: First plantar to digit II, laterally Second plantar to digit IV, medially Third plantar to digit V, medially	Sides of proximal phalanges of lateral three digits: First plantar to digit III, medially Second plantar to digit IV, medially Third plantar to digit V, medially	Similar to *Papio*
Nerve	Lateral plantar	Lateral plantar	Lateral plantar

BIBLIOGRAPHY

Alpers, B. J., R. G. Berry, and R. M. Paddison. 1959. Anatomical studies of the circle of Willis in normal brain. Arch. Neurol. Psychiat. (Chicago) 81:409-25.

Ariëns Kappers, C. V., G. C. Huber, and E. C. Crosby. 1936. The comparative anatomy of the nervous system of vertebrates, including man. New York: Macmillan.

Ashley-Montague, M. R. 1939. Anthropological significance of the musculus pyramidalis and its variability in man. Amer. J. Phys. Anthropol. 25:435-90.

Ashton, E. H., and C. E. Oxnard. 1958. Some variations in the maxillary nerve of primates. Proc. Zool. Soc. Lond. 131:457-70.

_____. 1963. The musculature of the primate shoulder. Trans. Zool. Soc. Lond. 29:553-650.

Atkinson, W. W., and H. Elftman. 1950. Female reproduction system of the gorilla. In The anatomy of the gorilla, ed. W. K. Gregory, pp. 205-7. New York: Columbia Univ. Press.

Barnett, C. H., and J. R. Napier. 1952. The rotatory mobility of the fibula in eutherian mammals. J. Anat. Lond. 86:11-21.

Batson, O. V. 1946. The adult thyroglossal duct. Anat. Rec. 94:499-50.

Benton, R. S., and J. A. Gavan. 1960. The concept of homology applied to the anterior superior iliac spine. Amer. J. Phys. Anthropol. 18:273-79.

Berringer, O. M., Jr., F. M. Browning, and C. R. Schroeder. 1968. An atlas and dissection manual of rhesus monkey anatomy. Tallahassee, Fla.: Anatomy Laboratory Aids.

Biegert, J. 1961. Volarhaut der Hände und Füsse. In Handbuch der Primatenkunde, 2/1, Lieferung 3. New York: S. Karger.

Bland-Sutton, J. 1884. On some points in the anatomy of the chimpanzee. J. Anat. and Physiol. 18:66-85.

Blount, R. F., and E. Lachman. 1966. The digestive system. In Morris' human anatomy, ed. B. J. Anson, pp. 1229-1384. 12th ed. New York: McGraw-Hill.

Bowden, R. E. M., Z. Y. Mahran, and M. R. Godding. 1960. Communication between the facial and trigeminal nerves in certain mammals. Proc. Zool. Soc. Lond. 135:587-611.

Boyden, E. A. 1955. The choledocho- and pancreatoco-duodenal junctions in the chimpanzee. Surgery 37:918-27.

_____. 1966. The pancreatic sphincters of the baboon as revealed by serial sections of the choledochoduodenal junction. Surgery 60: 1187-94.

Brodman, K. 1909. Vergleichende Lokalisationslehre der Grosshirnrinde. Leipzig.

Buettner-Janusch, J. 1966. A problem in evolutionary systematics: Nomenclature and classification of baboons, genus Papio. Folia Primat. 4:288-308.

Campbell, B. G. 1966. Human evolution: An introduction to man's adaptations. Chicago: Aldine.

Campbell, C. B. G. 1969. The visual system of insectivores and primates. Annals N. Y. Acad. Sci. 167:388-403.

Celemencki, J., and S. Zajac. 1968. Structure and topography of the great salivary glands in *Macacus cynomolgus*. Folia Morphol. 27:91-96.

Champneys, F. 1871. On the muscles and nerves of a chimpanzee *(Troglodytes niger)* and a *Cynocephalus anubis*. J. Anat. and Physiol. 7:176-211.

Chapman, W. L., Jr., and J. R. Allen. 1971. The fine structure of the thymus of the fetal and neonatal monkey *(Macaca mulatta)*. Z. Zellforsch. 114:220-33.

Chase, R. E., and C. F. De Garis. 1940. The brachial plexus in *Macacus rhesus,* compared with man. Amer. J. Phys. Anthropol. 27:223-54.

———. 1948. The subclavian and axillary arteries in *Macacus rhesus,* compared with man. Amer. J. Phys. Anthropol. 6:85-109.

Chouké, K. S. 1946. On incidence of foramen civinini and porus crotaphitoco-buccinatorius in American whites and Negroes: I. Observations in 1544 skulls. Amer. J. Phys. Anthropol. 4:203-25.

Connolly, C. J. 1936. The fissural pattern of the primate brain. Amer. J. Phys. Anthropol. 21:301-422.

———. 1950. External morphology of the primate brain. Springfield, Ill.: Charles C. Thomas Co.

Crosby, E. C., T. Humphrey, and E. W. Lauer. 1962. Correlative anatomy of the nervous system. New York: Macmillan.

De Garis, C. F. 1935. Patterns of the aortic arch in a series of 133 macaques. J. Anat. Lond. 70:149-58

DuBrul, E. L., and H. Sicher. 1954. The adaptive chin. Springfield, Ill.: Charles C. Thomas Co.

Elliot Smith, G. 1902. Descriptive and illustrated catalogue of the physiological series of comparative anatomy contained in the Museum of the Royal College of Surgeons of England. London: Taylor and Francis.

———. 1903. On the morphology of the brain in the mammalia, with special reference to that of lemurs. Trans. Linn. Soc. Lond. 8:312-432.

Erikson, G. E. 1963. Brachiation in the New World monkeys and in anthropoid apes. Symp. Zool. Soc. Lond. 10:135-64.

Francis, C. C. 1966. The nervous system (The peripheral nervous system). In Morris' human anatomy, ed. B. J. Anson, pp. 1022-1119. 12th ed. New York: McGraw-Hill.

Freedman, L. 1957. The fossil Cercopithecoidea of South Africa. Annals Transvaal Mus. 23:121-262. Cambridge: Cambridge Univ. Press.

Frey, H. 1923. Untersuchungen über die Scapula, speziell über ihre äussere Form und deren abhängigkeit von der Funktion. Zeitschr. f. Anat. u. Entwicklungsgesch. 68: 277-324.

Frick, H. V. 1960. Das Herz der Primaten. In Primatologia: Handbook of primatology, ed. H. Hofer, A. H. Schultz, and D. Starck, 3/2:163-272. New York: S. Karger.

Gardner, W. V. 1966. The endocrine glands and unclassified organs. In Morris' human anatomy, ed. B. J. Anson, pp. 1539-62. 12th ed. New York: McGraw-Hill.

Gasser, R. F., and A. G. Hendrickx. 1969. The development of the trigeminal nerve in baboon embryos (Papio sp.). J. Comp. Neur. 136:159-82.

Geist, F. D. 1933. Nasal cavity, larynx, mouth and pharynx. In The anatomy of the rhesus monkey, ed. C. G. Hartman and W. L. Straus, Jr., pp. 189-209. Baltimore, Md.: Williams and Wilkins.

George, R. M., Jr. 1968. The intrinsic back musculature of Macaca mulatta. Master's thesis, Dept. of Anatomy, Medical College of Virginia, Richmond.

Glidden, E. M., and C. F. De Garis. 1936. Arteries of the chimpanzee (Pan spec.). Amer. J. Phys. Anthropol. 58:501-27.

Gourmain, J. 1966. Le plexus lombosacré chez les primates. J. für Hirnforschung, ed. S. Heft. 4:315-41.

Grant, J. C. Boileau. 1962. An atlas of anatomy. 5th ed. Baltimore, Md.: Williams and Wilkins.

Gregory, W. K. 1916. Studies on the evolution of the primates. Bull. Amer. Mus. Nat. Hist. 35:239-355.

_____. 1949. The humerus from fish to man. Amer. Mus. Novitates No. 1400, pp. 1-54.

Grzybowski, J. 1926. Badamia filogenetyczne nad tetnica (a. coeliaca) i jej rozgalezieniami w szeregu naczelnych (L'artère coeliaque chez les primates). C .R. Soc. Sci. Varsouvie 19:165-94. Fr. abst.

Guilloud, N. B., and H. M. McClure. 1969. Air sac infection in the orang-utan (Pongo pygmaeus). In Recent advances in primatology, ed. C. Noback and W. Montagna, 3:143-47. New York: S. Karger.

Harris, W. 1939. The morphology of the brachial plexus with notes on the pectoral muscle and its tendon twist. London: Oxford Medical Publishers.

Hayek, H. von. 1960. Die Lunge und Pleura der Primaten. In Primatologia: Handbook of primatology, ed. H. Hofer, A. H. Schultz, and D. Starck, 3/2:588-624. New York: S. Karger.

Hayreh, S. S. 1964. The orbital vessels of rhesus monkeys. Exp. Eye Res. 3:16-30.

Hellman, M. 1928. Racial characters in human dentition. Proc. Amer. Philos. Soc. 67:157-74.

Hershkovitz, P. 1970. Primate chins. Bull. Field Mus. Nat. Hist. 41:6-10.

Hill, W. C. Osman. 1953. Man's ancestry: A primer of human phylogeny. Springfield, Ill.: Charles C. Thomas Co.

_____. 1957. Pharynx,oesophagus, stomach, small and large intestine form and position. In Primatologia: Handbook of primatology, ed. H. Hofer, A. H. Schultz, and D. Starck, 3/2:139-207. New York: S. Karger.

_____. 1959. The correct name of the olive baboon. J. Mammal. 40:143-44.

_____. 1966. Primates: Comparative anatomy and taxonomy, vol. 6: Cercopithecoidea. New York: Interscience Publishers.

_____. 1967a. The taxonomy of the genus *Pan*. In Progress in primatology, ed. D. Starck, R. Schneider, and H. J. Kuhn, 8:47-58. Stuttgart.

_____. 1967b. Taxonomy of the baboon. In The baboon in medical research, ed. H. Vagtborg, 2:3-11. Austin: Univ. of Texas Press.

_____. 1969. The vascular supply of the face in long-snouted primates. Z. Morph. Anthropol. 61:18-32.

_____. 1970. Primates: Comparative anatomy and taxonomy, vol. 8: Cynopithecinae. New York: Wiley-Interscience.

Hill, W. C. Osman, and R. E. Rewell. 1948. The caecum of primates: Its appendages, mesenteries, and blood supply. Trans. Zool. Soc. London 26:199-256.

Hilloowala, R. A. 1969. The laryngeal air sacs and air spaces in certain primates. Anat. Rec. 169:340. Abst.

_____. 1970. A comparative study of the primate hyoid bone. Anat. Rec. 166:319. Abst.

Hindze, B. 1930. Cerebral arteries of chimpanzee. Zeitschr. f. Morphol. u. Anthropol. 27:468-91.

Hofer, H. O. 1969. On the evolution of the craniocerebral topography in primates. Annal. N. Y. Acad. Sci. 162:15-24.

Hornbeck, P. V., and D. R. Swindler. 1967. Morphology of the lower fourth premolar of certain Cercopithecidae. J. Dent. Res. 46:979-83.

Howell, B., and W. L. Straus, Jr. 1933a. The spinal nerves. In The anatomy of the rhesus monkey, ed. C. G. Hartman and W. L. Straus, Jr., pp. 307-27. Baltimore, Md.: Williams and Wilkins.

_____. 1933b. The muscular system. In The anatomy of the rhesus monkey, ed. C. G. Hartman and W. L. Straus, Jr., pp. 89-175. Baltimore, Md.: Williams and Wilkins.

Hrdlička, A. 1920. Shovel-shaped teeth. Amer. J. Phys. Anthropol. 3:429-71.

Huber, E. 1931. Evolution of facial musculature and facial expression. Baltimore, Md.: Johns Hopkins Press.

Huelke, D. R. 1957. A study of the formation of the sural nerve in adult man. Amer. J. Phys. Anthropol. 15:137-47.

James, W. W. 1960. The jaws and teeth of primates. London: Pitman Medical Publishing Co.

Kassell, N. F., and T. W. Langfitt. 1965. Variations in the circle of Willis in *Macaca mulatta*. Anat. Rec. 152:257-64.

Kelemen, G. 1969. Anatomy of the larynx and the anatomical basis of vocal performance. In The chimpanzee: Anatomy, behavior and diseases of chimpanzees, ed. G. H. Bourne. New York: S. Karger.

Kerr, A. T. 1918. The brachial plexus of nerves in man, the variations in its formation and branches. Amer. J. Anat. 23:285-395.

Krogman, W. M. 1930. Studies in growth changes in the skull and face of Anthropoids. II. Ectocranial and endocranial suture closure in Anthropoids and Old World apes. Amer. J. Anat. 46:315-53.

Kusakabe, A., H. Shiozumi, S. Ounaka, and H. Mizoguti. 1965. Plexus brachialis of a chimpanzee *(Pan satyrus)*. Acta Anat. Nippon 40:183-91.

Lander, K. F. 1918. The pectoralis minor: A morphological study. J. Anat. 52:292-318.

Le Gros Clark, W. E. 1960. The antecedents of man: An introduction to the evolution of the primates. Chicago: Quadrangle Books.

Leichtz, J. D., T. W. Shields, and B. J. Anson. 1957. Variations pertaining to the aortic arches and their branches. Quart. Bull. Northwestern Univ. Med. Sch. 31:136-43.

Leppi, T. J. 1967. Gross anatomical relationships between primate submandibular and sublingual salivary glands. J. Dent. Res. 46:359-65.

Lewis, O. J. 1965. The evolution of the mm. interossei in the primate hand. Anat. Rec. 153:275-87.

Lightoller, G. S. 1928. The facial muscles of three orang-utans and two Cercopithecidae. J. Anat. 63:19-81.

Lineback, P. 1933. The vascular system. In The anatomy of the rhesus monkey, ed. C. G. Hartman and W. L. Straus, Jr., pp. 248-65. Baltimore, Md.: Williams and Wilkins.

Loth, E. 1907. Die Plantaraponeurose beim Menschen und den übringen Primaten. Korresp. Bl. Dtsch Ges. Anthropol. 38:169-93.

_____. 1949. Anthropological studies of muscles of living Negroes of Uganda. In Yearbook of physical anthropology, ed. G. W. Lasker and C. I. Shade, 5:220-31. New York: The Viking Fund.

Ludwig, F. J. 1957. The mandibular second premolars: Morphologic variation and inheritance. J. Dent. Res. 36:263-73.

McCormack, L. J., E. W. Cauldwell, and B. J. Anson. 1953. Brachial and antebrachial arterial patterns. Surg. Gyn. and Obst. 96:43-54.

McCoy, H. 1964. The regional anatomy of the temporal and infratemporal areas of the rhesus monkey *(Macaca mulatta)*. Master's thesis, Medical College of South Carolina, Charleston.

McCoy, H., D. R. Swindler, and J. W. Albers. 1967. The external carotid artery of the baboon and the rhesus monkey: Its branching pattern and distribution. In The baboon in medical research, ed. H. Vagtborg, 2:151-79. Austin: Univ. of Texas Press.

Manners-Smith, T. 1912. The limb arteries of primates. J. Anat. and Physiol. 7:95-172.

Maples, W. R. 1972. Systematic reconsideration and a revision of the nomenclature of Kenya baboons. Amer. J. Phys. Anthropol. 36:9-19.

Martin, C. P., and H. D. O'Brien. 1938. The coracoid process in the primates. J. Anat. 73:630-42.

Michels, N. A. 1955. Blood supply and anatomy of the upper abdominal organs. Philadelphia, Pa.: J. B. Lippincott.

Midlo, C., and H. Cummins. 1942. Palmar and plantar dermatoglyphics in primates. Philadelphia, Pa.: Wistar Institute of Anatomy and Biology.

Mijsberg, W. A. 1923. Uber den dau des Urogenitalapparates bei den mannlichen Primaten. Verhandl. Kon. Akad. Wet. Amsterdam 23:1-92.

Miller, R. 1934. Comparative studies upon the morphology and distribution of the brachial plexus. Amer. J. Anat. 54:143-75.

_____. 1947. The inguinal canal of primates. Amer. J. Anat. 80:117-42.

Moore, A. W. 1949. Head growth of the macaque monkey as revealed by vital staining, embedding and undecalcified sectioning. Amer. J. Orthodont. 35:654-71.

Morton, D. J. 1935. The human foot: Its evolution, physiology and functional disorders. New York: Columbia Univ. Press.

Napier, J. R. 1961. Prehensility and opposability in the hands of primates. Symp. Zool. Soc. Lond. 5:115-32.

_____. 1962. The evolution of the hand. Sci. Amer. 207:56-62.

Napier, J. R., and P. H. Napier. 1967. A handbook of living primates. New York: Academic Press.

Oxnard, C. E. 1963. Locomotor adaptions in the primate forelimb. Symp. Zool. Soc. Lond. 10:165-82.

_____. 1968. The architecture of the shoulder in some mammals. J. Morph. 126:249-90.

Platzer, W. 1960. Das Arterien und Venensystem. In Primatologia: Handbook of primatology, ed. H. Hofer, A. H. Schultz, and D. Starck, 3/2:273-387. New York: S. Karger.

Priman, J., and L. E. Etter. 1959. The pterygospinous and pterygoalar bars. Med. Radiogr. Photogr. 35:2-6.

Raven, H. C. 1950. Regional anatomy of the gorilla. In The anatomy of the gorilla, ed. W. K. Gregory, pp. 15-188. New York: Columbia Univ. Press.

Robinson, J. T., and E. F. Allin. 1966. On the Y of the Dryopithecus pattern of mandibular molar teeth. Amer. J. Phys. Anthropol. 25:323-24.

Rojecki, F. 1889. Sur la circulation artérielle chez le *Macacus cynomolgus* et le *Macacus sinicus* comparée à celle des singes anthropomorphes et de l'homme. J. Anat. Paris 25:343-86.

Ruge, G. 1887. Untersuchungen über die Gesichtsmuskulatur der Primaten. Leipzig.

Sakuma, F. 1961. Studies on the cerebral arteries of *Macacus cyclopsis*. Acta Med. Nagasakiensia 5:160-81.

Satoh, J. 1969. The m. serratus posterior superior in certain catarrhine monkeys and man, in particular the structure of the muscular digitations and the nerve supply. Okajimas Fol. Anat. Jap. 46:65-122.

_____. 1970. The m. serratus posterior inferior in monkey and man, in particular the structure of the digitations of this muscle and their nerve supply. Okajimas Fol. Anat. Jap. 47:19-61.

_____. 1971. The m. transversus thoracic in man and monkey. Okajimas Fol. Anat. Jap. 48:103-37.

Schaeffer, J. P., and A. J. Ramsay. 1966. The respiratory system. In Morris' human anatomy, ed. B. J. Anson, pp. 1385-1455. 12th ed. New York: McGraw-Hill.

Schultz, A. H. 1926. Fetal growth of man and other primates. Quart. Rev. Biol. 1:465-521.

_____. 1930. The skeleton of the trunk and limbs of higher primates. Human Biol. 2:303-438.

_____. 1936. Characters common to the higher primates and characters specific to man. Quart. Rev. Biol. 11:259-455.

_____. 1961. Vertebral column and thorax. In Primatologia: Handbook of primatology, ed. H. Hofer, A. H. Schultz, and D. Starck, 4:1-66. New York: S. Karger.

_____. 1969. The skeleton of the chimpanzee. In The chimpanzee: Anatomy, behavior and diseases of chimpanzees, ed. G. H. Bourne, 1:50-101. New York: S. Karger.

Schuman, E. L., and C. L. Brace. 1955. Metric and morphologic variations in the dentition of the Liberian chimpanzee: Comparisons with anthropoid and human dentitions. In The non-human primates and human evolution, ed. J. A. Gavan, pp. 61-90. Detroit, Mich.: Wayne State University Press.

Schwartz, D. J., and D. F. Huelke. 1963. Morphology of the head and neck of the macaque monkey: The muscles of mastication and the mandibular division of the trigeminal nerve. J. Dent. Res. 42:1222-33.

Seib, G. A. 1934. The azygos system of veins in American whites and American Negroes, including observations on the inferior caval system. Amer. J. Phys. Anthropol. 19:39-163.

Sigmon, B. A. 1969. The scansorius muscle in primates. Primates 10:247-61.

Sigmon, B. A., and J. T. Robinson. 1967. On the function of m. gluteus maximus in apes and in man. Amer. J. Phys. Anthropol. 27:245-46. Abst.

Sonntag, C. F. 1922. On the anatomy of the Drill *(Mandrillus leucophaeus)*. Proc. Zool. Soc. Lond. 1:429-53.

_____. 1923. On the anatomy, physiology and pathology of the chimpanzee. Proc. Zool. Soc. Lond. 1:323-429.

_____. 1924. The morphology and evolution of the apes and man. London: John Bale, Sons, and Davidson, Ltd.

Soutoul, J. H., A. LeGuyader, Y. Lanson, C. Dujardin, and J. Kekey. 1966. Le plexus lombaire des singes Cercopithéques d'Afrique. Arch. D'Anatomie Pathologique (Paris) 14:128-32.

Starck, D., and R. Schneider. 1960. Larynx. In Primatologia: Handbook of primatology, ed. H. Hofer, A. H. Schultz, and D. Starck, 3:423-575. New York: S. Karger.

Straus, W. L., Jr. 1929. Studies on primate ilia. Amer. J. Anat. 43:403-60.

_____. 1936. The thoracic and abdominal viscera of primates with special reference to the orang-outan. Proc. Amer. Philos. Soc. 76:1-85.

_____. 1949. The riddle of man's ancestry. Quart. Rev. Biol. 24:200-23.

_____. 1962. The mylohyoid groove in primates. Bibl. Primat. 1:197-216. New York: S. Karger.

_____. 1963. The classification of Oreopithecus. In Classification and human evolution, ed. S. L. Washburn, pp. 146-77. Chicago: Aldine Publ. Co.

Swindler, D. R., H. A. McCoy, and P. V. Hornbeck. 1967. The dentition of the baboon (Papio anubis). In The baboon in medical research, ed. H. Vagtborg, 2:133-51. Austin: Univ. of Texas Press.

Tandler, J. 1899. Zur vergleichenden Anatomie der Kopfarterien bei den Mammalia. Denkschr. Akad. Wiss. Wien. 67:677-784.

Thorington, R. W., Jr., and C. P. Groves. 1970. An annotated classification of the Cercopithecoidea. In Old World monkeys: Evolution, systematics and behavior, ed. J. P. Napier and P. H. Napier, pp. 629-47. New York: Academic Press.

Tilney, F. 1928. The brain from ape to man. New York: Hoeber.

Tuttle, R. H. 1965. A study of the chimpanzee hand with comments on hominoid evolution. Ph.D. dissertation, Dept. of Anthropology, University of California, Berkeley.

Uhlmann, K. V. 1968. Hüft-und Oberschenkelmuskulatur, Systematische und vergleichende Anatomie. In Primatologia: Handbook of primatology, ed. H. Hofer, A. H. Schultz, and D. Starck, 5:1-422. New York: S. Karger.

Urbanowicz, Z., and S. Zaluska. 1969. Formation of the lumbar plexus in man and macaca. Folia Morphol. 28:256-71.

Vidic, B. 1970. The connections of the intra-osseous segment of the facial nerve in baboon (Papio sp.) Anat. Rec. 168: 477-90.

Voneida, T. J. 1966. The central nervous system. In Morris' human anatomy, ed. B. J. Anson, pp. 913-1021. 12th ed. New York: McGraw-Hill.

Waldhausen, J. A., F. L. Abel, and W. L. Pearce. 1967. Portalsystemic venous shunts in hemorrhagic shock in the dog and monkey. Annals Surg. 166:183-89.

Washburn, S. L. 1950. The analysis of primate evolution with particular reference to the origin of man. In Cold spring harbor symposia on quantitative biology: Origin and evolution of man, 15:67-78. Lancaster, Pa.: Science Press.

Waterman, H. C. 1929. Studies on the evolution of the pelvis of man and other primates. Bull. Amer. Mus. Nat. Hist. 58:585-642.

Watts, J. W. 1933. A comparative study of the anterior cerebral artery and the circle of Willis in primates. J. Anat. 68:534-50.

_____. 1934. Ligation of the anterior cerebral artery in monkeys. J. Nerv. and Ment. Dis. 79:153-58.

Weinstein, J. D., and T. R. Hedges, Jr. 1962. Studies of intracranial and orbital vasculature of the rhesus monkey (Macaca mulatta). Anat. Rec. 144:37-41.

Wells, L. H. 1935. A peroneus tertius muscle in a Chacma baboon (Papio porcarius). J. Anat. Lond. 69:508-14.

Whipple, I. L. 1904. The ventral surface of the mammalian chiridium. Zeitschr. f. Morphol. u. Anthropol. 7:261-368.

Wislocki, G. B. 1933. The reproductive systems. In The anatomy of the rhesus monkey, ed. C. G. Hartman and W. L. Straus, Jr., pp. 231-47. Baltimore, Md.: Williams and Wilkins.

Wojtowicz, Z., T. Sadowski, and D. Kurek. 1969. The external ocular muscles in Macacus rhesus. Folia Morphol. 28:235-40.

Wood Jones, F. 1948. Hallmarks of mankind. London: Baillière, Tindall and Cox.

Zuckerkandl, E. 1895. Zur Anatomie und Entwickelungsgeschichte der Arterien des Unterschenkels und des Fusses. Arb. Anat. Inst. Wiesbaden 5:207-91.

Zuckerman, S. 1926. Growth changes in the skull of the baboon Papio porcarius. Proc. Zool. Soc. Lond. 2:843-73.

_____. 1938. Observations on the autonomic nervous system and on vertebral and neural segmentation in monkeys. Trans. Zool. Soc. Lond. 23:315-78.

INDEX